Certified Nurse Educator (CNE®) and Certified Nurse Educator Novice (CNE®n) Review

Ruth A. Wittmann-Price, PhD, RN, CNS, CNE, CNEcl, CHSE, ANEF, FAAN, is a professor and chair of undergraduate nursing at Jefferson College of Nursing in Center City, Philadelphia. Ruth has been an obstetrical/women's health nurse for 42 years. Dr. Wittmann-Price received her AAS and BSN degrees from Felician College, Lodi, New Jersey, and her MS as a perinatal clinical nurse specialist (CNS) from Columbia University, New York, New York. She completed her PhD in nursing at Widener University, Chester, Pennsylvania, and received the Dean's Award for Excellence. Ruth developed a mid-range nursing theory, "Emancipated Decision-Making in Women's Health Care," and has tested her theory in four research studies. International researchers are currently using her theory as the foundation for their studies. Her theory is being used by researchers at the University of Limpopo, South Africa, in their campaign, "Finding Solutions for Africa," which helps women and children. Dr. Wittmann-Price has taught all levels of nursing students over the past 24 years and has completed international service-learning trips. Currently, she teaches Doctor of Nursing Practice students as well as undergraduate maternal-child health. Dr. Wittmann-Price coedited or authored 16 books, contributed many chapters, and written numerous articles. She has presented her research regionally, nationally, and internationally. Dr. Wittmann-Price was inducted into the National League for Nursing Academy of Nurse Educator Fellows in 2013 and became a fellow in the American Academy of Nursing in October 2015.

Maryann Godshall, PhD, CNE, CCRN, CPN, is an associate clinical professor at Drexel University College of Nursing and Health Professions in Philadelphia, Pennsylvania. She obtained her BSN from Allentown College of St. Francis DeSales, Center Valley, Pennsylvania, and her MSN from DeSales University, Center Valley, Pennsylvania. She has a postmaster's degree in nursing education from Duquesne University, Pittsburgh, Pennsylvania. She completed her PhD at Duquesne University (2014), where her research topic was "Exploring Learning of Pediatric Burn Patients Through Storytelling." Dr. Godshall has been a nurse for more than 28 years and has worked in pediatric critical care, inpatient pediatrics, pediatric rehabilitation nursing, and adult medical surgical nursing. She holds certifications in both pediatrics (CPN) and pediatric critical care (CCRN) and has taught in both the university and hospital settings. Dr. Godshall is coeditor of The Certified Nurse Educator (CNE) Review Manual (2017; Springer Publishing Company), and author of Fast Facts of Evidence-Based Practice, Third Edition (2020; Springer Publishing Company). She has published chapters in several books and textbooks, including Maternal–Child Nursing Care: Optimizing Outcomes for Mothers, Children and Families, Second Edition (2016), NCLEX-RN® EXCEL (2010; Springer Publishing Company), and Disaster Nursing: A Handbook for Practice (2009). She has also written many journal articles. She is a question item writer and is published in Rudd & Kocisko's Davis Edge for Pediatric Nursing, 2nd Ed. (F.A. Davis, 2018). In 2008, Dr. Godshall won the Nightingale Award of Pennsylvania Nursing Scholarship. Dr. Godshall has presented nursing and education topics both nationally and internationally. Most recently, "Moral Distress, Compassion Fatigue and Burnout in Nursing" at The International Nursing Conference, Rome, Italy, October 23, 2019.

Linda Wilson, PhD, RN, CPAN, CAPA, NPD-BC, CNE, CNEcl, CHSE-A, FASPAN, ANEF, FAAN, is an assistant dean for continuing education, simulation, and events, and a clinical professor at Drexel University, College of Nursing and Health Professions, Philadelphia, Pennsylvania. Dr. Wilson completed her BSN at College Misericordia, Dallas, Pennsylvania; her MSN in critical care and trauma at Thomas Jefferson University, Philadelphia, Pennsylvania; and her PhD in nursing research at Rutgers University, Newark, New Jersey. Dr. Wilson has a postgraduate certificate in epidemiology and biostatistical methods from Drexel University and a postgraduate certificate in pain management from the University of California, San Francisco School of Medicine. Dr. Wilson also completed the National Library of Medicine/Marine Biological Laboratory Biomedical Informatics Fellowship and the Harvard University Institute for Medical Simulation's Comprehensive Workshop and Graduate Course in Medical Simulation. Dr. Wilson has several certifications, including certified post anesthesia nurse (CPAN), certified ambulatory perianesthesia nurse (CAPA), American Nurses Credentialing Center (ANCC) board certification (NPD-BC) in nursing professional development, certified nurse educator (CNE), certified academic clinical nurse educator (CNEcl), and certified healthcare simulation educator advanced (CHSE-A). Dr. Wilson served as the president of the American Society of Perianesthesia Nurses (2002–2003), and has served as an ANCC Commission on Accreditation Appraiser Site surveyor since 2000. In 2014, Dr. Wilson was inducted into the National League for Nursing (NLN) Academy of Nurse Educator Fellows (ANEF) and was also inducted as a Fellow in the American Academy of Nursing (FAAN).

Certified Nurse Educator (CNE®) and Certified Nurse Educator Novice (CNE®n) Review

Fourth Edition

Ruth A. Wittmann-Price, PhD, RN, CNS, CNE, CNEcl, CHSE, ANEF, FAAN

Maryann Godshall, PhD, CNE, CCRN, CPN

Linda Wilson, PhD, RN, CPAN, CAPA, NPD-BC, CNE, CNEcl, CHSE-A, FASPAN, ANEF, FAAN

Editors

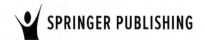 SPRINGER PUBLISHING

Springer Publishing Company, LLC
11 West 42nd Street, New York, NY 10036
www.springerpub.com
connect.springerpub.com/

Acquisitions Editor: Jaclyn Koshofer
Compositor: Integra

ISBN: 9780826156440
ebook ISBN: 9780826156457
DOI: 10.1891/9780826156457

23 24 25 26 27 / 7 6 5 4 3

The author and the publisher of this Work have made every effort to use sources believed to be reliable to provide information that is accurate and compatible with the standards generally accepted at the time of publication. The author and publisher shall not be liable for any special, consequential, or exemplary damages resulting, in whole or in part, from the readers' use of, or reliance on, the information contained in this book. The publisher has no responsibility for the persistence or accuracy of URLs for external or third-party Internet websites referred to in this publication and does not guarantee that any content on such websites is, or will remain, accurate or appropriate.

LCCN: 2021912955

Contact sales@springerpub.com to receive discount rates on bulk purchases.

Publisher's Note: **New and used products purchased from third-party sellers are not guaranteed for quality, authenticity, or access to any included digital components.**

Printed in the United States of America by Hatteras, Inc.

Contents

Contributors

Diane M. Billings, EdD, RN, FAAN, ANEF Chancellor's Professor Emeritus, Indiana University School of Nursing, Indianapolis, Indiana

Frances H. Cornelius, PhD, MSN, RN-BC(informatics), CNE, ANEF Assistant Dean for Teaching, Learning and Engagement, Clinical Professor, College of Nursing and Health Professions, Drexel University, Philadelphia, Pennsylvania

Anita Fennessey, DrNP, RN, CNE Assistant Professor, Thomas Jefferson University, Horsham, Pennsylvania

Tracy P. George, DNP, APRN-BC, CNE Associate Professor of Nursing, Coordinator of Bachelor of General Studies Program, Amy V. Cockroft Fellow 2016-2017, Francis Marion University, Florence, South Carolina

Karen K. Gittings, DNP, RN, CNE, CNEcl, Alumnus CCRN Professor of Nursing and Dean, School of Health Sciences, Associate Dean, Associate Professor, School of Health Sciences, Francis Marion University, Florence, South Carolina

Mary Ellen Smith Glasgow, PhD, RN, ANEF, FAAN Dean and Professor, School of Nursing and Vice Provost for Research, Office of Research and Innovation, Duquesne University, Pittsburgh, Pennsylvania

Maryann Godshall, PhD, CNE, CCRN, CPN Associate Clinical Professor of Nursing, College of Nursing and Health Professions, Drexel University, Philadelphia, Pennsylvania

Susan H. Kelly, EdD, MSN, RN, CMSRN, CNE, CHSE Clinical Assistant Professor and Director of Undergraduate Adjunct Faculty and Clinical Affairs, Nursing, Duquesne University, Pittsburgh, Pennsylvania

Ruth Ann Kiefer, DrNP, RN, CRRN, CNE Assistant Professor, Thomas Jefferson University, Horsham, Pennsylvania

Marylou K. McHugh, EdD, RN, CNE Associate Clinical Professor, Division of Graduate Nursing, Advanced Role MSN Department, College of Nursing and Health Professions, Drexel University, Philadelphia, Pennsylvania

Carol Okupniak, DNP, RN, BC-NI, CHSE Associate Clinical Professor of Nursing, Thomas Jefferson University, Philadelphia, Pennsylvania

Kathryn M. Shaffer, EdD, RN, CNE, CCFP Associate Professor, Thomas Jefferson University, Philadelphia, Pennsylvania

Dorie Weaver, DNP, MSN, FNP-BC, CNE Assistant Professor of Nursing and Coordinator of the Nurse Educator Program, Francis Marion University, Florence, South Carolina

Linda Wilson, PhD, RN, CPAN, CAPA, NPD-BC, CNE, CNEcl, CHSE-A, FASPAN, ANEF, FAAN Assistant Dean for Continuing Education, Simulation and Events, Clinical Professor, College of Nursing and Health Professions, Drexel University, Philadelphia, Pennsylvania

Ruth A. Wittmann-Price, PhD, RN, CNS, CNE, CNEcl, CHSE, ANEF, FAAN Professor of Nursing, Chair Undergraduate Programs, Center City Thomas Jefferson University, Philadelphia, Pennsylvania

Ksenia Zukowsky, PhD, CRNP, APRN, NNP-BC Associate Professor, Chair Graduate Programs, Thomas Jefferson University, Philadelphia, Pennsylvania

Foreword

The critical role of nurses in healthcare has been highlighted day after day during the COVID-19 pandemic. Nurses are on the frontline planning and delivering care to patients in crisis situations but have an equally important role in the community to keep the public safe. To prepare a sufficient number of nurses to meet these healthcare needs, both in hospitals and in the community, schools of nursing need well-prepared nurse educators. Studies continue to document the high number of qualified applicants to nursing programs being turned away because of a lack of faculty to teach them, among other factors. The faculty shortage has occurred for a number of reasons, including fewer graduate students preparing for educator roles to replace the number of faculty who are retiring, difficulties in recruiting clinicians to teach in schools of nursing because of the lower salaries of faculty compared with healthcare settings, and new career paths for nurses.

Accompanying the shortage of nurse educators is the recognition that nursing education has a body of knowledge to be learned and core competencies to be developed for expert teaching. Nurse educators need an understanding of learning theories, clinical judgment and higher-level thinking, motivation, and deep learning, among other concepts. These theories and concepts provide educators with a framework for how best to facilitate students' learning and development of competencies. Nurse educators may teach small and large groups of learners, in the classroom and online environment, in simulation and skills laboratories, and in clinical practice. They need to be effective across all of these environments, and that requires skill in selecting appropriate teaching methods for the outcomes to be achieved and developing active learning strategies. The rapid advances and constant changes in technology create opportunities and challenges for teaching. Successful integration of technology in the nursing curriculum requires competencies for the teacher.

To guide students in achieving the course outcomes, educators need to understand the relationship of those outcomes and the course in which they teach to the overall curriculum. All nursing faculty should know general concepts of curriculum development and their roles and responsibilities in planning and revising the curriculum and courses within it.

Educators not only teach, but they also are responsible for evaluating students' learning and clinical competencies. Much of this evaluation is formative, providing feedback to students on their progress and guiding their continued learning. At certain points in time, however, the evaluation is summative, and educators need to understand these differences. Nursing faculty members not only evaluate student learning and development but also evaluate the program, curriculum, courses, resources, and other aspects to ensure a high-quality education for students. This evaluation is done within a quality improvement framework.

Nurse educators function within institutions and need to understand the environment in which they teach and its effects on their roles and responsibilities. The mission and goals of the setting influence the educator's role. Differences across schools of nursing in expectations of faculty, criteria for appointment and advancement, and requirements for tenure and promotion are striking. To be successful, the teacher needs to understand those expectations and requirements.

Across all settings, the nurse educator is a leader and change agent, participating in efforts to improve nursing education, developing educational innovations, and gaining leadership skills. Once prepared as a nurse educator, one's own learning and professional development continue. Educators need to expand their own knowledge and skills and be committed to participating in career development activities. As faculty members foster the value of lifelong learning among students, so too are faculty lifelong learners. Decisions about educational practices should be based on sound evidence generated through research that is of high quality. The role of the nurse educator as scholar not only includes conducting research and disseminating findings but also approaching one's teaching by questioning current practices and searching for evidence to answer those questions.

Many healthcare fields offer certifications to acknowledge expertise in a specialty area of practice or role. Similar to certifications in clinical specialties, certification in nursing education is a means for teachers to demonstrate their knowledge about nursing education and expertise in the educator role. The National League for Nursing offers certification in nursing education through its Certified Nurse Educator (CNE) examination. That examination assesses the teacher's knowledge about learning and teaching strategies, learner development and socialization, assessment and evaluation, curriculum development and evaluation, quality improvement as a nurse educator, scholarship in nursing education, and the faculty member's role within an institutional environment and academic community. The CNE examination serves as a means of documenting advanced knowledge, expertise, and competencies in the role of nurse educator.

This book was developed as a resource for nurse educators to prepare themselves to take *and pass* the CNE examination. It includes valuable information for this purpose and also serves as a review of important principles for effective teaching in nursing. The book describes the concepts and principles that define nursing education, describes the core competencies of nurse educators, and provides a perspective of expert teaching in nursing. Case studies and practice questions are included in each chapter to guide application of the concepts and content in the chapter and serve as a review. There also is a comprehensive examination with answers at the end of the book, which is of much value as a review for the CNE examination. This book is a critical resource for nurse educators in preparing for the CNE examination and for aspiring teachers in nursing.

Marilyn H. Oermann, PhD, RN, ANEF, FAAN
Thelma M. Ingles Professor of Nursing
Director of Educational Research
Duke University School of Nursing
Durham, North Carolina
Editor-in-Chief, *Nurse Educator* and *Journal of Nursing Care Quality*

Preface

Through teaching we can touch more patients than ever possible with our own two hands.
—*Ruth A. Wittmann-Price*

The first three editions of this book assisted many nurse educators in becoming certified. We decided to update and expand the content to keep up with the ever-changing discipline of nursing education. This fourth edition includes much of the information provided in the first three editions, but we have integrated remote learning philosophies, techniques, and best practices due to the current educational environment caused by the COVID-19 pandemic. This book also incorporates the current National League for Nursing (NLN) Certified Nurse Educator (CNE) test plan and has many new chapter practice questions as well as a 150-question test. Other topics that are prominent in the nursing literature have been added, including flipped classes, vulnerable populations, global learning activities, civic engagement, and online learning. Nurse educators continue to understand and remain passionate about teaching the next generation of nurses. Witnessing a student or colleague become excited about new information, techniques, or skills is extremely gratifying. The classroom, internet learning environment, skills laboratory, simulation laboratory, virtual laboratories, and clinical realms all fall within the expertise of the nurse educator. These realms are parts of larger systems that nurse educators navigate successfully to accomplish their goal of professional development in graduates from their programs. In any one classroom, online session, laboratory, or clinical setting, facilitating the education of others is not only a rewarding experience but a role that greatly impacts the future of healthcare.

In the past, nurse educators had no special education about teaching. Nurse educators were content experts who learned the pedagogy by trial and error. Now, nursing education is recognized as a specialty unto itself that contains a distinct body of knowledge. Like nursing, it is also an applied science. This book highlights areas outlined by the NLN as essential knowledge needed for the nurse educator to excel in the field and pass the CNE examination.

The competencies for nurse educators listed at the beginning of each chapter are taken from the NLN website. Competency is defined by WordNet® 3.0. (n.d.) as "the quality of being adequately or well qualified physically and intellectually." Competence can be viewed as a minimal skill set or level that must be achieved to pass. Excellence means "possessing good qualities in high degree" (WordNet® 3.0., n.d.), and the CNE publicly designates that distinction upon nurse educators.

The CNE was created by our nursing leaders to recognize and capture excellence in nursing education. Since the first examination was offered to 174 candidates as a pencil-and-paper test in Baltimore, MD, on September 28, 2005, thousands of nurse educators have passed the exam (NLN, 2021). Those nurse educators proudly display the CNE certification after their names.

To prepare nurse educators for the certification examination, the NLN provides resources that can be accessed from their informative website (http://www.nln.org/facultycertification/index.htm). This book was created because many nurse educators have asked us how we prepared for the first examination in Baltimore in 2005.

This book is a supplement to the materials already available from the NLN, and it is developed independently from the NLN in order to further assist nurse educators in gaining confidence about taking the examination. This book is modeled after the NLN's most recently published test plan. Many of the areas in the test plan overlap; therefore, you may find places in this book that are cross-referenced. Cross-referencing replicates the nature of nursing education; it is an interwoven realm of content, context, and process—all of which affect learning outcomes. We hope this book captures the essence of information needed for nurse educators to move to a recognized level of excellence. We have put additional references and Teaching Gems in place for those who would like further explanation and exploration of topics and encourage you to investigate these. We have searched for evidence to support our content and, where applicable, have inserted research into each chapter and clearly designated Evidence-Based Teaching Practice boxes to help the reader focus on the evidence discovered by fellow educators. We have also provided case studies at the end of each chapter to promote educational decision-making and provided sample test questions that may be similar to those encountered during the CNE examination.

The Introduction covers some of the specifics of the CNE examination, describes recertification, and reviews test-taking skills.

Chapter 1 reviews how a nurse educator facilitates learning by assessing the learning needs and skills of the students. It also reviews learner outcomes and teaching strategies and how to adapt them to the student's own experiences. This is important to assess in order to develop an appropriate teaching plan. Another area discussed is how the nurse educator models the role of nurse for the student and helps the student to become motivated and enthusiastic about learning.

Chapter 2 discusses learning strategies. Active and passive learning strategies are reviewed, and advantages and disadvantages of each strategy are considered.

Chapter 3 discusses technology in the realm of nursing education. This topic has grown immensely and now needs its own chapter. Technology is used to facilitate learning, and this is done by using new innovations that engage the learner along with Web 2.0 tools and Web 3.0 functionality of the World Wide Web.

Chapter 4 is dedicated to online teaching, an ever-needed medium for facilitating learning for all levels of nursing students. Online teaching is just as much an art and science as live classroom teaching. Often, nurse educators are the leaders in their educational organizations in online learning.

Chapter 5 demonstrates the competencies needed by nurse educators to facilitate learning in the nursing skills lab. This is an important area of foundational learning for students, which is included in most nursing curricula.

Chapter 6 discusses clinical education and the importance of coaching students in facilitating knowledge of professionalism, skill, and interdisciplinary competencies.

Chapter 7 is devoted to in-person and virtual simulation and follows the clinical education chapter because the two methods of facilitating learning are very much intertwined. Best practices in human patient simulator (HPS) simulation, standardized patient (SP) simulation, and debriefing are discussed. The new opportunities for certification in simulation are also introduced.

Chapter 8 is devoted to socialization skills of students intraprofessionally and interprofessionally and speaks to the ever-increasing diversity in culture and styles that affect nursing education. Another important aspect of Chapter 9 is the examination of resources for students who are at risk for any number of individual reasons that affect them perceptually, cognitively, physically, or culturally. Incivility is addressed in relation to today's teaching environment.

Chapter 9 also deals with the second NLN competency for nurse educators, socialization of learners, which is accomplished by describing global learning and civic engagement. Encouraging learners to understand civic engagement and have a global view of healthcare is important in today's world of connectedness.

Chapter 10 discusses evaluation strategies used by nurse educators and how they balance the aspects of admission, progression, and retention to ensure good program outcomes. Effective evaluation tools are extremely important in promoting student success and public safety.

Chapter 11 addresses the larger institutional considerations of curriculum design and evaluation. How courses are developed within a curriculum and how the curriculum flows are analyzed. This chapter discusses how the curriculum interfaces with the mission of the institution and the community.

Chapter 12 highlights professional development of nurse educators and how educators navigate their roles and become mentors to the next generation of nurse educators. For educators, learning is lifelong and has increased in intensity exponentially with the accelerating advancements in information and technology. This chapter provides the nurse educator with ideas on how to keep up-to-date and remain involved in the field of nursing education.

Chapter 13 speaks to the nurse educator's role as a leader who interfaces with the larger community of academics and administrators. This chapter examines nursing's place in the larger systems as well as how nurse educators can effect change in those systems.

Chapter 14 dissects the scholarship needed for nurse educators to stay on top of their game. "Publish or perish" is a phenomenon known to academics that is applicable to nurse educators in an academic setting. This chapter discusses different types of scholarship and professional plans for becoming proficient at publishing and emphasizes the importance of disseminating nursing knowledge.

Chapter 15 discusses interdisciplinary collaboration within the institution for nurse educators. Nursing has a longer history of using standalone schools than it does being part of a larger educational community. Nurse educators have assimilated into the larger community as experts in a field that has the unique components of clinical and didactic education. The professionalism that we bring to the larger academic community has enhanced the standings of many institutions and colleges. Nursing is a visible professional entity that collaborates and contributes to the overall mission of the institution of nursing and to society.

Chapters 16 and 17 include a comprehensive examination and the answers to the chapter questions and the comprehensive examination. These practice questions will assist you to answer correctly on the actual CNE examination.

We have developed this fourth edition to assist nurse educators to prepare for the CNE examination. Many nurse educators have used previous editions of this book to successfully pass the examination. Our hope is that this is an effective tool to help you reach your goal of recognized excellence. We applaud your efforts as colleagues in the quest to educate the next generation of nurses. We thank you for your efforts to recognize excellence in our field.

Ruth A. Wittmann-Price
Maryann Godshall
Linda Wilson

REFERENCES

Competency. (n.d.). In WordNet® 3.0. http://dictionary.reference.com/browse/competency

Excellence. (n.d.). In WordNet® 3.0. http://dictionary.reference.com/browse/excellence

National League for Nursing. (2021). Certification for nurse educators (CNE). http://www.nln.org/facultycertification/index.htm

Acknowledgments

The three coeditors would like to acknowledge Dr. Frances H. Cornelius for all the excellent information she continues to contribute to this book.

Thank you to all of my students over the years who have taught and continue to teach me a tremendous amount about nursing, life, and humility.

—*Ruth A. Wittmann-Price*

Thank you to all my current and former students who motivate me in my drive for excellence. Their hunger for knowledge and learning makes me passionate to continue my role as an educator. I would also like to acknowledge the nurses and doctors I have worked with over the years. They have been teaching me and sharing their passion for caring for our sickest of patients. Lastly, I would like to express my gratitude to the patients from infant to adult and their families who have allowed me to come into their lives at the scariest of times and help them through their journey. It is because of them I want to educate and inspire the next generation of nurses. You are all forever in my heart. May this book help prepare the next generation of nurse educators.

—*Maryann Godshall*

To H. Lynn Kane, Helen "Momma" Kane, Linda Webb, and Elizabeth Diaz, thank you for your amazing friendship and for being my family. To Lou Smith, Evan Babcock, Steve Johnson, and Trish Costa-DePena, thank you for your wonderful friendship and support. To Fabien Pampaloni, thank you for your endless help, friendship, and support.

—*Linda Wilson*

Pass Guarantee

If you use this resource to prepare for your exam and you do not pass, you may return it for a refund of your full purchase price. To receive a refund, you must return your product along with a copy of your original receipt and exam score report. Product must be returned and received within 180 days of the original purchase date. This excludes tax, shipping, and handling. One offer per person and address. Refunds will be issued within 8 weeks from acceptance and approval. This offer is valid for U.S. residents only. Void where prohibited. To initiate a refund, please contact customer service at CS@springerpub.com.

Introducing the CNE® and the CNE®n Exams and Blueprints

Ruth Ann Kiefer

Nursing is an art: and if it is to be made an art, it requires an exclusive devotion as hard a preparation, as any painter's or sculptor's work; for what is the having to do with dead canvas or dead marble, compared with having to do with the living body, the temple of God's spirit? It is one of the Fine Arts: I had almost said, the finest of Fine Arts.
—Florence Nightingale (1860)

▶ LEARNING OUTCOMES

Identify the processes to best prepare for The Certified Nurse Educator (CNE) or The Certified Nurse Educator Novice (CNEn) examinations

- Utilize the tips for success to promote understanding and learning of key concepts
- Demonstrate time-management skills to enhance studying
- Integrate standards from practice into information that is outlined in the CNE and CNEn test blueprints
- Improve comprehension by eliminating anxiety related to test taking
- Utilize technology to track competencies in preparation for completion of the 5-year recertification activity record

● INTRODUCTION

Nurse educator certification comes at a time in history when nursing is actively recruiting advanced practiced nurses into the educational realm. The U.S. Bureau of Labor Statistics (2020) predicts a 7% growth in the employment of RNs from 2019 to 2029. This increase is the direct result of growing chronic conditions, such as diabetes and obesity, the emphasis on preventive care, and the demand for healthcare services from baby-boom populations. Nursing will continue to expand as healthcare continues to branch out into community-based primary care and outpatient sites. However, job availability is directly related to the region, number of graduates per year, and the increase in the number of experienced nurses who could have retired but continue to work because of the state of the economy and the diverse employment opportunities in healthcare. Additionally, COVID-19 has placed an enormous strain on the U.S. healthcare system, and nurses are needed to care for the millions of patients affected (Stribling et al., 2020).

There is an increased demand for nurse practitioners (NPs) in response to the healthcare movement into the community and the concentration on health promotion and health maintenance as well as on sick-care services. According to the American Nurses Association, NPs play a pivotal role in the future of healthcare services as primary care providers. The growing emphasis on prevention and public health will continue to create excellent job opportunities for NPs.

The Tri-Council for Nursing, an alliance of the American Association of Colleges of Nursing (AACN), the American Nurses Association, the American Organization of Nurse Executives, and the National League for Nursing (NLN), determined that a more highly educated nursing workforce is critical to delivering safe and effective patient care. This was supported by the Institute of Medicine's (IOM; 2010) Future of Nursing report and is promoted by healthcare leaders in academia and clinical practice. The evidence-based recommendations in the IOM report call for preparing at least 80% of the RN workforce at the baccalaureate level by 2020. This change in RN preparation has also been encouraged by the nation's Magnet®-designated hospitals (American Nurses Credentialing Center, 2020). According to the AACN data from 2020, this mandate has resulted in a 0.6% increase in RNs enrolling in RN to BSN programs to build on their initial education at the associate degree or diploma level making this the 15th consecutive year of increase in RN to BSN program completion.

WHY BECOME A CNE OR CNEn?

A substantial increase in student nurses is only one factor that summons the urgency for CNE or CNEn. Another contributing factor, adding to the faculty shortage, is the demographics of the current teaching faculty. Based on the NLN Faculty Census 2019, 50.2% of full-time nurse educators across all ranks are between 46 and 60 years of age. The national nurse faculty vacancy rate is 7.2% (NLN, 2020).

Becoming a CNE or a CNEn can also enhance the quality of nursing education, which is the foundation needed to promote the culture of safe and effective patient-centered care. At the present time, multiple innovative methods to facilitate learning are being utilized, such as enhancing critical thinking and clinical reasoning in the classroom, integrating evidence-based research, utilizing information technology, expanding hands-on service-learning experiences through global initiatives, certification programs for online educators, and providing an interprofessional healthcare team approach through simulations. The other important aspect of nursing education is incorporating strategies to effectively assess and evaluate the learner within the theoretical and clinical components.

A retrospective analysis study examined the results of a sample of educators taking the CNE examination. Highest level of education and institutional affiliation were statistically correlated to pass rates. Faculty development, experience, and advanced education are recommended on the journey to seeking certification (Lundeen, 2018).

Many colleges and schools of nursing are recruiting expert nurse clinicians and advanced practice RNs (APRNs) to assist in filling their vacant academic and clinical nurse educator roles. This recruitment process has been fostered by state and foundational funds to supplement nurse educator programs at the master's and doctoral levels. The role development that many nurse educators undergo involves a difficult process of struggling to evolve from being an expert clinician to being a novice educator. Nursing literature provides ample documentation to demonstrate that being an expert clinician does not provide an educator with the skill set needed to become a successful teacher. Through additional studies that lead to certification in nursing education, expert clinicians can become comfortable in their new role as nurse educators and build their new practice, preparing the next generation of nurses while using proven teaching and learning principles.

> **TEACHING GEM** Effective nurse educators are dependent upon knowledge, support, and the willingness to incorporate inclusive teaching strategies as they prepare to teach the diverse learner in diverse learning environments (Levey, 2016).

Indeed, nurse educators with years of experience can validate their expertise and knowledge through certification. These educators are an invaluable resource to the current system, and certified educators are surely needed as mentors, role models, and visionaries to assist future nurse educators. Educators who complete the core competencies of a CNE and CNEn are needed to move the profession forward. The following list outlines just a few ways in which that progression will manifest itself:

- Assisting with preparation to create interactive learning environments in both face-to-face and virtual settings.
- Using versatile education styles to provide quality education for diverse populations of learners.
- Developing higher level and alternate format test questions.
- Understanding test-item analysis that results in appropriate decision-making.

The CNE also has an in-depth understanding of the need to balance teaching, research/scholarship, and service, which has become an expectation in nursing academia (Wittmann-Price, 2012). The CNE is still a relevant examination and certification today, after two decades, due to content revision of the test plan and updating the examination items to maintain currency and rigor (Simmons & Christensen, 2018).

The CNEn examination is for nurse educators with less than three years of teaching and encourages beginning educators to strive for teaching excellence. The focus of the CNEn is teaching learning strategies rather than career advancement. This focus makes sense for beginning nurse educators who are developing and fine tuning courses to engage students in the learning process.

REACH FOR ACADEMIC EXCELLENCE, BECOME A CNE OR CNEn

Academic excellence often is encouraged through an atmosphere that influences educators to challenge themselves to reach beyond their normal expectations. Nurse educators who support an atmosphere of excellence can thrive, and their success will raise the bar of academic standards within the discipline. Becoming certified as a nurse educator allows faculty to better understand its multifaceted role. This role includes teaching, communicating with learners and colleagues, using information resources, understanding professional practice within the college of nursing and the university, functioning as a change agent, and engaging in scholarly activities. The role is stimulating and encourages educators to be innovative and collaborative in the academic environment.

- Nurse educators who have validated their expertise have the ability to prepare learners who are competent and confident nurses.
- Research and scholarship advanced through publications and presentations will provide a positive impact on pedagogy.
- Involvement in service, such as professional societies or committees at the program, department, college, or university level, will enhance the ability to collaborate and network within the academic community.

Your decision to take the CNE or CNEn certification examination is a challenging one, which will allow you to test your proficiency as a nurse educator.

If peer review is used in the college or university where you teach, consider this as a positive force that will impact your development as a nurse educator.

EVIDENCE-BASED TEACHING PRACTICE

Poindexter, Lindell, and Hagler (2019) quantitatively studied the perceived value of the CNE by administering the Perceived Value of Certification Tool for Academic Nurse Educators (PVCT-ANE) with certified and noncertified nursing faculty and administrators ($N = 718$) was conducted. The results demonstrated that the CNE was valued for the following reasons:

- Denoting specialized knowledge
- Promoting a professional standard
- Demonstrating competence in nursing education
- Increased professional credibility

TEACHING GEM A great way to display the scholarship of teaching for a midlevel career nurse educator is to create a new nursing elective course that will enhance the curriculum.

The following chapters in this CNE and CNEn preparation guide present a content review for each of the content areas that appear on the CNE examination. The NLN designates which content area is most important by assigning a percentage of the test to that area. The test plan can be easily found on the NLN site in the most current CNE Handbook and CNEn Handbook (NLN, 2021).

 ## PREPARING FOR THE CNE EXAMINATION

▶ SETTING UP A STUDY SCHEDULE

When you create a study schedule, begin prioritizing the order in which you study the content by using the CNE blueprint. Create a chart and divide your total studying time into eight sections and break up the total studying time into percentages that correlate with the topic's content percentage. The highest percentages of content covered in the examination and the related chapters in this book are as follows:

- Area 1—facilitate learning (22%; Chapters 2–8)
- Area 3—use assessment strategies (19%; Chapter 11)
- Area 4—participate in curriculum design and evaluation of program outcomes (17%; Chapter 12)

The next-highest percentages of content covered in the examination are:

- Area 2—facilitate learner development and socialization (15%; Chapters 9 and 10)
- Area 6—engage in scholarship, service, and leadership (15%), which includes
  - Area 6A—function as a change agent and leader (Chapter 14)
  - Area 6B—engage in scholarship of teaching (Chapter 15)
  - Area 6C—function effectively within the institutional environment and the academic community (Chapter 16)

■ Area 5—pursue continuous quality improvement in the academic nurse educator role (12%; Chapter 13)

Employing the aforementioned strategy will help ensure that you will have time to review the areas that represent the highest percentage of questions on the CNE examination. It is also very helpful to attend a CNE review course either in person or via webcast. The course will provide a concentrated review of information such as test development and item analysis, learning needs of special groups, curriculum development, teaching styles, and evaluation of program outcomes. The course presents an opportunity to practice items with educators who are certified and allows time to ask questions. Taking the course will impact your understanding of the key concepts.

For nurse educators taking the CNEn examination the study strategy will be slightly different.

■ Area 1—Facilitating learning will encompass 39% of the exam.
■ Area 2—Facilitating Learner Development and Socialization is 11%,
■ Area 3—Use of Assessment Strategies is 15%,
■ Area 4—Participate in Curriculum Design and Evaluation of Program Outcomes is 5%,
■ Area 5—Function as a Change Agent and Leader - 7%,
■ Area 6—Pursue Continuous Quality Improvement in the Role of Nurse Educator - 8 %,
■ Area 7—Engage in Scholarship - 4%
■ Area 8—Function within the Educational Environment - 11%.

Therefore, the nurse educators taking the CNEn should concentrate on Areas 1, 3, 2, and 8.

Key topics for inclusion in your review include those in Table 1.

Table 1 Key Topics to Include in Your Review

Teaching styles—authoritarian, Socratic, heuristic, and behavioral	Teaching–learning process
Active learning	Cooperative learning and testing
Self-directed learning	Planning clinical learning experiences
Critical thinking activities—classroom and clinical	Characteristics of learners (cultural, traditional, non-traditional, and educationally disadvantaged)
Domains—cognitive, psychomotor, and affective	Promotion of professional responsibility by self-assessment and peer review
Graduation and retention rates	Academic appeals process
Bloom's taxonomy	Test blueprint
Norm- and criterion-referenced tests	Formative and summative evaluation
Test validity	Test reliability
Item discrimination ratio	Point-biserial correlation
Item difficulty	Program standards—federal laws, state regulations, professional accreditation—the Commission on Collegiate Nursing Education (CCNE) and the Accreditation Commission for Education in Nursing (ACEN)
Credentialing—American Association of Colleges of Nursing (AACN)	Curriculum—mission statement, conceptual framework, level objectives, behavioral objectives, and evaluation of learning outcomes (theoretical and clinical)

(continued)

Table 1 Key Topics to Include in Your Review (*continued*)

Curriculum evaluation—internal and external	Family Educational Rights and Privacy Act (FERPA)/Buckley Amendment
Audio conferencing	Video streaming
Synchronous and asynchronous methods of instruction	Types of leadership
Scholarship of discovery	Scholarship of teaching
Scholarship of practice (application)	Scholarship of integration

EVIDENCE-BASED TEACHING PRACTICE

Research predicts that by the year 2025 artificial intelligence (AI) healthcare spending will reach billions of dollars. This technological investment will revolutionize nursing care as innovative robotics are launched into acute care and community settings. These innovations will inform nursing education, and modalities will have to be adjusted to accommodate innovative learning (Robert, 2019).

▶ PLANNING AND REGISTERING FOR THE CNE EXAMINATION USING THE NLN WEBSITE TO ESTABLISH YOUR ELIGIBILITY

Verify that you meet the eligibility requirements to take the examination. These requirements are listed on the NLN website.

- Access the NLN website: www.nln.org.

Click on "Certification for Nurse Educators."

- Print the Certified Nurse Educator CNE or CNEn 2021 Candidate Handbook (NLN, 2021) or current edition, which includes the detailed test blueprint (outlines specific information under each of the six content areas) and list of recommended texts and journals.
- Order the Self-Assessment Examination (SAE).
- This 65-item practice examination has multiple-choice questions with available rationales. Although it is half the length of the certification examination, it correlates with the content categories and cognitive complexity item distribution in the certification examination. The score report, calculated in each of the six areas, can be used to focus your review. Candidates have access to the examination for 60 days from the date of purchase. (Note: There is a fee for this optional practice test.)
- Register to take the examination.
- Registration deadlines can be found on the website, so make sure you register in advance because you will need this confirmation prior to scheduling the test location, date, and time. The notice of eligibility may take up to 3 weeks to arrive after completing the registration.
- Current fees are available on the NLN website.
- Your faculty administrator can provide you with information about reimbursement for the examination fee.

NUTS AND BOLTS OF THE CNE EXAMINATION

▶ BECOME FAMILIAR WITH THE CNE EXAMINATION

- The examination has 150 items; 130 are operational, and 20 are pre-test items that do not count toward the score.
- Items contain four options of multiple-choice questions that are within the cognitive levels of recall, application, and analysis.
- Three hours are allotted to complete the examination, which includes a short tutorial.
- This allows approximately 72 seconds for each question.
- Avoid rapid guessing on the examination.
- Read questions carefully and answer items at a consistent pace.
- Focus on important words in the question to improve your focus.
- Answer all questions to increase your chance of being successful.

EXAMINATION ITEMS REQUIRING ADDITIONAL TIME

- Information about learner grades that require math calculations.
- Information about test item analysis that requires a comparison of data.

▶ BECOME FAMILIAR WITH ELECTRONIC TESTING ADVANTAGES

- If you are unsure of an answer, you can bookmark the question or write the number of the question on the small whiteboard provided by the testing center and return to it when you have completed the remainder of the examination.
- Arrows, to page forward or backward during the examination, provide the ability to return to a question and change the answer. Only change answers if there is a good rationale to do so; changing answers does not negatively affect grades as so often believed (Blakeman & Laskowski, 2020; George et al., 2016).

TIPS FOR SUCCESS

▶ INCORPORATE STRATEGIES TO EASE THE FEAR OF TEST ANXIETY

It is normal for a nurse educator to feel anxious about taking the CNE examination.

- Anxiety is a natural response to the new challenges in our lives.
- Some anxiety will produce a heightened awareness and may improve test taking, whereas anxiety that is uncontrolled will impede the ability to think critically.
- Everyone who takes tests experiences anxiety; however, recognizing and controlling anxiety is an important key.

Some strategies that can be used to ease test anxiety include the following:

1. Reducing anxiety related to time constraints

- Schedule the examination when you have a semester that is less stressful.

- Start a study group with other educators and plan to meet once a week for 2 hours.
- Use the detailed test plan to divide assignments.
  - Each faculty member can complete an assignment and share notes with the group.
  - Faculty members can also share the sources of information recommended by the NLN.

2. Reducing anxiety related to not having recent experience in test taking

- After reviewing the content for the examination, complete as many test questions as possible, including the practice examination from the NLN.
- Self-evaluation will assist you in refocusing on specific content.
- Practice will increase your confidence.

3. Reducing anxiety related to previous experience with testing difficulty

- Stop negative thoughts that begin with "what if."
- Strategies, such as positive self-talk, daily exercise, yoga, and meditation, have all been proven to decrease anxiety.
- Practice these strategies on a regular basis so that decreasing anxiety becomes easy to achieve.
- Engage in activities that you find relaxing in the evening prior to the examination, such as watching a movie or going to dinner with friends.

EVIDENCE-BASED TEACHING PRACTICE

Testing anxiety can be reduced by guided imagery, guided reflection, music, aromatherapy, and relaxation breathing. Also, study and focus groups can be of assistance before a testing situation (Broderson, 2017).

 # UTILIZE LEARNING STRATEGIES

▶ REMEMBER BY COMPARISON

An example of remembering by comparison is determining what information is the same and what is different among a variety of areas of information. This learning strategy focuses on the differences. An example of this learning strategy using Boyer's model of scholarship is remembering that all four types of scholarship include peer-reviewed articles, research, and grant awards. However, there are distinct differences among the four areas as described here.

Scholarship of Discovery

The scholarship of discovery is the discovery of new knowledge (Boyer, 1990). A scientific finding is integrated into the application and integration process of healthcare. Examples are peer-reviewed publications of research, theory, or philosophical essays and grant awards in support of research or scholarship. Discovery includes primary empirical research, historical research, theory development, and testing. It includes work that receives state, regional, national, and international recognition.

Scholarship of Teaching

The scholarship of teaching has transpired into an active learning environment in which the nurse educator uses a variety of teaching methods to provide learners with the ability to discuss, collaborate, and explore. The curriculum has been developed to reflect a global, diverse population. Examples are peer-reviewed publications of research related to teaching methodology or learning outcomes and grant awards in support of teaching and learning. It includes state, regional, national, and international recognition.

Scholarship of Practice (Application)

The scholarship of application is the ability to apply theory to practice. This process of clinical reasoning and intervention results in positive patient outcomes. It can also be related to defining and resolving health problems of a community. Examples are peer-reviewed publications of research, case studies, technical applications or other practice issues, and grant awards in support of practice. It includes state, regional, national, and international recognition.

Scholarship of Integration

The scholarship of integration is becoming common practice as it involves providing an interprofessional healthcare team approach for critical analysis and integration of ideas to research complex health problems. Because of the dynamics and experience of various disciplines, the result is a comprehensive holistic solution. Examples are peer-reviewed publications of research, policy analysis, case studies, integrative reviews of literature, interdisciplinary grant awards, copyrights, licenses, patents, and products for sale.

Publication of nursing knowledge is an expectation of a nurse educator's role and can be accomplished through persistence in writing and the mindset that dissemination is a responsibility. Just like all other skills, practice with the assistance of mentors is invaluable for the writing process (Oermann & Hays, 2015).

TEACHING GEM   Nick (2016) discusses the need for nurse educators to "go global." There is a great need for international professional development about many nurse educator topics such as clinical trends, evidence-based practice, online searching of databases, and learning active teaching–learning strategies.

▶ DEVELOP MNEMONIC DEVICES

Develop mnemonics if a memory aid is needed; however, using mnemonics may be less useful in some situations in which it may be easier to just remember the facts. For example, when the nurse educator is developing a test, the BOBCAT mnemonic can provide guidance to develop the test appropriately. This mnemonic stands for

- Blueprint
- Objectives of the course content
- Bloom's taxonomy
- Client needs categories (National Council of State Boards of Nursing [NCSBN], 2016)
- Analysis of data
- Test results and changes for the future

In summary: A blueprint is developed from the objectives of the course. Bloom's taxonomy is used to develop questions at higher cognitive levels such as application and analysis. Client needs areas of NCLEX-RN® (National Council Licensure Examination for Registered Nurses; NCSBN, 2020) are necessary to guide educators teaching in an undergraduate prelicensure program to construct questions in the eight areas, such as management of care, safety and infection control, health promotion and maintenance, and reduction of risk potential, to name a few. Analysis of data is performed, and test results are determined. After the results of the test are reviewed, revisions to items should be completed so they can be used in the future.

▶ RELATE INFORMATION TO BE LEARNED TO INFORMATION ALREADY MASTERED

Learning new information is easier if it can be related to information or facts that are already understood. An example of this learning strategy is illustrated next. Many times, test validity and test reliability become confused. If you understand what test validity means, you only need to add to your memory the information about reliability.

- Validity means the test is measuring the information it is supposed to measure. It is "valid." The test blueprint is used to developed questions related to the objectives of the course; this ensures validity.
- Reliability refers to the consistency of the test scores. The test's reliability can be improved by making changes to the items so that they are more discriminating.

▶ CORRELATE TESTING WITH PRACTICE

Examine your own activities as an educator and relate them to the content in the questions. This will be helpful in developing a complete understanding of the information. You will find that your experience will be very helpful in answering questions. Many examples of how to correlate your own experience with the content to be learned are presented in Table 2.

Table 2 Correlating Experience

Question Content	Educator Experience
Create opportunities for the learners to develop their own critical thinking skills	Learners can develop critical thinking skills by participating in the following assignments: writing a teaching plan, developing a concept map, discussing a case study, completing an exercise in delegation or prioritization in the clinical area, or making decisions in the simulation laboratory
Use information technologies to support the teaching–learning process	Specific materials may be taught more effectively by using technology. It may be advantageous for learners to create a video in response to a clinical situation, participate in synchronous *or asynchronous* discussions, work in a group in a virtual classroom environment, or develop a Wikipedia article

(continued)

Table 2 Correlating Experience (*continued*)

Question Content	Educator Experience
Respond effectively to unexpected events that affect the clinical and/or classroom instruction	Collect all the information, including anecdotal records if the event occurred at the clinical site. Clarify professional behavior as outlined in the Code of Ethics for Nurses with Interpretive Statement and Nursing: Scope and Standards of Practice Utilize conflict resolution, if indicated. Refer the student to the Student Conduct Committee, if indicated
Identify learning styles and unique learning needs of students from culturally diverse backgrounds	Many students speak English as a second language (ESL). The development of communication and active learning in the classroom may assist these students with understanding information such as: 1. Discussing cultural beliefs related to a specific disease, as this can impact client care in the clinical setting 2. Using a team approach by having students in small groups answer questions in class 3. Gaming, such as playing Jeopardy in the classroom, to review content
Provide input for the development of nursing program standards and policies regarding: 1. Admission 2. Progression 3. Graduation	If you have not had the opportunity to work with the admissions, academic progression, or graduation committees in your college of nursing, then request permission to review the minutes or attend meetings. Involvement in these committees promotes a clear understanding of the process Admission criteria are usually posted on the school's website and include Scholastic Aptitude Test scores, entrance examination scores, grade point average (GPA), and Test of English as a Foreign Language (TOEFL) requirements for students born in non-English-speaking countries The progression committee determines whether a student should be permitted to continue in the program after failure of a course or courses. The committee may overturn a decision if the student had extenuating circumstances, such as a serious illness or death in the family. The students may also go through the academic appeals process to overturn a grade they believe to be inaccurate. The committee also takes into account the student's grades in prerequisite and corequisite courses when making a decision

(*continued*)

Table 2 Correlating Experience (*continued*)

Question Content	Educator Experience
	Graduation occurs when the learner completes the minimum number of credits specified for the degree and his or her GPA is within the program standards. A student must also complete the clinical requirements for courses with a satisfactory rating in the clinical component
Participate in curriculum development or revision	Read and compare the mission statements and philosophy statements of the university and the college of nursing Review the level objectives and the behavioral objectives in the nursing program curriculum. Level objectives are reflective of the progressive competence of the students within the goals and philosophy of the program. Behavioral objectives drive the design for the courses with a focus on learning outcomes The curriculum is updated as needed *and should be reviewed annually* to incorporate changes in the student body and the community, the use of technology, and current healthcare trends. The goal is to improve program outcomes
Use feedback gained from self, peer, and learner evaluations to improve role effectiveness	Self-evaluation can assist faculty members in determining their own needs, such as preparation for class, organization, teaching strategy development, and test development Learners may have a need for the enhancement of information or clinical opportunities that are not recognized by the educator. Student evaluations can be used to improve the course Peer evaluations can be helpful; however, they can also cause conflict among faculty members. The educator should have specific guidelines designated for the evaluation, and the date of the didactic evaluation should be decided by both faculty members
Use legal and ethical principles to influence, design, and implement policies and procedures related to learners, educators, and the educational environment	Legal issues can include: 1. Co-signing documentation in the clinical area 2. Providing care that results in an injury to the client or the learner 3. Completion of an incident report 4. Cheating during an examination 5. Plagiarism on a class assignment 6. Dismissal of a student from the program The college should have policies addressing these issues

(*continued*)

Table 2 Correlating Experience (*continued*)

Question Content	Educator Experience
	In addition, students are protected by the U.S. Constitution's Bill of Rights. The First Amendment protects freedom of religion, press, speech, and the right to assemble. The Fourth Amendment provides protection against unreasonable search and seizure
Use evidence-based resources to improve and support teaching	Evidence-based resources can be used in the classroom or clinical setting by 1. Scheduling an assignment in which one group of learners takes a turn discussing a research article related to the content presented in the classroom that week 2. Providing evidence-based articles to learners in the clinical area who have down time; the learner(s) will take time to review the article and present the information during the post conference period
Participate in departmental and institutional committees	Examples of committees within the nursing department include faculty affairs, student affairs, scholarship and innovation, educator resources, curriculum, and technology. Some examples of committees within an institution include faculty and governance, faculty finance, green initiative, and sustainability

◎ **Critical Thinking Question**

What should a novice nurse educator look for when searching and interviewing for an academic position?

EVIDENCE-BASED TEACHING PRACTICE

Fitzgerald, Mcnelis, and Billings (2020) studied course descriptions in 529 schools of nursing education to determine if the NLN Core Competencies for Academic Nurse Educators and CNE preparation was present were present found that four core competencies were present in over 85% of course descriptions and four NLN competencies were not well represented and existed in less than 50% of course descriptions. This study highlights the need to include the NLN core competencies for Academic Nurse Educators and prepare nurse faculty for the CNE Certification.

EVIDENCE-BASED TEACHING PRACTICE

Byrne and Welch (2016) studied the motivation of nurse educators to take the CNE examination and variables that predicated success. Statistical analysis did not demonstrate any significant difference in test scores when comparing roles (faculty vs. new graduate) and years of teaching, indicating the need for future research related to significant variables that predict test success.

● HOW TO RENEW YOUR CERTIFICATION AFTER 5 YEARS

After you pass the CNE examination, you will feel elated and glad you will not need to think about it for another 5 years. However, you will have to think about it if you are going to record renewal credits (RCs).

There are two options for renewal:

1. Document 75 RCs that must be related to at least six of the NLN nurse educator core competencies. The credits earned must be distributed over the 5-year renewal period.
2. Register and pass the CNE or CNEn exam prior to the expiration date located on your certificate.

Simplify the recertification process with three steps:

1. Download the activity record form from the NLN (2020) website after you pass the examination. Complete the form when you meet any of the competencies. Each competency includes the specific activity, date, RC, and the outcome. It is much easier to complete the form immediately instead of trying to locate the information years later. RC is awarded when organized professional activities are employed to enhance professional development as a nurse educator. The educator must have submissions in at least six competencies in order to reflect the full academic role.

RC conversion examples:

One university college course (three semester hours) = 15 RC

One continuing education unit (CEU) = 1 RC

One hour of faculty development or scholarship = 1 RC

Access the NLN website for a full list of activities, the credit conversion table, and sample completion form. Please check the NLN website frequently for updated criteria.

2. Keep the hard copies of certificates of attendance in a folder. Scan these documents into a folder in your electronic PDF documents, so you have an additional copy in case the original copies become lost or damaged within the 5 years. These supporting documents only need to be sent if requested by the Academic Nurse Educator Certification Program (ANECP). The NLN Certification Program randomly selects a percentage for audit.
3. Submit the information approximately by September 30 of the year the RCs are due. The certification period begins on the date you passed the examination. The certification period ends on the expiration date located on the current CNE certificate, but RCs must be submitted by September 30 of the year the recertification is due.

If you fail to satisfy the recertification requirements prior to the conclusion of the cycle, you will be placed on an inactive list and you will receive a suspension notice. During the suspension period, faculty who are suspended may not represent themselves as certified by the NLN.

Table 3 can assist you with determining the activities that meet each competency. Please note that activities for recertification may overlap with more than one competency.

Table 3 Examples of Activities for Each Competency

Competency	Activities May Include But Are Not Limited to
Facilitate learning	■ Creating innovative teaching–learning activities—collaborative ventures with community partners ■ Using evidence-based practice or information technology
Facilitate learner development and socialization	■ Assist students to develop as nurses and integrate expected values and behaviors; an example would be development of a simulation experience ■ Identify individual learning styles and needs for culturally diverse, at risk, or physically challenged learners ■ Assist learners to engage in thoughtful constructive self- or peer evaluation
Use assessment and evaluation strategies	■ Create appropriate assessment instruments to evaluate learner outcomes ■ Design tools for assessing clinical practice ■ Provide input for the development of program policies regarding admission, progression, or graduation
Participate in curriculum design and evaluation of program outcomes	■ Design curricula that reflect trends while preparing graduates to function in the healthcare environment ■ Develop or update courses to reflect the theoretical framework of curricula ■ Support educational goals through community partnership
Pursue continuous quality improvement in the nurse educator role	■ Develop and maintain competence in the multidimensional role; examples would be attending conferences, seminars, workshops ■ Mentor and support faculty colleagues in the role of academic nurse educators ■ Engage in activities that promote role socialization; an example would be participation in a nursing organization ■ Use feedback from self, peers, learners, and/or administration for improvement
Function as a change agent and leader	■ Provide an active service within a nursing service organization, association, or committee ■ Work within a special panel or think tank for an educational issue ■ Represent nursing education within an intradisciplinary work group
Engage in scholarship	■ Develop an area of expertise within the academic educator role ■ Share expertise with colleagues; examples would be publications or presentations
Function within the educational environment	■ Collaborate with other disciplines to enhance the academic environment ■ Participate in committee work on the departmental or institutional level

Source: NLN (2021).

CASE STUDIES

CASE STUDY 1

Olivia is an APRN with 4 years of experience as a clinical educator in women's health. Olivia recently took a full-time position in a small private college and is responsible for the didactic portion of the women's health course. Olivia is feeling overwhelmed with preparing information for class and developing questions for examinations. Olivia is concerned because the learners do not agree with the correct answers on exams. Olivia fears that discussing this information with her mentor will indicate that she is unsuccessful in her new role.

> Should Olivia discuss this issue with her mentor?
> How should Olivia approach this issue with the learners?
> What data should Olivia be viewing to determine whether the questions are discriminating?

CASE STUDY 2

The nurse educator has 10 years of experience in critical care nursing and has worked for 3 years in quality improvement. The nurse educator accepted a position in a midsized university and developed some learner-centered activities for the class. The program director believes that the nurse educator should lecture to be sure the learners are provided with the information and then use the learner-centered activities if time allows.

> How should the nurse educator respond to the program director?
> How can the nurse educator evaluate whether the learner-centered activities have positive outcomes?

REFERENCES

American Nurses Association. (2020). The nursing workforce 2014: Growth, salaries, education demographics & trends. http://www.nursingworld.org/-mainmenucategories/thepracticeofprofessionalnursing/workforce/fast-facts-2014-nursing-workforce.pdf

American Nurses Credentialing Center. (2020). Magnet recognition overview. http://www.nursecredentialing.org/Magnet/ProgramOverview

Blake, J. R. & Laskowski, P. S. (2020). Beliefs and experiences of nurse educators regarding changing answers on examinations. *Nursing Education Perspectives*, 41(2), 97–102. 10.1097/01.NEP.0000000000000497

Boyer, E. (1990). *Scholarship reconsidered: Priorities of the professoriate*. Carnegie Foundation for the Advancement of Teaching.

Broderson, L. D. (2017). Interventions for test anxiety in undergraduate nursing students: An integrative review. *Nursing Education Perspectives*, 38(3), 131–137.

Byrne, M. & Welch, S. (2016). CNE certification drive and exam results. *Nursing Education Perspectives*, 37(4), 221–223. 10.5480/14–1408

Fitzgerald, A., McNelis, A. M. & Billings, D. M. (2020). NLN Core Competencies for Nurse Educators: Are they present in the course descriptions of academic nurse educator programs? *Nursing Education Perspectives*, 41(1), 4–9. 10.1097/01.NEP.0000000000000530

George, T., Muller, M. A., & Bartz, J. D. (2016). A mixed-methods study of prelicensure nursing students changing answers on multiple choice examinations. *Journal of Nursing Education, 55*(4), 220–223. 10.3928/01484834–20160316–07

Institute of Medicine. (2010). *The future of nursing: Leading change, advancing health.* National Academies Press. http://www.nationalacademies.org/HMD/Reports/2010/The-Future-of-Nursing-Leading-Change-Advancing-Health.aspx

Levey, J. A. (2016). Measuring nurse educators' willingness to adopt inclusive teaching strategies. *Nursing Education Perspectives, 37*(4), 215–220.

Lundeen, J. (2018). Analysis of first-time unsuccessful attempts on the certified nurse educator examination. *Nursing Education Perspectives, 37*(4), 215–220.

National Council of State Boards of Nursing. (2020). Test plans. https://www.ncsbn.org/test-plans.htm

National League for Nursing. (2021). Certified Nurse Educator (CNE) 2021 candidate handbook. http://www.nln.org/docs/default-source/default-document-library/cne-handbook-2021_revised_07-01-2021.pdf?sfvrsn=2

National League for Nursing. (2021). Certified Nurse Educator Novice (CNEn) 2021 candidate handbook. http://www.nln.org/Certification-for-Nurse-Educators/cne-n/cne-n-handbook

National League for Nursing. (2020). Renewal. http://www.nln.org/certification/recertification/index.htm

Nick, J. M. (2016). Tips for nurse educators who want to go global. *Reflections on Nursing Leadership, 42*(1), 1–4.

Oermann, M. H. & Hays, J. (2015). *Writing for publication in nursing* (3rd ed.). Springer Publishing.

Poindexter, K., Lindell, D., & Hagler, D. (2019). Measuring the value of academic nurse educator certification: Perceptions of administrators and educators. *Journal of Nursing Education, 58*(9), 502–509. 10.3928/01484834–20190819–02

Simmons, L. & Christensen, L. (2018). Development of the Certified Nurse Educator Certification Exam: A spotlight on competencies, scoring, and security. *Nursing Education Perspectives, 39*(3), 196. 10.1097/01.NEP.0000000000000333

Stribling, J., Clifton, A., McGill, G., & Vries, K. (2020). Examining the UK Covid-19 mortality paradox: Pandemic preparedness, healthcare expenditure, and the nursing workforce. *Journal of Advanced Nursing, 76*(12): 3218–3227. 10.1111/jan.14562

U.S. Bureau of Labor Statistics, U.S. Department of Labor. (2020). Occupational outlook handbook: Registered nurses. http://www.bls.gov/ooh/healthcare/-registered-nurses.htm

Wittmann-Price, R. A. (2012). *Fast facts for developing a nursing academic portfolio.* Springer Publishing.

Facilitate Learning

Ruth A. Wittmann-Price and Ksenia Zukowsky

Strive for excellence, not perfection.
—H. Jackson Brown, Jr.

▶ LEARNING OUTCOMES

This chapter addresses the Certified Nurse Educator and Certified Nurse Educator Novice Exams Content Area 1: Facilitate Learning. For the CNE exam this area is 22% of the examination, approximately 33 questions and for the CNEn examination this area is 39% of the examination or approximately 59 questions.

- Discuss the theoretical and philosophical underpinnings of nursing education
- Compare behaviorism and constructivism
- Describe learning and motivation
- Contrast andragogy with pedagogy
- Evaluate the evidence on critical thinking and metacognition
- Demonstrate learning session organization and management

● INTRODUCTION

Nursing education today is more exciting and challenging than ever before. Gone are the days of a homogeneous classroom of learners who respond unquestioningly to lockstep teaching and learning methods. Now nurse educators facilitate learning for students of all ages; from many different lifestyles, ethnic, and cultural backgrounds; with different generational characteristics; and, most importantly, with different learning styles. Additionally, nurse educators have to adjust to environmental and social issues such as pandemics, protests, and natural disasters, and keep the students engaged and focused on the learning outcomes. The overarching goal is that every learner deserves nurse educators who can best facilitate the learner's journey toward becoming a successful, professional nurse. Educational expertise is needed to assist students to become competent and caring professional nurses. To accomplish the goal of successful career transitions from learner to nurse or from nurse to advanced practice nurse, faculty must facilitate the development of clinical judgment and inspire lifelong learning. Nurse educators who understand the basics in teaching-learning principles, evaluation and assessment methods, and curriculum development and design can best prepare nursing professionals who provide quality, value-based patient care to meet the needs of the ever-changing and challenging healthcare environment.

EDUCATIONAL PHILOSOPHIES

A positive learning environment must be established to facilitate students' knowledge acquisition. This is accomplished when the learning environment is built on sound philosophical foundations. These foundations assume that nursing education is:

- Never stagnant and change as the larger social system matures and changes,
- Provide the foundations on which learning theories and educational pedagogies are built, and
- Considers a philosophy that addresses why we teach, how we teach, and what the goals of education are for learners and society (Yeom et al., 2018).

 ## CRITICAL THINKING

If **ontology** is concerned with becoming and what is actual and real and **epistemology** is concerned about theories of knowledge, how do these two concepts interact in your teaching philosophy (Yeom et al., 2018)?

Teaching philosophies of academic nurse educators are developed over time, and each nurse educator has a personal philosophy. Personal philosophies are developed from experiences and reflection. Educational philosophies and are used in the development of professional portfolios and form the basis of why and how nurse educators facilitate learning (Younas, 2018).

 ## LEARNING THEORIES

"**Teaching** is what the educator provides the learner in terms of goals, methods, objectives, and outcomes. **Learning** refers to the processes by which the learner changes skills, knowledge, and dispositions through a planned experience" (Kaakinen & Arwood, 2009, p. 1). How people learn and how they store, connect, discover, and retrieve information and skills have been well studied and formalized into many theoretical frameworks. These frameworks try to explain the connection between knowledge and the human brain, a truly interesting subject that affects learners every day.

Educational philosophy guides learning theories, and there is some overlap in terms and ideas from among them. Philosophies are driven by **metaphysics**, the study of what is real; **epistemology**, the study of what is knowledge and truth; and **axiology**, the study of what is good (Meleis, 2018). Theories have more defined concepts and are more applicable to the teaching situation than philosophies are. The learning theories discussed today in nursing are mainly **constructivism** and **behaviorism** (Barbour & Schuessler, 2019). In Table 1.1, philosophical foundations are broken down into brief descriptions of general philosophies, sometimes referred to as "worldviews," educational philosophies, and the corresponding teaching–learning theories.

Table 1.1 Worldview Philosophies, Educational Philosophies, and Teaching–Learning Theories

Worldview Philosophies	Educational Philosophies	Teaching–Learning Theories
Traditional Philosophies and Theories		
Idealism (Plato, Socrates) ■ The ideal vision is important ■ People would like to live in a perfect world	**Perennialism** (Thomas Aquinas) ■ Traditional educational style (teacher-centered) ■ Liberal art education is valued ■ Studies should include great thinkers of the past ■ Prepare learners for adult life ■ Reading, writing, and arithmetic are important (the 3 r's)	**Information Processing** (Gagne, 1970) ■ Describes how information is received, stored, and processed in the mind as part of cognitive growth ■ Learning is a function of the brain (brain-based learning) ■ Humans process information and store it in memory ■ Memory is achieved by sensory input, which goes to short-term memory (working memory), which is then stored, if significant, in long-term memory, in which information may be forgotten but is never lost completely
Realism (Positivism) (Aristotle) ■ The world is orderly ■ Science can be viewed objectively and analyzed ■ Develop knowledge that is value and context-free (Mann, 2011)	**Essentialism** (Bagley, Hirsh) ■ Traditional educational approach that develops learners' minds through knowledge passed to the learner from the educator ■ A core curriculum is valued, as are democracy and cultural heritage ■ Physical world is the true reality ■ Learners should appreciate the masterworks of art and literature ■ Learners need critical thinking skills to help society ■ Teacher-directed learning	**Behaviorism** (Pavlov, Watson, Skinner) ■ Stimulus and response are the basis for learning ■ The environment develops the person ■ Requires behavior modification and class management ■ Positive reinforcement is used to encourage acceptable behavior ■ Generated the idea of "programmed learning" ■ Tyler (1949) introduced behavioral objectives in education ■ Faculty decides on the educational experience ■ Nursing education is still steeped in behaviorism today (lockstep curriculum and pre-determined objectives) **Social Learning Theory or Social Cognitive Theory** (Bandura, 1997) ■ Perception of confidence in oneself in the situation (self-efficacy) ■ Positive expectations are the incentives ■ Bandura's term *reciprocal determinism* means that the world and the person's behavior cause each other ■ Feedback to the learner is important ■ Self-efficacy is based on four principles: 1) Enactive mastery experiences or the learner's own history of successes

(continued)

Table 1.1 Worldview Philosophies, Educational Philosophies, and Teaching–Learning Theories (continued)

Worldview Philosophies	Educational Philosophies	Teaching–Learning Theories
Realism (Positivism) (Aristotle) (cont.)	Essentialism (Bagley, Hirsh) (cont.)	Behaviorism (Pavlov, Watson, Skinner) (cont.) 2) Vicarious experiences or the observed behaviors of a role model being successful at a task 3) Verbal persuasion or telling someone that he or she will be successful 4) Physiological states or the person's "gut feeling" that he or she can succeed (Hawker et al., 2021; Mann, 2011)
Poststructuralism or Modern Philosophies and Theories		

Pragmatism (Dewey, Pierce)
■ Ideas can be tested scientifically
■ The human experience is important
■ Influenced by social reform and the growth of citizenship in early 19th century
	Progressivism (Dewey)
	■ School mimics society
	■ Real-life curriculum and problem-solving exercises are the most important
	■ Attend to and optimize inquisitive, active learning
	■ Experiential learning takes place in the learning session
	■ Learners have choices about what to learn
	■ Learners are engaged in group and peer learning
	■ Education experiences are learner-centered
		Constructivism (Piaget, Vygotsky)
		■ "Active" learning theory
		■ Learning is built by the learner and is built on previous knowledge and in the reality of the learner
		■ Attributes of constructivism include:
		  ● Learning is actively constructed through interaction with the environment, and it is marked by reflection and actions
		  ● The learner tries to make sense out of his or her perceptions and experiences (Mann, 2011)
		  ● Doing is learning
		  ● Social negotiation is a part of learning
		  ● Supports multiple perspectives on subjects
		  ● Taking ownership of learning is important
		  ● Be self-aware and reflective in the knowledge-acquisition process
		  ● The goals are problem-solving, reasoning, critical thinking, and the active and reflective use of knowledge
		  ● Most important, it is learner-focused (Lai & Bower, 2020)
		
		Piaget (1972) described cognitive learning as a process of:
		■ Accommodation
		■ Assimilation
		■ Equilibration
		
		Knowles's (1980) adult learning theory (andragogy)
		■ Supports constructivism because it also builds on the learner's previous experiences (more information about andragogy can be found later in this chapter)

(continued)

Table 1.1 Worldview Philosophies, Educational Philosophies, and Teaching–Learning Theories *(continued)*

Worldview Philosophies	Educational Philosophies	Teaching–Learning Theories
		Situated Learning Theory ■ Closely linked with constructivism ■ Reality based ■ Learner is an active participant in learning ■ Especially helpful when applied to clinical practice (O'Brien & Battista, 2020) **Experiential Learning Theory** Experimental learning theory (ELT) is a framework for learning whereby students reflect on what they are doing. It is usually hands-on and the outcome is minimized and the process is what is reflected upon. It is defined as "the process whereby knowledge is created through the transformation of experience. Knowledge results from the combination of grasping and transforming experience" (Kolb, 1984, p. 41)
Existentialism (Kierkegaard, Satre) ■ Seeks individual meaning in life ■ Schools hold social ideals ■ Perception of the individual is reality ■ No one can know us as we know ourselves ■ Education of the whole person is the goal ■ Subject matter takes second place to the development of a positive self-concept, self-knowledge, and self-responsibility	**Reconstructionism/Critical Theory** (Habermas, Freire) ■ School is important for social change ■ School alone can prepare a learner for life ■ Includes the way educators construct or influence learning ■ Contains not only knowledge but also considers power ■ It includes constructing privilege, social identity, and cultural practices (Saar-Heiman, & Gupta, 2020)	There are four major concepts within the theory: ■ Concrete experience (CE) or those experiences built from reality ■ Abstract conceptualization (AC) or thinking about an experience ■ Reflective observation (RO) or taking in the experience ■ Active experimentation (AE) using hands-on experiences to learn (Kolb, Boyatzis, & Mainemelis, 1999) **Humanism** (Rogers, Maslow) ■ Human beings are autonomous, and the dignity of human beings is most important ■ Self-actualization and education lead to individual happiness ■ A nursing approach can be found in Bevis and Watson's (1989) *Toward a Caring Curriculum* **Narrative Pedagogy** (Diekelmann, 2005) A phenomenological pedagogy ■ Focus is on the meaning and significance of teaching through phenomenology pedagogies such as narratives and storytelling

(continued)

Table 1.1 Worldview Philosophies, Educational Philosophies, and Teaching–Learning Theories (*continued*)

Worldview Philosophies	Educational Philosophies	Teaching–Learning Theories
■ Learners have great latitude in choosing subject matter	**Emancipatory Education** (Freire, 1970) ■ Education is a microsystem of society ■ Educators are cultural workers who profess freedom through an equalized learning session ■ Both educators and students are learners through true dialogue **Feminism** ■ Personal knowledge is a true knowledge ■ Power in the learning session must be analyzed ■ No human being should be marginalized ■ Places a great emphasis on empowerment and the learners' voices ■ Empirical knowledge is only one type of knowledge ■ Also uses narrative pedagogy (Burton, 2020)	■ Builds experiences that stray from a formal, competency-based, outcome education format ■ Develops deeper thinking and finds meaning in lived experiences ■ Bases understanding on interpreting, not memorizing ■ Students and faculty learn from each other (Brady & Asselin, 2016)

Source: Adapted from Chinn, P. (2007). Philosophical foundations for excellence in nursing. In B. Moyer & R. A. Wittmann-Price (Eds.). *Nursing education: Foundations of practice excellence* (pp. 15–28). Philadelphia, PA: F. A. Davis.

Critical Thinking Question
What belief(s) or philosophies speak to you as an academic nurse educator?

THEORY OF MEANINGFUL LEARNING

Sousa, Formiga, Oliveira, Costa, and Soares (2015) describe "meaningful learning" as a learning theory that was developed by Ausubel (1962), which describes how learning must make sense personally to the learner. The **Theory of Meaningful Learning** proposes that knowledge must be interesting to the learner and be grounded in past experiences. The learner uses knowledge to develop new and unique meaning. The theory discusses the receptiveness of the learner and discovery. Active teaching strategies increase individualized knowledge discovery. The Theory of Meaningful Learning is akin to the constructivist theoretical assumptions. Meaningful learning can occur face-to-face and online (Petrovic et al., 2020).

EVIDENCE-BASED TEACHING PRACTICE

Reiger et al. (2020) used a constructivist grounded theory to study how arts-based pedagogy fostered meaningful learning for nursing students ($n = 30$) and nurse educators ($n = 8$). Four sources of data were collected including, a socio-demographic questionnaire, semi-structured interviews, photo/art elicitation, and field notes. The findings revealed that 80% of students navigated the creative process through interactive phases and valued the learning. The findings highlighted multi-level enabling and restraining factors for student involvement in creative learning and inform nursing education of modifiable factors to increase student engagement and learning using art-based pedagogy.

 TEACHING GEM   When a class begins with learning objectives (behaviorism) and reviews the anatomy and physiology before the patient condition (constructivism) is discussed, two learning theories are integrated.

MODELS SPECIFIC TO NURSING

There are two classic nursing models that have been significant in nursing education for the past several decades and are widely used as the theoretical foundations for many nursing studies and curricula, and learning activity development. They are Barbara Carper's (1978) "ways of knowing" and Patricia Benner's (1982) "novice to expert theory." Both will be reviewed in brief.

Carper (1978) described four ways that nurses understand practice situations, and they are:

1. Empirical or scientific knowledge (includes evidence-based practice [EBP])
2. Personal knowledge or understanding of how you would feel in the patient's position

3. Ethical knowledge or attitudes and understanding of moral decisions

4. Aesthetic knowledge or understanding the situation of the patient at the moment

Munhall (1993) added the fifth way of knowing: **unknowing** or understanding that the nurse cannot know everything about the patient and must place himself or herself in a position willing to learn from the patient's perspective.

EVIDENCE-BASED TEACHING PRACTICE

Starkweather et al. (2019) studied inter and intraprofessional collaborations to advance biobehavioral symptom science. The study was guided by Carper's patterns of knowing. The researchers found that strategic partnerships across nursing associations and organization can help to build collaborations to advance biobehavioral symptom science by sharing workgroups, data, and research results. Inter and intraprofessional teams use multiple ways of knowing that nurses often use to produce new knowledge, develop innovations, and apply knowledge and innovation to practice.

Benner (1982) described five levels of nursing expertise patterned on studies of how nurses grow in their role, and they include:

Novice—a beginner with no experience

- Relies on general rules to help perform tasks
- Rules are context-free, independent of specific cases, and applied universally
- Behavior is limited and inflexible

Advanced beginner—a person who is at the point of demonstrating acceptable performance and

- Has gained prior experience in actual situations to recognize some patterns
- Uses principles based on experiences that begin to be formulated to guide actions

Competent—typically a nurse with 2 to 3 years' experience in the same role and

- Is aware of long-term goals
- Has a perspective about planning care with conscious, abstract, and analytical thinking
- Has greater efficiency and organization

Proficient—a nurse who perceives and understands situations as a whole and

- Understands patients holistically and has improved decision making
- Learns from experiences what to expect in certain situations
- Can be flexible and modify plans

Expert—a nurse who no longer relies on principles, rules, or guidelines to understand patient needs and determine actions and

- Has an intuitive grasp of practice situations
- Is flexible and highly proficient

EVIDENCE-BASED TEACHING PRACTICE

Graf et al. (2020) completed a narrative critical literature review with the goal of finding the best fit for graduate nursing students' transitioning into the practice environment. The review was based on four theories, including Kramer's reality shock theory, Benner's novice to expert theory, Bridges's transition theory, and Duchscher's stages of transition theory. The researchers found that Duchscher's stages of transition theory best describe the experiences of registered nursing transition into practice. Duchscher's stages of transition theory application can assist in explaining the challenges of new graduates.

Dr. Patricia Benner has also been the primary author of a literature review and analysis contained in the book *Educating Nurses: A Call for Radical Transformation* (2009), which was funded by the Carnegie and Atlantic philanthropies. After a thorough historical and current review of nursing education, the following significant recommendations were made and are still applicable today:

- Use teaching to integrate knowledge into the practice setting
- Decrease the division between didactic and clinical knowledge
- Emphasize clinical reasoning and multiple ways of thinking along with critical thinking
- Focus on the formation of professional identity along with socialization

---

TEACHING GEM   The recommendations from Benner (2009) are being realized throughout nursing education, such as the National Council State Boards of Nursing (2020) emphasis on clinical decision-making in the "Next Generation NCLEX-RN Examination."

DEEP, SURFACE, AND STRATEGIC LEARNING

Deep learning is a term first described by Marton and Saljo (1976) to refer to a learning approach and type of knowledge acquisition. The approach a learner takes to information presented in the learning session can be classified into three types of learning styles: deep, surface, and strategic.

1. A deep learning approach is accomplished when a learner addresses material with the intent to understand both the concepts and meaning of the information.

    - The learner relates new ideas to existing experiences and formulates links in long-term memory.
    - The motivation for a deep learning approach is primarily intrinsic, created from the learner's interest and desire to understand the relevance of the information to applied practice.
    - A type of deep learning is utilizing tangible everyday household objects to link new concepts to promote deep learning in an effort to link the concept to long-term memory (Wittmann-Price & Godshall, 2009).

2. A surface learning, or atomistic, approach facilitates learning by:

    - Memorization of facts and details. Surface learning is similar to rote learning in that the learner assimilates information presented at face value.
    - Motivation for surface learning, which is primarily extrinsic, is driven by either the learner's fear of failing or the desire to complete the course successfully.

3. A strategic learning approach; using this learning approach, the learner does what is needed to complete a course. Strategic learning is a mixture of both deep and surface learning techniques (Wittmann-Price & Godshall, 2009).
   ■ All three approaches to learning can be measured by the Approaches and Study Skills Inventory for Students (ASSIST; Ramsden & Entwistle, 1981).

Interactive teaching techniques enhance deep learning by increasing student engagement (Shustack, 2019).

EVIDENCE-BASED TEACHING PRACTICE

D'Souza and colleagues (2019) used a cross-sectional survey to study the educational environment in undergraduate nursing education and learning approaches used by students (N = 252) in relation to academic outcome. The results showed that nursing students had a positive perception of the environment and there was a positive, significant correlation with academic outcomes (rs = 0.348, p = .001). Results demonstrated a weak positive relation between deep learning and learning approaches with the academic outcome (rs = 0.159, p = .012 and rs = 0.204, p = .001), denoting that students use varied learning approaches and facilitating understanding of the approaches may enhance deep learning.

 MOTIVATIONAL THEORIES

Not only do nurse educators need to know how learners acquire information, but they also need to know why they learn. What are learners' motivating factors? Motivation has been linked to learner retention and success. Many variables affect motivation; motivation can be influenced by the need for achievement or curiosity, or it can be a function of the situation at hand or a person's ability. A learner's **locus of control** can be **extrinsically** or **intrinsically motivated**. Motivation includes a student's goals, beliefs, perceptions, and expectations (Li, 2020).

▶ ARCS MODEL

Keller (1987) talks about the factors that educators can implement to motivate learners in the **ARCS model**. The model is still useful today and can be used as a guide for in-class and online.

A—Attention (keeping the learner's attention through stimulus changes in the didactic or clinical setting)
R—Relevance (make the information relevant to the learner's goals)
C—Confidence (make expectations clear so the learner will engage in learning)
S—Satisfaction (have appropriate consequences for the learner's new skills)

EVIDENCE-BASED TEACHING PRACTICE

Kaulback (2020) quantitatively studied the relationship between baccalaureate nursing students' (N = 124) self-directed learning (SDL) and lifelong learning. The results demonstrated a positive correlation between SDL and intent for life-long learning, which included interpersonal communication, planning and implementing, self-monitoring, and learning motivation.

▶ BROPHY MODEL

Brophy (1986) listed the following methods by which motivation is formed:

- Modeling
- Communication of expectations
- Direct instruction
- Socialization by parents and educators

▶ VROOM'S EXPECTANCY MODEL

Vroom's expectancy model (VEM) describes what people want and whether they are positioned to obtain it. The Vroom model describes three concepts:

1. Force (F)—the amount of effort a person will put into reaching a goal
2. Valence (V)—how attractive the goal is to the person
3. Expectancy (E)—the possibility of the goal being achieved

The VEM model is $F = V \times E$ (Vroom, 1964).

▶ BELONGINGNESS

Belongingness is conceptually related to motivation. Students, like all people, have a need to belong or be part of the group. Belongingness is instrumental in students' achievement, retention, self-esteem, self-directed learning (SDL), and self-efficacy. Without belongingness, students are at risk for attrition (Ashktorab et al., 2015). Vinales (2015) describes nursing students' belongingness in relation to building empowerment through increasing competency and confidence using a nurse role model. Hasanvand, Ashktorab, and Seyedfatemi (2014) report that students will conform to the norm in clinical learning experiences in order to gain a feeling of belongingness. Levett-Jones and Lathlean (2008) have completed landmark studies on belongingness and have identified themes about learning, which assist learners to either succeed or disengage; these are listed in Exhibit 1.1.

Exhibit 1.1 Themes About Learning

Theme A = Motivation to learn—being accepted and valued as a learner
Theme B = SDL assists in building confidence
Theme C = Anxiety is a barrier to learning
Theme D = Confidence to ask questions

EVIDENCE-BASED TEACHING PRACTICE

Daniels and colleagues (2020) developed a "belongingness" tool and piloted the instrument with undergraduate medical students ($N = 181$) to assess their participation in a community of practice. The tool is reliable and valid to assess variations in student learning experiences that may impact their academic success. Lottes (2008) uses a formula that she calls **FIRE UP** to enhance learners' motivation. This motivational strategy is shown in Exhibit 1.2.

▶ CHANGE

Change and motivation are interwoven concepts—one is dependent on the other. Change (learning new information, skills, or values) does not happen unless a learner is motivated; therefore, an unmotivated learner most likely will not change. Change theories are well described in Chapter 14.

Exhibit 1.2 Lotte's FIRE UP Motivational Strategy

F: be Funny—Use light entertainment to increase attention I: be Interesting—Use graphics to help learners focus R: be Real—Remember that you were a nursing student once E: Engage them—Use active learning techniques U: be Unique—Use an individual style in the learning session P: be Passionate—Of course, love what you do

Source: Lottes (2008). Reprinted with permission of SLACK Inc.

◎ **Critical Thinking Question**

What was your motivation for going back to school to become a nurse educator or for studying for the Certified Nurse Educator examination? Was it intrinsically or extrinsically motivated?

▶ PEDAGOGY AND ANDRAGOGY

Pedagogy is generally defined as the art and science of teaching. It refers to the manner in which educators instruct, and its development was intended for children. **Andragogy** refers to the art and science of teaching adults (Knowles, 1980). Differences in the learning styles of students are discussed in detail in Chapter 9. Table 1.2 discusses the differences between andragogy and pedagogy.

Table 1.2 Andragogy and Pedagogy

Educational Element	Andragogy	Pedagogy
Demands of learning	Learners have life demands besides school	Learners can devote more time to the demands of learning because responsibilities are minimal
Role of instructor	Learners are autonomous and self-directed Educators facilitate the learning but do not supply all the facts	Teacher centered because the educator directs the learning Often uses surface learning
Life experiences	Learners have a tremendous amount of life experience Learners connect the learning to their knowledge base Learners must recognize the value of the learning	Learners do not have the knowledge base to make the connections between new knowledge and life experiences without facilitation

(continued)

Table 1.2 Andragogy and Pedagogy *(continued)*

Educational Element	Andragogy	Pedagogy
Purpose for learning	Learners have a goal in sight for their learning	Learners cannot always see the long-term necessity of information
Permanence of learning	Learning is self-initiated and tends to last a long time	Learning is compulsory and tends to disappear shortly after instruction

 ## TEACHING STYLES AND EFFECTIVENESS

Every academic nurse educator has his or her own style of teaching; teaching styles have been classified by many different methods. Nurse educators rarely subscribe to just one teaching style. Most educators use a variety of styles, even within a single learning session. This mixed approach can appeal to a variety of learning styles and can improve learning outcomes. Reflecting on the type of style that you use most encourages self-understanding and may serve to improve your effectiveness.

Several attributes contribute to teaching effectiveness. Nurse educator attributes that students assess as positive include communication, accessibility, and faculty knowledge about the subject matter (Saini et al., 2020).

EVIDENCE-BASED TEACHING PRACTICE

Saini and colleagues quantitatively studied students ($N = 192$) perceptions of faculty. Participants identified important attributes of faculty as:

1. 92.7% identified self-confidence as important.
2. 86.5% identified speaking style as important.
3. 86.5% identified the ability to clarify information.
4. 86.4% identified scientific area of expertise.
5. 85.5% identified method teaching.
6. 84.4% identified mastery of scientific material.

▶ ONLINE TEACHING PRESENCE

Due to changing times, there is increased current research about faculty presence online.

Online teaching presents challenges for faculty, and students have identified that faculty presence is an important piece of academic satisfaction. Online presence, besides cognitive presence related to content and expertise, and identity presence related to faculty's self as an expert, there needs to be a "social presence." Social presence provides the learner with the perception that on the other end of the internet there is a live person that cares about their success. Social presence is enhanced through responsiveness, feedback, clarity, and active teaching-leaning strategies (Andel et al., 2020).

EVIDENCE-BASED TEACHING PRACTICE

Yilmaz (2020) studied teaching, social presence, and cognitive presence using a randomized control study with university students ($N = 104$) and found that the data collected with the Community of Inquiry Scale, the Reflective Thinking Scale, and a semi-structured student opinion form revealed that sending feedback on individual assignments had a statistically significant effect on the students' perceptions of community of inquiry and reflective thinking skills.

> **EVIDENCE-BASED TEACHING PRACTICE**
>
> Palese and colleagues (2020) studied the educational activities that are "missed" or delayed in nursing programs and included clinical rotations, classroom teaching, and students' overall learning experience. Indirectly the researchers identified other missed experiences such as faculty professional development. This research was conducted by focus groups ($N = 32$), and the themes included impact on the quality of nursing education and the faculty–student relationship suffers.
>
> Following are some of the ways teaching styles are categorized. Also included are good teaching behaviors and personality traits for educators that experts consider most effective.

▶ GRASHA'S CLASSIFICATION OF TEACHING STYLES

Grasha's (1996) classification defines teaching styles as expert, formal authority, demonstrator, facilitator, and delegator. The characteristics of each teaching style are unique and are listed in Table 1.3.

Table 1.3 Grasha's Teaching Styles

Style	Characteristics
Expert	Educator uses his or her vast knowledge base to inform learners and challenges them to be well prepared. This can be intimidating to the learner
Formal authority	This style puts the educator in control of the learners' knowledge acquisition. The educator is not concerned with student–teacher relationships but rather focuses on the content to be delivered
Demonstrator or personal model	The educator coaches, demonstrates, and encourages a more active learning approach
Facilitator	Learner-centered; active learning strategies are encouraged. The accountability for learning is placed on the learner
Delegator	The educator role is that of a consultant, and the learners are encouraged to direct the entire learning process

Source: Grasha (1996). Reprinted with permission of Carol Grasha.

▶ QUIRK'S CLASSIFICATION OF TEACHING STYLES

Quirk (1994) categorizes teaching styles into four distinct types:

1. Assertive—an assertive style is usually content-specific and drives home information.
2. Suggestive—educator uses experiences to describe a concept and then requests the learners research more information on the subject.
3. Collaborative—educator uses skills to promote problem-solving and a higher level of thinking in the learners.
4. Facilitative—educators using this style often challenge the learners to reflect and use affective learning. Educators challenge learners to ask ethical questions and to demonstrate skill with interpersonal relationships and professional behavior.

▶ KELLY'S TEACHING EFFECTIVENESS

Kelly (2008) also studied learners' perceptions of teaching effectiveness and found that the three most important attributes were:

1. Teacher knowledge
2. Feedback
3. Communication skills

▶ HOUSE, CHASSIE, AND SPOHN'S TEACHING BEHAVIORS

House, Chassie, and Spohn (1999) provide examples of the following behaviors and their effect on learners:

- Making eye contact can encourage learner participation in class.
- Positive facial expressions that elicit a positive learner response, such as head nodding, can assist learners in feeling comfortable speaking in class, whereas negative gestures, such as frowning, can discourage learner class participation.
- Vocal tone is very important and can easily portray underlying feelings and encourage or discourage learner participation.

▶ CHOO'S CHARACTERISTICS OF EDUCATORS

Choo (1996) lists some of the characteristics of educators that are positive and promote learning:

- Values learning
- Exhibits a caring relationship
- Provides learner independence
- Facilitates questioning
- Tries different approaches
- Accepts the differences among learners

▶ KOSHENIN'S POSITIVE TEACHER–LEARNER RELATIONSHIP ATTRIBUTES

Koshenin (2004) identified five themes in the mentoring teacher–learner relationship that are worthy of note, because they can be conceptually transferred into the learning session. They are as follows:

- Worry about the learner's adjustment
- The pervasive experience of the relationship
- The feeling of mutual learning
- Worry about the learning results
- Disappointment in the lack of cooperation between the school and field (or within the larger organization of academia)

▶ HICKS AND BURKUS' MASTER TEACHERS

Hicks and Burkus (2011) describe attributes of "master teachers," which include:

- Clear communication—oral and written
- Positive role modeling
- Professionalism demonstrated in lifelong learning and scholarship
- Reflective practice and making adjustments for improvement
- Use of philosophical, epistemological, and ontological influences in their practice of education

▶ STORY AND BUTTS' FOUR "Cs"

Story and Butts (2010) discuss teaching delivery in the framework of the important four "Cs":

1. Caring—learners need to know that educators truly care about them
2. Comedy—humor is used to "demystify" the heavy content proposed to learners in the learning session
3. Creativity—creative learning activities, such as food examples and role-play, are integrated into the lessons
4. Challenge—maintain high expectations, and the learners will reach them

▶ MANN'S 11 PRACTICAL TIPS

A. S. Mann (2004) provides 11 practical tips for new college educators, which are designed to assist with their transition into academia. They are as follows:

1. Do not use a red pen to correct work.
2. Provide breaks for long classes.
3. Review test answers in writing, if requested.
4. Take roll call to emphasize the importance of being present.
5. Set boundaries.
6. Evaluate the advice of others and be yourself.
7. Write down your expectations.
8. Do not change textbooks during a course.
9. Attend any and all services you can about teaching.
10. Teach to the learners' level.
11. Prepare for the next year every year.

▶ THE MYERS–BRIGGS TYPE INDICATOR

The educator's personality also affects instruction. The Myers–Briggs Type Indicator (MBTI) measures Jung's (1921) 16 personality types by classifying them into four bipolar dimensions.

1. Extroversion/introversion
2. Sensing/intuition
3. Thinking/feeling
4. Judgment/perception

Besides cognitive evaluations of grades and standardized test scores, students' personality types may indicate success in higher education. Noncognitive indicators can be another variable to predict educational success. Using the MBTI as a reflection mechanism to enhance communication, leadership, and conflict-resolution skills in nursing (Childs-Kean et al., 2020).

EVIDENCE-BASED TEACHING PRACTICE

Devries and Beck (2020) studied the Myers-Briggs Type Indicator (MBTI) personalities of undergraduate students who choose a healthcare profession (recreational therapy) and found that approximately 60% of students identified as one of three personality types (ESFJ, ENFJ, or ENFP). This study demonstrates that personality type has implications for students and faculty.

Silver, Hanson, and Strong (1996) developed a Teaching Style Inventory (TSI) based on Jung's theory of psychological types or personality types. It tests the educator's propensity for one of four types:

1. Sensing thinking (ST)—prefers to collect, organize, and explain
2. Sensing feeling (SF)—prefers reciprocal learning
3. Intuitive thinking (NT)—prefers to master content
4. Intuitive feeling (NF)—prefers analytical content and organization

● FACULTY INCIVILITY

Incivility penetrates all aspects of nursing, and most educational and healthcare organizations have adopted a zero-tolerance policy. Incivility has been defined as behaviors that include disrespect and promote conflict. Incivil behavior increases stress among the members of a group. Incivility and workload stress often go hand-in-hand. Civility can be a learned skill that can be assisted by a mentor (Clark & Dunhma, 2020).

Incivil behaviors can take many forms, including:

- Complaining
- Lying
- Gossiping
- Using abusive language
- Insubordination
- Scapegoating

Additionally, incivility can produce fear and humiliation and can impair clinical judgment and learning. Incivility can reduce psychological safety and increase cognitive load (Clark & Fey, 2020). Incorporating moral resilience in students is an effective method for faculty to assist students to build confidence and guard against incivility in academia and the clinical environment (Baker & Cummings, 2020).

> **EVIDENCE-BASED TEACHING PRACTICE**
>
> Rose and colleagues (2020) used virtual simulation with nursing students ($N = 53$) to determine if virtual reality simulation increased awareness of civility and incivility. The researchers found that virtual simulation is an effective tool to raise awareness of incivility.

Zsohar and Smith (2006) have composed a list of the "top-10 don'ts" for teaching, as these very well may be perceived as being incivil to learners.

1. Don't be late for class.
2. Don't pretend knowledge.
3. Don't read or repeat information that is easily accessible to the learner.
4. Don't bring personal baggage into class.
5. Don't come unprepared with excuses for lack of preparation.
6. Don't be confrontational.
7. Don't interrupt.
8. Don't devalue the content taught by colleagues.
9. Don't be inconsistent with expectations.
10. Don't forget to be passionate about teaching.

Learner incivility toward nurse educators is addressed in Chapter 9.

LEARNING OUTCOMES VERSUS LEARNING OBJECTIVES

Historically, nursing education has used objectives for learning since Tyler's landmark book, *Basic Principles of Curriculum and Instruction* (1949), encouraged educators to develop behavioral objectives to organize their teaching. Therefore, objectives are part of the behavioral paradigm. To standardize the format of objectives, educators have incorporated the action verbs outlined in Bloom's taxonomy, which has since been revised.

Most teaching sessions begin with objectives or learning outcomes to frame the content or experience. **Objectives** and **learning outcomes** are two terms used often in nursing education; the differences between the terms may, on the surface, be slight, but they depict two approaches to evaluating learning that have emerged in recent years.

1. An objective speaks to the process; therefore, it is teacher-centric.
2. An outcome, on the other hand, speaks to the product; thus, it is learner-centric (Wittmann-Price & Fasolka, 2010).

Changing from objectives to outcomes is truly more of a conceptual change than an operational change. Some nurse educators have simply switched words but not their thought processes. Others believe that neither objectives nor outcomes give us the freedom needed to encourage learners to think critically (Bevis & Watson, 1989;

Diekelmann, 1997). Nursing education leaders have rightfully questioned the use of objectives within today's postmodern educational philosophy environment because:

- All learning is not displayed in behavior.
- By predetermining objectives or outcomes, the depth and breadth of the learners' experiences may be squelched.

It is difficult at best to package the human intellect into a modifiable mold for convenience in grouping, evaluating, and justifying what is being taught or presented and what a learner carries forth from experience.

Developing learning outcomes is done on many levels in academia. Outcomes are more general at the institutional level, and more specifically at the course level. Learning outcomes will vary depending on the level for which they are being developed: the entire school, a program, levels within a program, and the course-specific level. Clinical courses can have two sets of outcomes: one set for the theory portion of the course and the second set for the clinical portion. Because most educational institutions still describe learning in terms of outcomes, sample formulas used to write the objectives are depicted in Table 1.4.

Table 1.4 Learning Outcomes

Antecedent	Learner	Verb Describing Behavior	Content	Context	Criteria
By the end of this session	The learner will	Demonstrate	Sterile gloving	In clinical settings	100% of the time
By the end of this session	The learner will	Compare	Different cultures	Related to childbearing experiences	By Interviewing two culturally different patients

---

EVIDENCE-BASED TEACHING PRACTICE

Hampton and colleagues (2020) qualitatively studied faculty ($N = 100$) satisfaction and self-efficacy and its effect on achieving student learning outcomes in an online learning environment. The study found that faculty that were satisfied teaching online and had self-efficacy related to the online modality promoted student achievement of the learning outcomes.

▶ BLOOM'S TAXONOMY

Bloom's *Taxonomy of Educational Objectives* (Bloom, Englehart, Furst, Hill, & Drathwohl, 1956) describes an end behavior (see Table 1.5). The taxonomy uses "behavioral terms" to divide learning into leveled achievement, from knowledge acquisition to the synthesis of new ideas (Novotny & Griffin, 2006).

Table 1.5 Bloom's Taxonomy

Level	Concept	Verbs Used When Writing Learning Outcomes
Creating (formerly called *synthesis*)	Judgment, selection	Design, assemble, construct, conjecture, develop, formulate, author, investigate
Evaluating (formerly called *evaluation*)	Productive thinking, novelty	Appraise, argue, defend, judge, select, support, value, critique, weigh
Analyzing (formerly called *analysis*)	Induction deduction, logical order	Differentiate, organize, relate, compare, contrast, distinguish, examine, experiment, question, test
Applying (formerly called *application*)	Solution, application	Execute, implement, solve, use, demonstrate, interpret, operate, schedule, sketch
Understanding (formerly called *comprehension*)	Memory, repetition, description	Classify, describe, discuss, explain, express, identify, indicate, locate, report, restate, review, select, translate
Remembering (formerly called *knowledge*)	Explanation, comparison, illustration	Arrange, define, duplicate, label, list, memorize, name, order, recognize, relate, recall, repeat, reproduce, state

▶ LEARNING DOMAINS

Learning is discussed as a process that takes place in three domains: cognitive, affective, and psychomotor. Quality and Safety Education for Nurses (QSEN) competencies include the same domains with different labels cognitive (knowledge), attitude (affective), and skills (psychomotor) (Haley & Palmer, 2020). Learners in nursing programs are evaluated for growth in all three domains. Bloom's taxonomy (see Table 1.5) identifies learning mainly in the cognitive domain. Psychomotor domains are not difficult to evaluate because they produce an observable behavior change. Many times this change is related to procedures and skills. The affective domain of learning is more difficult to assess because it is related to judgment and values (Partusch, 2007). Wong and Driscoll (2008) describe the learning development of the affective domain in stages, which are:

1. Receiving—when learners attend, listen, watch, and recognize
2. Responding—when learners answer, discuss, respond, reply, and participate
3. Valuing—when learners accept, adopt, initiate, or have a preference
4. Organizing—this is conceptualized as formulating, integrating, modifying, and systematizing
5. Internalizing—this occurs when learners commit, exemplify, and incorporate into practice

EVIDENCE-BASED TEACHING PRACTICE

Hanshaw and Dickerson (2020) completed a meta-analysis ($N = 20$) about high-fidelity simulation learning's effect on increasing leaves of thinking in undergraduate pre-licensure baccalaureate nursing students. Bloom's Taxonomy was used as the outcome measure, and the study examined Remembering/Understanding/Applying (knowledge/skills), Analyzing/Perception, and Evaluating/Creating outcomes. The results indicate that further studies are needed to relate higher levels of thinking and competence from education to clinical practice.

▶ GAGNE'S CONDITIONS OF LEARNING

Gagne (1970) reinforced the need for objectives by stating that objectives are the second event in the nine conditions of learning (Table 1.6). Gagne characterized objectives as a useful step to inform a learner of what is to be achieved. Gagne's steps for instruction are a classic list of tasks that is still referenced today.

Table 1.6 Gagne's Conditions of Learning

Instructional Event	Operationalization of Event
1. Gain attention of the learner	Stimuli activate receptors
2. Inform learners of objectives	Sets expectations for the learner
3. Stimulate recall of prior learning	Activates short-term memory and the retrieval of information by asking questions
4. Present the content	Presents content with features that can be remembered
5. Provide "learning guidance"	Assists the learner to organize the information for long-term memory
6. Elicit performance (practice)	Asks learners to perform to enhance encoding and verification
7. Provide appropriate feedback	Encourages performance
8. Assess performance	Evaluates learning
9. Enhance retention and transfer	Review periodically to decrease memory loss of information

EVIDENCE-BASED TEACHING PRACTICE

Rourke, Leong, and Chatterly (2018) used Gagne's Condition-based Learning Theory and included 4 practices outlined by Gagne; (1) presenting information, (2) eliciting performance, (3) providing feedback, and (4) assessing learning to assess 25 studies' instructional interventions. The results demonstrated that less than 50% of the studies elicited performance or provided feedback to students. The results suggest that instruction that uses less than the 4 outlined Gagne practices may have less educational impact. Further studies are needed to assess instructional implementation.

DEVELOPING A LESSON PLAN

Lesson plans are not often spoken about in higher education to the same extent they are in primary education. In higher education, lesson plans often simply consist of a chart showing what learning the educator expects to facilitate during a specific time period and how that learning facilitation is going to be accomplished. Yet, lesson plans are very valuable and provide structure to the learning session. Lesson plans can be general or very detailed and include even the technology resources needed for a learning session. Most importantly, lesson plans can assist to keep the learning session on time (Osinski & Turrise, 2020).

An example of a lesson plan is shown in Exhibit 1.3.

Exhibit 1.3 Lesson Plan

Learning Outcomes	Related Course Objectives	Content Outline	Time	Assignment	Teaching Strategy	Equipment Needed	Evaluation
Discuss hyperbilirubinemia in the preterm infant	Understand the physiological needs of the high-risk infant	1. Physiological jaundice 2. Pathological jaundice 3. Diagnostic tools 4. Nursing interventions	45 minutes	Case study using bilirubin graph	Lecture with case study and clicker questions	Audience response system (project Bilirubin graphs) for each learner	Five multiple-choice or alternative type questions on test 3
Compare Rh and ABO blood group incompatibilities	Understand the physiological needs of the high-risk infant	1. Rh sensitivity 2. ABO matching	30 minutes	None	Powerpoint presentation then use quick Jeopardy game	Easel and flip chart for game	Three multiple-choice or alternative type questions on test 3

EVIDENCE-BASED TEACHING PRACTICE

Vaccaria et al. (2020) successfully used a lesson plan model for laboratory skills training for undergraduate nursing students. The implementation study was done through 7 phases: (1) literature review, (2) work process, (3) division of tasks, (4) validation, (5) pilot test, (6) revision, and (7) dissemination. The results increased the effectiveness of the teaching-learning process for faculty and students.

● COMPETENCY-BASED EDUCATION (CBE)

Today's healthcare environment increasingly calls for more positive and efficient outcomes. The 1999 Institute of Medicine (IOM) report "To Err is Human" underscored the need for better patient outcomes nurse educators understand that positive patient/client care outcomes occur when interventions being taught are based on best practices. Best practices are developed and nurtured during the educational processes.

Much literature has been written about the education to practice gap (Leggett, 2015). CBE is gaining momentum in academia as a method to close the ever-widening education to practice gap. The goal of healthcare education is to graduate competent and caring providers. CBE is outcomes-based and a method to improve healthcare quality (Sargeant, Wong, & Campbell, 2018). There are 4 essential components of CBE:

1. CBE is responsive to society because graduates have skills needed as practicing professional nurses.
2. Curriculum design is based on abilities or competencies.
3. CBE is focused on outcomes that can be assessed by multiple evaluation methods (Sargeant, Wong, & Campbell, 2018).
4. CBE is learner-centered and congruent with constructivism, in which students understand the educational goals and independently construct knowledge themselves to reach the goals.

Components that are not elements of CBE that may have been emphasized in traditional educational models, include:

- Time-based goals, and
- Content coverage without specific outcomes (Gruppen et al., 2016).

In CBE, nursing students are encouraged to work at their own pace to accomplish the abilities and skills needed for their profession. CBE promotes student accountability because the responsibility of mastering skills is placed on the student (Touchie & Cate, 2016). CBE builds the learning and the curriculum around the competencies that are identified as needed for the professional. Competencies are not just hands-on nursing skills; they include knowledge and professional attitude.

According to Covert, Sherman, Miner, and Lichtyeld (2019), competencies have 5 characteristics:

1. Focus on the performance of the end-product or instructional goal.
2. Reflect what is learned in the instructional program.
3. Be expressed in terms of measurable behavior.
4. Use a standard for judging competence independent of others' performance.
5. Inform learners and other stakeholders about what is expected of them (p. 321).

● CRITICAL THINKING, METACOGNITION, AND CLINICAL REASONING

Critical thinking, as an educational concept, can be traced back to 1941, when Glaser defined composites of knowledge. Other historical developments about the concept of critical thinking include:

- In 1989, NLN recognized the inclusion of critical thinking as a specific criterion for the accreditation of nursing programs.
- Miller and Malcolm (1990) adapted Glaser's definition into a model for critical thinking and advised educators to pay closer attention to learners' mental processes.
- In the early days of concept development, educators were concerned with finding an appropriate definition for **critical thinking** in order to evaluate its development within learners.
- A multitude of definitions arose, and some of the more prominent ones are listed in Table 1.7.

Table 1.7 Descriptions of Critical Thinking

Author	Description of Critical Thinking
Facione, Facione, and Sanchez (1994)	Critical thinking is the process of purposeful, self-regulating judgment
Paul and Elder (2007)	Attitudes are central, rather than peripheral, to critical thinking, as are independence, confidence, and responsibility, which are needed to arrive at one's own judgment
Bandman and Bandman (1995)	Critical thinking is the rational examination of ideas, inferences, assumptions, principles, arguments, conclusions, issues, statements, beliefs, and actions. It covers scientific reasoning and includes the nursing process, decision-making, and reasoning in controversial issues. It also includes deductive, inductive, informal, and practical reasoning

Nurse educators can *role-model critical thinking* and *create opportunities for learners to develop their own critical thinking skills* by asking higher-level questions and "thinking out loud," or dialoguing about an issue from different perspectives in order to synthesize a solution. The authors of *The ISNA Bulletin* (Indiana State Nurses Foundation & Indiana State Nurses Association, 2014) define attributes or characteristics that enhance and deter critical thinking; these are listed in Table 1.8.

Table 1.8 Attributes or Characteristics that Enhance and Deter Critical Thinking

Characteristics of Critical Thinking	Characteristics That Deter Critical Thinking
■ Universal intellectual standards are upheld and include: ● Clarity ● Accuracy ● Precision ● Relevance ● Depth ● Breath ● Logic ■ Intellectual humility as opposed to intellectual arrogance ■ Intellectual courage as opposed to intellectual cowardice ■ Intellectual empathy as opposed to intellectual narrow-mindedness ■ Intellectual autonomy as opposed to intellectual conformity ■ Intellectual integrity as opposed to intellectual hypocrisy ■ Intellectual perseverance as opposed to intellectual laziness ■ Confidence in reason as opposed to distrust of reason and evidence ■ Fair-mindedness as opposed to intellectual unfairness ■ Reasoning ■ Divergent thinking ■ Creativity ■ Clarification	■ Egocentrism fallacy ● It's true because I believe it. ● It's true because we believe it. ● It's true because I want to believe it. ● It's true because I have always believed it. ● It's true because it is in my selfish interest to believe it. ● Omniscience fallacy ■ Omnipotence fallacy ■ Invulnerability fallacy ■ The halo effect

Source: Indiana State Nurses Foundation & Indiana State Nurses Association. (2014). Developing a nursing IQ—Part 1. Characteristics of critical thinking: What critical thinkers do, what critical thinkers do not do. ISNA *Bulletin*, 41(1), 6–14.

Ritchie and Smith (2015) propose that critical thinking is the seventh "C" needed in community health nursing along with:

1. Care
2. Compassion
3. Competence
4. Communication
5. Courage
6. Commitment
7. Critical thinking

Walker (2003) reviewed some of the teaching strategies that enhance critical thinking and suggests that they include:

- Questioning that promotes the evaluation and synthesis of facts
- Learning session discussions and debates with open negotiation
- Short, focused writing assignments, such as
  - Summarize five major points in a chapter
  - Discuss the essence of the chapter using a metaphor
  - Explain the chapter to your neighbor, who has a high school education
  - How does the chapter affect your life, personally or professionally?
- Using case studies—use of case studies has been reported as a learning strategy to increase critical thinking skills (Popil, 2012)
  - Reflective journaling (Raterink, 2016)
  - Analytical writing (Price, 2015)
  - Concept mapping (Hundial, 2020)

EVIDENCE-BASED TEACHING PRACTICE

Christenson (2020) completed a systematic review related to Emotional intelligence (EI) and critical thinking (CT) in undergraduate nursing students. The themes identified were: (1) EI and CT are interdependent; (2) EI and CT are critical for success in nursing education; and (3) nursing education should foster EI and CT.

Assessment of learners' critical thinking skills has been completed by use of several different tools. Two of the most widely used tools are:

- The California Critical Thinking Disposition Inventory; this tool evaluates seven "habits of the mind":
  1. Truth-seeking
  2. Open-mindedness
  3. Analyticity
  4. Systematicity
  5. Self-confidence
  6. Inquisitiveness
  7. Cognitive maturity

- The Watson-Glaser Critical Thinking Appraisal (1964); this tool offers three different forms of the instrument, and the newest version has 16 scenarios and 40 items. There are five subcategories:
  1. Inference
  2. Recognition of assumptions
  3. Deduction
  4. Interpretation
  5. Evaluation (Romeo, 2010)

EVIDENCE-BASED TEACHING PRACTICE

Ahmady and Shahbazi (2020) used a quasi-experimental design to study the impact of social problem-solving training on nursing students' ($N = 40$) critical thinking and decision-making. The researchers used a demographic questionnaire, social problem-solving inventory-revised, California critical thinking test, and decision-making questionnaire. The results suggest that the social problem-solving course positively affected the students' social problem-solving, decision-making, and critical thinking skills.

▶ MINDFULNESS

Mindfulness is a term related to critical thinking. *The ISNA Bulletin* (Indiana State Nurses Foundation & Indiana State Nurses Association, 2014) defines **mindfulness** as: "You are engaged with a certain activity, focused and actively thinking about whatever it is you are undertaking at the moment" (p. 6).

EVIDENCE-BASED TEACHING PRACTICE

Yildirim and colleagues (2020) completed a randomized control study about Mindfulness-based Stress Reduction program used on nursing students. The intervention for the intervention groups was done in 90- to 95-minute sessions twice a week for 12 weeks. The results suggest that the mindfulness-based stress reduction program reduces the stress experienced by students during nursing education. The program had the following positive student effects:

- Increased mindfulness
- Strengthened coping mechanisms
- Increased self-confidence
- Increased optimism
- Decreased helplessness

▶ METACOGNITION

Metacognition is a concept that is from critical thinking. "Metacognition is an active process of knowing, or being acutely aware of one's cognitive state with the ability to complete a given task" (Hsu & Hsieh, 2014, p. 234). Metacognition refers to evaluating your own learning and ideas and being able to change them to understand and promote your own learning success.

EVIDENCE-BASED TEACHING PRACTICE

Schuler and Joohyun (2019) used a structured debriefing and studied its effect on nursing students' metacognitive skills in a mixed-method pilot study. The results indicated that students who used the structured debriefing increase their metacognition over time.

CLINICAL REASONING

Also identified as an effective teaching style is the use of methods that enhance clinical reasoning. Good clinical reasoning skills are a goal for every graduate and are emphasized on licensure examinations to promote patient safety and positive patient outcomes. There are teaching methods such as concept mapping, questioning, case studies, and vignettes that increase in complexity that assist the development of clinical reasoning (Deschenes et al., 2020). Additionally important in the development of clinical reasoning is the guidance from academic clinical faculty and preceptors in the clinical learning environment. Barriers to clinical reasoning have also been identified and should be avoided when possible. Barriers include traditional classroom environments and teaching methods, large student to faculty ratios, uncivil clinical learning experience environments, and students' attributes and attitudes towards learning (Wong & Kowitlawakul 2020).

EVIDENCE-BASED TEACHING PRACTICE

Alexander (2020) completed a double-blind, randomized control trial to explore the impact of purposeful simulation role assignment, using preferred learning styles, on prelicensure nursing students' clinical reasoning. The results demonstrated that assigning student roles in the simulation laboratory based on their learning styles increased clinical reasoning. An example is providing active learners a direct care provider role and reflective learners an observer role.

EVIDENCE-BASED TEACHING PRACTICE

The foundations of evidence-based teaching practice (EBTP) are analogous to EBP. Nurse educators use the same method of synthesizing and appraising evidence in order to draw a conclusion or develop an opinion that is grounded and derived from logical, common ideas in the literature (Hicks & Butkus, 2011).

Kalb, O'Conner-Von, Brockway, Rierson, and Sendelbach (2015) surveyed nursing education program administrators and faculty ($N = 551$) in a national study on the use of EBTP in their programs. EBTP was considered in the areas of teaching, learning, and program development. Participants all perceived EBTP as an important element in their teaching, and EBTP needs to be continuously emphasized and resourced. Few studies about the use of EBTP have been done in the past 5 years.

Ferguson and Day stated in 2005, and it still holds true today, that nursing education still needs much more quantitative and qualitative research to improve the science of nursing education. EBTP is based on four elements:

1. Evidence—both quantitative and qualitative
2. Professional judgment—nurse educators' decision-making ability
3. Values of learners as clients—using judgment appropriately by getting to understand learners
4. Resource issues—money, time, and space

EVIDENCE-BASED TEACHING PRACTICE

Simmonds et al. (2020) completed a literature review ($N = 46$) about EBTP practices that assist undergraduate nursing students to develop a professional nursing identity. The themes from the review reveal that there is a range of contexts in which nursing students learn and that identity formation is multidimensional. Also, identity formation may be dependent on pedagogical methodologies ad student learning outcomes. Additional studies are needed to better understand evidence-based teaching practices that support professional identity development in undergraduate nursing students.

EVIDENCE-BASED TEACHING PRACTICE

Chicca (2020) reviewed the evidence for the use of the clinical preceptorship model for und undergraduate nursing education. The author found that even though the preceptorship model is heralded as the pinnacle of clinical learning experiences, there is a lack of robust evidence for using this model.

Faculty development about identifying and using EBTP is a need in many nursing programs. Understanding the significance and the need to use best practices in teaching is a nursing educational priority. Mentorship into the faculty role by seasoned faculty who have been seeking out and using EBTP is essential for a successful learning environment (Anderson et al., 2020).

EVIDENCE-BASED TEACHING PRACTICE

Tucker (2020) developed an EBTP model for faculty succession planning in order to successfully retain, develop, and recruit academic nurse leaders using evidence and best practices. The research involves a case study in which the developed model was used to promote faculty success.

 # LEARNING ENVIRONMENT MANAGEMENT

The underpinning of positive class or online management is respect for the learners. Once an atmosphere of trust and respect is established, there should be very few learning environment management issues. Class management is also very different today when compared to the past because of large cohort sizes and new technologies. Chickering and Gamson's (1987) seven principles of good teaching practice are as follows:

1. Encourage contact between learners and educators
2. Develop reciprocity and cooperation among learners
3. Encourage active learning
4. Give prompt feedback
5. Emphasize time on task
6. Communicate high expectations
7. Respect diverse talents and ways of learning

Learning session management also includes deterring cheating. Learners who are dishonest in the educational setting are likely to be dishonest in the clinical setting (Pittman et al., 2020). Some EBTP to deter academic dishonesty include:

- Publishing detailed integrity policies
- Ensuring students and faculty know the policies
- Providing test security
- Using proctors or remote proctoring
- Using high-level test questions
- Ensuring personal property is not out in the open

According to Mulligan (2007), there are four pillars of class management:

Pillar 1: Educators should use instructional strategies (active learning strategies) that motivate and keep learners interested and engaged.

Pillar 2: Educators need to use instructional time wisely and take a proactive approach to teaching by making the learners accountable for their learning.

Pillar 3: Social behaviors that need attention and correction should be done immediately, face to face, and privately.

Pillar 4: Educators need to create a flexible environment that adjusts to the learners' needs. For example, a learner with attention deficits may be less disruptive if placed up front and center.

Learning environment management is important to maintain a positive culture because poor learning environment management is akin to students perceiving faculty as incivil (Cain, 2017).

Learners' use of technology in the class has also become a concern for nurse educators. Establishing "ground rules" early in the course and communicating them clearly may assist in maintaining learning environment management. Educational technology is addressed in Chapter 3.

● CLOSING AND NOT JUST "ENDING" A COURSE

"So the course is over. I enter my office, turn on the light, and begin to consider how I will facilitate closure for the next group of students. Just like caring for a patient, the process starts well before I ever meet them" (Yonge, Lee, & Luhanga, 2006, p. 151).

● CASE STUDIES

CASE STUDY 1.1

A new faculty member joins at a small baccalaureate school of nursing. The new faculty member is full time, tenure track, and working on a doctoral degree. The new faculty member is assigned a mentor and a 12-credit semester teaching assignment, which is normal for many institutions. The new faculty member meets with the assigned mentor, who goes over the for the learning session that the new faculty member will be. The mentor asks the new faculty member why there are so many assignments in a clinical course. The new faculty member states that their belief is that the learners' writing skills are lacking and they need writing assignments.

If you were the mentor and saw a novice place 50% of the clinical course grade on writing assignments, how would you handle it?

CASE STUDY 1.2

A seasoned faculty member has been placed in the accelerated prelicensure learner curriculum. There are a large number of learners, and the faculty member has 10 clinical groups with seven different adjunct instructors as part of their responsibility. The faculty member uses the same syllabus used for the traditional prelicensure undergraduates, whom they taught successfully last semester. An assignment on the syllabus of the accelerated prelicensure learners is to pick a patient and create a complete care plan for the patient, including assessment, diagnoses, planning implementation, and evaluation format. The rubric states that the plan should be in American Psychological Association (APA) format and approximately 10 to 12 pages long. The majority of learners complete the assignment on time. At the end of the semester, the faculty member is taken aback that the learners had so many negative comments about the care plan assignment.

If you were the faculty member, how would you alter the assignment yet still ensure that you meet the course learning outcomes of developing a plan of care for a complex patient?

1. The nurse administrator observes a new faculty member in a face-to-face learning session. The faculty member uses active learning strategies and provides the students with time to ask questions. Two students in the back of the class continue to look at the mobile phone devices in their laps and exchange comments to each other. Constructive advice about the observational experience that the nurse administrator should provide to the faculty member is:

   A. Address the behavior after the class is over
   B. Ask all students to put their phones at the front of the classroom on the table
   C. Provide additional active learning activities to keep all students engaged strategies
   D. Request the students sit up front with a seat in between them

2. The nurse educator is developing a test and would like to increase the level of the question using Bloom's taxonomy. Which of the following question(s)/statement(s) is written at the highest level of Bloom's taxonomy?

   A. Which procedure demonstrates appropriate nursing care for a patient with deep vein thromboses?
   B. Differentiate the appropriate discharge education for a patient with deep vein thromboses
   C. What is the correct description of the appropriate initial nursing care for a patient with deep vein thromboses?
   D. Select the priority nursing care for a patient with deep vein thromboses.

3. A nurse educator has submitted a syllabus with the following student learning outcomes. Which learning outcome is written at the highest level of Bloom's taxonomy?

   A. Demonstrate caring to geriatric patients
   B. Discuss common health care concerns of geriatric patients
   C. Appraise literature about geriatric patients' home safety
   D. Implement a plan of care for a geriatric patient

4. During a curriculum meeting, the Certified Healthcare Simulation Educator (CHSE) states, "This semester we will do objective structured clinical examinations (OSCEs) and students will be assessed on their performance." The philosophical foundations for this analysis would best fit:

   A. Narrative pedagogy
   B. Behaviorism
   C. Constructivism
   D. Feminism

1. A) Address the behavior after the class is over

Addressing the behavior as soon as possible is the first action that should be taken to limit incivility. The faculty member is already providing active learning strategies, and changing the environment is not the first step to correct learning session management.

2. D) Select the priority nursing care for a patient with deep vein thromboses

Select is on the evaluative level of Bloom's Taxonomy. Demonstrate is on the application level, differentiate is on the analysis level, and describe is on the understanding level.

3. C) Appraise literature about geriatric patients' home safety

Appraise is on the evaluative level, discuss is understanding, implement is application as is demonstrated.

4. B) Behaviorism

Behaviorism is the theory that learning is demonstrated in behavior, narrative pedagogy is learning through words and stories, constructivism is building knowledge on past experiences, and feminism is looking through a lens of inequality.

5. A nursing program is moving toward a competency-based educational system. A faculty member needs more understanding of competency-based education when they state:

   A. Competencies are pre-determined by professional standards
   B. Students can be provided formative evaluation to assist them to reach competency
   C. Competencies are only used in the psychomotor domain of learning
   D. Students can achieve competencies at their own pace

6. A novice nurse educator is interested in the Theory of Meaningful Learning and finds the following true:

   A. The activities have to be well-planned by the faculty
   B. The content has to be new to learners
   C. The student discovers the constructs
   D. Learning is futuristic

7. A faculty member promotes deep learning by:

   A. Using medication flashcards
   B. Using mnemonics for sequences
   C. Starting with the overall concept
   D. Discussing common lab values

8. A nurse faculty is implementing strategies to improve undergraduate students' clinical reasoning. The best strategy to implement is:

   A. Concept mapping
   B. Traditional care planning
   C. Observation in a clinical setting
   D. Group projects

(See answers next page.)

5. C) Competencies are only used in the psychomotor domain of learning

Competencies are used in all three domains; cognitive, psychomotor, and affective. Students should be provided with formative evaluations to assist them to reach competency, and they can reach competencies at their own pace. Competencies are pre-determined by professional standards such as safe medication administration.

6. C) The student discovers the constructs

Meaningful Learning has receptiveness and discovery by the learner, is built on past experiences, and is student-centered. Content should be interesting to the learner.

7. C) Starting with the overall concept

Deep learning promotes understanding concepts and not just details that can be remembered with flashcards, mnemonics, or memorized values.

8. A) Concept mapping

Concept mapping assists critical thinking and clinical reasoning because students have to connect concepts that have consequences on each other such as medication and system functioning. Tradition care planning is often linear and group projects many times provide students with a piece of the issue. Observation in clinical may or may not be effective depending on the situation.

9. A new faculty member is chronically late for meetings and often does not answer electronic messages in a timely manner. The faculty member does a good job teaching and contributes to committee work. The nurse administrator should address this behavior because it may be interpreted as:

A. Faculty to student incivility
B. Student to faculty incivility
C. Faculty to faculty incivility
D. Faculty to administration incivility

10. A nurse administrator tracks the attrition rates of nursing students and finds that minority students are dismissed during their junior year at twice the number of nonminority students. The faculty discusses strategies for decreasing minority student attrition and decides the best method would be:

A. Re-examine the admission criteria
B. Start a one-to-one faulty–student tutoring program
C. Identify high-risk students in their sophomore year and offer to have them go part-time their junior year
D. Establish a minority student nursing organization that meets monthly and provides social events and mentoring

(See answers next page.)

9. C) Student to faculty incivility
This would be construed as faculty-to-faculty incivility because it is issued with peer environment, not student. It is not incivility to administration because committee work is peer-driven.

10. D) Establish a minority student nursing organization that meets monthly and provides social events and mentoring
A minority nurse's association group and mentoring will increase belongingness. Admission criteria should be the same for all students. One-to-one faulty tutoring may not be helpful if there is a lack of minority faculty members. Asking students to go part-time usually jeopardizes financial aid.

⬤ REFERENCES

Ahmady, S., & Shahbazi, S. (2020). Impact of social problem-solving training on critical thinking and decision making of nursing students. *BMC Nursing, 19*(1), N.PAG-N. PAG. 10.1186/s12912-020-00487-x

Alexander, E, (2020). Purposeful simulation role assignment. *Clinical Simulation in Nursing, 48*, 1–7. 10.1016/j.ecns.2020.07.008

Andel, S. A., de Vreede, T., Spector, P. E., Padmanabhan, B., Singh, V. K., de Vreede, G. (2020). Do social features help in video-centric online learning platforms? A social presence perspective. *Computers in Human Behavior, 113*, N.PAG-N.PAG. 10.1016/j. chb.2020.106505

Anderson, C. M., Campbell, J., Grady, P., Ladden, M., McBride, A. B., Montano, N. P., & Woods, N. F. (2020). Transitioning back to faculty roles after being a Robert Wood Johnson Foundation Nurse Faculty Scholar: Challenges and opportunities. *Journal of Professional Nursing, 36*(5), 377–385. 10.1016/j.profnurs.2020.02.003

Ashktorab, T., Hasanvand, S., Seyedfatemi, N., Zayeri, F., Levett-Jones, T., & Pournia, Y. (2015). Psychometric testing of the Persian version of the Belongingness Scale— Clinical placement experience. *Nurse Education Today, 35*(3), 439–443. 10.1016/j. nedt.2014.11.006

Ausubel, D. P. (1962). A subsumption theory of meaningful verbal learning and retention. *Journal of General Psychology, 66*, 213–244.

Baker-Townsend, J., & Cummings, C. Incorporating moral resilience into an undergraduate nursing program. *Archives of Psychiatric Nursing, 34*(5), 391–393. 10.1016/j.apnu.2020.06.001

Bandman, E. L., & Bandman, B. (1995). *Critical thinking in nursing* (2nd Ed.). Norwalk, CT: Appleton & Lange.

Bandura, A. (1997). *Self-efficacy: The exercise of control.* New York, NY: W. H. Freeman.

Barbour, C., & Schuessler, J. B. (2019). A preliminary framework to guide implementation of The Flipped Classroom Method in nursing education. *Nurse Education in Practice, 34*, 36–42. 10.1016/j.nepr.2018.11.001

Benner, P. (1982). From novice to expert. *American Journal of Nursing, 82*(3), 402–407.

Bevis, E., & Watson, J. (1989). *Toward a caring curriculum: A new pedagogy for nursing.* New York, NY: National Nursing League Publications.

Bloom, B., Englehart, M., Furst, E., Hill, W., & Drathwohl, D. (Eds.). (1956). *Taxonomy of educational objectives.* New York, NY: Longmans, Green.

Brady, D. R. & Asselin, M. E. (2016). Exploring outcomes and evaluation in narrative pedagogy: An integrative review. *Nurse Education Today, 45*, 1–8. 10.1016/j. nedt.2016.06.002

Brophy, J. (1986). *On motivating students. Occasional paper no. 101.* East Lansing: Institute for Research on Teaching, Michigan State University.

Burton, C. W. (2020). Paying the caring tax: The detrimental influences of gender expectations on the development of nursing education and science. *Advances in Nursing Science, 43*(3), 266–277. 10.1097/ANS.0000000000000319

Cain, L. B. (2017). Relationship between age, gender, and incivility in online registered nurses to bachelor of science in nursing degree classes. *Relationship Between Age, Gender & Incivility in Online Registered Nurses to Bachelor of Science in Nursing Degree Classes*, 1–1.

Carper, B. A. (1978). Fundamental patterns of knowing in nursing. *Advances in Nursing Science*, 1(1), 13–24.

Chicca, J. (2020). Should we use preceptorships in undergraduate nursing education? *Nursing Forum*, 55(3), 480–484. 10.1111/nuf.12452

Chickering, A. W., & Gamson, Z. F. (1987). Seven principles for good practice in undergraduate education. *Wingspread Journal*, 9(2), 1–7.

Childs-Kean, L., Edwards, M., & Smith, M. D. (2020). A Systematic review of personality framework use in health sciences education. *American Journal of Pharmaceutical Education*, 84(8), 1–9.

Chinn, P. (2007). Philosophical foundations for excellence in nursing. In B. Moyer & R. A. Wittmann-Price (Eds.). *Nursing education: Foundations of practice excellence* (pp. 15–28). Philadelphia, PA: F. A. Davis.

Choo, L. A. (1996). Reflections: Learning at work. *Professional Nurse, Singapore*, 23(3), 8–11.

Christianson, K. L. (2020). Emotional intelligence and critical thinking in nursing students: Integrative review of literature. *Nurse Educator*, 45(6), E62–E65.

10.1097/NNE.0000000000000801

Clark, C. &. Dunham, M. (2020). Civility mentor: A virtual learning experience. *Nurse Educator*, 45(4), 189–192. 10.1097/NNE.0000000000000757

Clark, C. & Fey M. K. (2020). Fostering civility in learning conversations: Introducing the PAAIL Communication Strategy. *Nurse Educator*, 45(3), 139 -143.10.1097/NNE.0000000000000731

Covert, H., Sherman, M., Miner, K., & Lichtyeld, M. (2019). Core competencies and a workforce framework for community health workers: A model for advancing the profession. *American Journal of Public Health*, 109(2), 320–327. Http://dx.doi.org/10.2105/AJPH.2018.304737

Daniels, R., Harding, A., Smith, J. R., & Gomez-Cano, M. (2020). Development and validation of a tool to measure belongingness as a proxy for participation in undergraduate clinical learning. *Education for Primary Care*, 31(5), 311–317. 10.1080/14739879.2020.1782272

Deci, E., Eghrari, H., Patrick, B. C., & Leone, D. R. (1994). Facilitating internalization: The self-determination theory perspective. *Journal of Personality*, 62(1), 119–142. 10.1111/j.1467-6494.1994.tb00797.x

Devries, D. & Beck, T. (2020). Myers-Briggs type indicator profile of undergraduate therapeutic recreation students. *Therapeutic Recreation Journal*, 54(3), 243–258. 10.18666/TRJ-2020-V54-I3-9510

D'Souza, P., Jenevive, J., & Nayak, S. G. (2019). Impact of educational environment and learning approaches on academic outcome of undergraduate nursing students. *International Journal of Caring Sciences*, 12(3), 1530–1536.

Diekelmann, N. L. (1997). Creating a new pedagogy for nursing. *Journal of Nursing Education*, 36(4), 147–148.

Diekelmann, N. L. (2005). Engaging the students and the teacher: Co-creating substantive form with narrative pedagogy. *Journal of Nursing Education*, 44(6), 249–252.

Deschenes, M., Goudreau, J., & Fernandez, N. (2020). Learning strategies used by undergraduate nursing students in the context of a digitial educational strategy based on script concordance: A descriptive study. *Nurse Education Today, 95*, N.PAG-N.PAG. 10.1016/j.nedt.2020.104607

Facione, N. C., Facione, P. A., & Sanchez, C. A. (1994). Critical thinking disposition as a measure of Competent judgment: The development of the California Critical Disposition Inventory. *Journal of Nursing Education, 33*, 345–350.

Freire, P. (1970). *Pedagogy of the oppressed.* New York, NY: Continuum.

Ferguson, L., & Day, R. A. (2005). Evidence-based nursing education: Myth or reality? *Journal of Nursing Education, 44*(3), 107–115.

Gagne, R. (1970). *The conditions of learning* (2nd ed.). New York, NY: Holt, Rinehart and Winston.

Graf, A. C., Jacob, E., Twigg, D., & Nattabil, B. (2020). Contemporary nursing graduates' transition to practice: A critical review of transition models. *Journal of Clinical Nursing, 29*(15/16), 3097–3107. Http://dx.doi.org.proxy1.lib.tju.edu/10.1111/jocn.15234

Grasha, A. F. (1996). *Teaching with styles.* Pittsburgh, PA: Alliance Publishers.

Gruppen, L. D., Burkhardt, J. C., Fitzgerald, J. T., Funnell, M., Haftel, H. M., Lypson, M. L. et al. (2016). Competency-based education: Programme design and challenges to implementation. *Medical Education, 50*, 532–539. Http://dx.doi.org/10.1111/medu.12977

Haley, B., & Palmer, J. (2020). Escape tasks: An innovative approach in nursing education. *Journal of Nursing Education, 59*(11), 655–657. 10.3928/01484834-20201020-11

Hampton, D., Culp-Roche, A., Hensley, A., Wilson, J., Otts, J., Thaxton-Wiggins, A., Fruh, S., & Moser, D. K. (2020). Self-efficacy and satisfaction with teaching in online courses. *Nurse Educator, 45*(6), 302–306. 10.1097/NNE.0000000000000805

Hanifi, N., Parvizy, S., & Joolaee, S. (2013). Motivational journey of Iranian bachelor of nursing students during clinical education: A grounded theory study. *Nursing & Health Sciences, 15*(3), 340–345. 10.1111/nhs.12041

Hanshaw, S. L., & Dickerson, S. S. (2020). High fidelity simulation evaluation studies in nursing education: A review of the literature. *Nurse Education in Practice, 46*, N.PAG-N.PAG. 10.1016/j.nepr.2020.102818

Hasanvand, S., Ashktorab, T., & Seyedfatemi, N. (2014). Conformity with clinical setting among nursing students as a way to achieve belongingness: A qualitative study. *Iranian Journal of Medical Education, 14*(3), 216–231.

Hawker, C. O., Merkouris, S. S., Youssef, G. J., & Dowling, N. A. (2021). Exploring the associations between gambling cravings, self-efficacy, and gambling episodes: An Ecological Momentary Assessment study. *Addictive Behaviors, 112*, N.PAG-N.PAG. 10.1016/j.addbeh.2020.106574

Hicks, N. A., & Burkus, E. (2011). Knowledge development for master teachers. *Journal of Theory Construction and Testing, 15*(2), 32–35.

House, B. M., Chassie, M. B., & Spohn, B. B. (1999). Questioning: An essential ingredient in effective teaching. *Journal of Continuing Education in Nursing, 21*(5), 196–201.

Hsu, L., & Hsieh, S. (2014). Factors affecting metacognition of undergraduate nursing students in a blended learning environment. *International Journal of Nursing Practice, 20*(3), 233–241. 10.1111/ijn.12131

Hundial, H. (2020). The Safe Care Framework™: A practical tool for critical thinking. *Nurse Education in Practice, 48,* N.PAG-N.PAG. 10.1016/j.nepr.2020.102852

Indiana State Nurses Foundation & Indiana State Nurses Association. (2014). Developing a nursing IQ—Part 1. Characteristics of critical thinking: What critical thinkers do, what critical thinkers do not do. *ISNA Bulletin, 41*(1), 6–14.

Institute of Medicine (IOM) Committee on Quality of Health Care in America (2000). Washington, DC: Academies Press. Https://www.ncbi.nlm.nih.gov/pubmed/25077248

Jung, C. G. (1921). Psychological types. In R. F. C. Hull (Ed.), *The collected works of C. G. Jung* (Vol. 6, Bollingen Series XX, H. G. Baynes, Trans.). Princeton, NJ: Princeton University Press.

Kaakinen, J., & Arwood, E. (2009). Systematic review of nursing simulation literature for use of learning theory. *International Journal of Nursing Education Scholarship, 6*(1), 1–20. 10.2202/1548-923X.1688

Kalb, K. A., O'Conner-Von, S. K., Brockway, C., Rierson, C., & Sendelbach, S. (2015). Evidence-based teaching practice in nursing education: Faculty perspectives and practices. *Nursing Education Perspectives, 36*(4), 212–219. 10.5480/14-1472

Keller, J. M. (1987). Development and use of the ARCS model of motivational design. *Journal of Instructional Development, 10*(3), 2–10.

Kelly, C. (2008). Students' perceptions of effective clinical teaching revisited. *Nurse Education Today, 27*(8), 885–892.

Knowles, M. (1980). *The modern practice of adult education.* Chicago, IL: Follett.

Kolb, D. A. (1984). *Experiential learning: Experience as the source of learning and development.* Upper Saddle River, NJ: Prentice-Hall.

Kolb, D. A., Boyatzis, R. E., & Mainemelis, C. (1999). *Experiential learning theory: Previous research and new directions.* Cleveland, OH: Department of Organizational Behavior, Weatherhead School of Management, Case Western Reserve University. Retrieved from http://www.d.umn.edu/~kgilbert/educ5165-731/Readings/experiential-learning-theory.pdf

Koshenin, L. (2004). A nurse's role in mentoring a foreign student. *Sairaanhoitaja, 77*(11), 18–21.

Kaulback, M. K. (2020). Correlating self-directed learning abilities to lifelong learning orientation in baccalaureate nursing students. *Nurse Educator, 45*(6), 347–351. 10.1097/NNE.0000000000000803

Lai, J. W. M. & Bower, M. (2020). Evaluation of technology use in education: Findings from a critical analysis of systematic literature reviews. *Journal of Computer Assisted Learning, 36*(3), 241–259. 10.1111/jcal.12412

Leggett, T. (2015). Competency-based education: A brief overview. *Radiation Therapist, 24*(1), 107–110.

Levett-Jones, T., & Lathlean, J. (2008). Belongingness: A prerequisite for nursing students' clinical learning. *Nurse Education in Practice, 8*(2), 103–111.

Li, L., Gao, F., & Guo, S. (2020). The effects of social messaging on students' learning and intrinsic motivation in peer assessment. *Journal of Computer Assisted Learning, 36*(4), 439–448. Http://dx.doi.org.proxy1.lib.tju.edu/10.1111/jcal.12409

Lottes, N. C. (2008). FIRE UP: Tips for engaging student learning. *Journal of Nursing Education, 47*(7), 331–332.

Mann, A. S. (2004). Eleven tips for the new college teacher. *Journal of Nursing Education, 43*(9), 389–390.

Mann, K. V. (2011). Theoretical perspectives in medical education: Past experience and future possibilities. *Medical Education, 45*, 60–68. 10.1111/j.1365-2923.2010.03757.x

Marton, F., & Saljo, R. (1976). On qualitative differences in learning: I—Outcome and process. *British Journal of Educational Psychology, 46*(1), 4–11.

Meleis, A. I. (2018). *Theoretical nursing: Development and progress.* Wolters Kluwer. ISBN: 978-0-06-000042-4

Miller, M. A., & Malcolm, N. S. (1990). Critical thinking in the nursing curriculum. *Nursing & Health Care, 11*(2), 67–73

Miner, A., Mallow, J., Theeke, L., & Barnes, E. (2015). Using Gagne's 9 events of instruction to enhance student performance and course evaluations in undergraduate nursing course. *Nurse Educator, 40*(3), 152–154. 10.1097/NNE.0000000000000138

Mulligan, R. (2007). Management strategies in the educational setting. In B. Moyer & R. A. Wittmann-Price (Eds.), *Teaching nursing: Foundations of practice excellence* (pp. 109–125). Philadelphia, PA: F. A. Davis.

Munhall, P. L. (1993). Unknowing: Toward another pattern of knowing in nursing. *Nursing Outlook, 41*(3), 125–128.

National League for Nursing. (2021). Certified Nurse Educator (CNE) 2021 candidate handbook. Http://www.nln.org/docs/default-source/default-document-library/cne-handbook-2021_revised_07-01-2021.pdf?sfvrsn=2

National League for Nursing. (2021). Certified Nurse Educator Novice (CNEn) 2021 candidate handbook. Http://www.nln.org/Certification-for-Nurse-Educators/cne-n/cne-n-handbook

National Council State Boards of Nursing (2020). *Next generation NCLEX news.* Https://www.ncsbn.org/NGN_Summer20_Eng_05.pdf

Nesje, K. (2015). Nursing students' prosocial motivation: Does it predict professional commitment and involvement in the job? *Journal of Advanced Nursing, 71*(1), 115–125. 10.1111/jan.12456

Novotny, J., & Griffin, M. T. (2006). *A nuts-and-bolts approach to teaching nursing.* New York, NY: Springer Publishing.

O'Brien, B. C. & Battista, A. (2020. Situated learning theory in health professions education research: a scoping review. *Advances in Health Sciences Education, 25*(2), 483–509. 10.1007/s10459-019-09900-w

Osinski, J. & Turrise, S. L. (2020). Creating a tutorial for locating clinical practice guidelines. *Nurse Educator, 45*(6), 315–315. 10.1097/NNE.0000000000000835

Palese, A. Cracina, A., Marini, E., Caruzzo, D., Fabris, S., Mansutti, I., Mattiussi, E., Morandidi, M., Moreales, R., Venturini, M., Achil, I., & Danielis, M. (2020). Missed nursing education: Findings from a qualitative study. *Journal of Advanced Nursing, 76*(12), 3506–3518. 10.1111/jan.14533

Partusch, M. (2007). Assessment and evaluation strategies. In B. A. Moyer & R. A. Wittmann-Price (Eds.), *Nursing education: Foundations of practice excellence* (pp. 213–227). Philadelphia, PA: F. A. Davis.

Paul, R., & Elder, L. (2007). Critical thinking: The nature of critical and creative thought. *Journal of Developmental Education, 32*(2), 34–35.

Petrovic, K. A., Hack, R., & Perry, B. (2020). Establishing meaningful learning in online nursing postconferences: A literature review. *Nurse Educator, 45*(5), 283–287. 10.1097/NNE.0000000000000762

Piaget, J. (1972). *The psychology of the child.* New York, NY: Basic Books.

Pittman, O., & Barker, E. (2020). Academic dishonesty: What impact does it have and what can faculty do? *Journal of the American Association of Nurse Practitioners, 32*(9), 598–601. 10.1097/JXX.0000000000000477

Popil, I. (2012). Promotion of critical thinking by using case studies as teaching method. *Nurse Education Today, 31*(2), 204–207. 10.1016/j.nedt.2010.06.002

Price, B. (2015). Applying critical thinking to nursing. *Nursing Standard, 29*(51), 49–58. 10.7748/ns.29.51.49.e10005

Quirk, M. E. (1994). *How to learn and teach in medical school: A learner-centered approach.* New York, NY: Charles C. Thomas.

Ramsden, P., & Entwistle, N. J. (1981). Effects of academic departments on students' approaches to studying. *British Journal of Educational Psychology, 51*, 368–383.

Raterink, G. (2016). Reflective journaling for critical thinking development in advanced practice registered nurse students. *Journal of Nursing Education, 55*(2), 101–104. 10.3928/01484834-20160114-08

Reiger, K. L., Chernomas, W. M., McMillan, D. E., & Morin, F. L. (2020). Navigating creativity within arts-based pedagogy: Implications of a constructivist grounded theory study. *Nurse Education Today, 91*, N.PAG-N.PAG.

Http://dx.doi.org.proxy1.lib.tju.edu/10.1016/j.nedt.2020.104465

Ritchie, G., & Smith, C. (2015). Critical thinking in community nursing: Is this the 7th C? *British Journal of Community Health, 20*(12), 578–579. 10.12968/bjcn.2015.20.12.578

Romeo, E. M. (2010). Quantitative research on critical thinking and predicting nursing students' NCLEX-RN performance. *Journal of Nursing Education, 49*(7), 378–386.:10.3928/01484834-20100331-05

Rose, K. A., Jenkins, S. D., Astroth, K. S., Woith, W., & Jarvill, M. (2020). Testing a web-based intervention to improve awareness of civility and incivility in Baccalaureate nursing students. *Clinical Simulation in Nursing, 48*, 46–54. 10.1016/j.ecns.2020.08.011

Rourke, L., Leong, J., & Chatterly, P. (2018). Conditions-Based Learning Theory as a framework for comparative-effectiveness reviews: A worked example. *Teaching & Learning in Medicine, 30*(4), 386–394. 10.1080/10401334.2018.1428611

Saar-Heiman, Y., & Gupta, A. (2020). The poverty-aware paradigm for child Protection: A critical framework for policy and practice. *British Journal of Social Work, 50*(4), 1167–1184. 10.1093/bjsw/bcz093

Saini, N. K., Sethi, G. K., & Chauhan, P. (2019). Assessing the student's perception on teacher's characteristics for effective teaching. *International Journal of Nursing Education, 11*(1), 90–95. 10.5958/0974-9357.2019.00028.X

Sargeant, J., Wong, B. M., & Campbell, C. M. (2018). CPD of the future: A partnership between quality improvement and competency-based education. *Medical Education 52*, 125–135. Http://dx.doi.org/10.1111/medu.13407

Schuler, M. S., & Joohyun, C. (2019). Exam wrapper use and metacognition in a fundamentals course: Perceptions and reality. *Journal of Nursing Education, 58*(7), 417–421. 10.3928/01484834-20190614-06

Shustack, L. (2019). The sinking ship: An innovative strategy for teaching research sampling. *Journal of Nursing Education, 58*(9), 554–554. Http://dx.doi.org.proxy1.lib.tju.edu/10.3928/01484834-20190819-13

Silver, H., Hanson, J. R., & Strong, R. W. (1996). *Teaching styles & strategies (Unity in diversity series, Manual no. 2).* Alexandria, VA: Silver and Strong.

Simmonds, A., Nunn, A., Gray, M., Hardie, C., Mayo, S., Peter, E., & Richards, J. (2020). Pedagogical practices that influence professional identity formation in baccalaureate nursing education: A scoping review. *Nurse Education Today*, 93, N.PAG-N.PAG. (1p) 10.1016/j.nedt.2020.104516

Sousa A. T. O., Formiga, N. S., Oliveira, S. H. S., Costa, M. M. L., & Soares, M. J. G. O. (2015). Using the theory of meaningful learning in nursing education. *Revista Brasilieira de Enfermagem, 68*(4), 626–635. 10.1590/0034-7167.2015680420i

Starkweather, A. R., Colloca, L., Dorsey, S. G., Griffioen, M., Lyon, D., & Renn, C. (2019). Strengthening inter- and intraprofessional collaborations to advance biobehavioral symptom science. *Journal of Nursing Scholarship, 51*(1), 9–16. Http://dx.doi.org.proxy1.lib.tju.edu/10.1111/jnu.12456

Stonecypher, K., & Willson, P. (2014). Academic policies and practices to deter cheating in nursing education. *Nursing Education Perspectives, 35*(3), 167–179. 10.5480/12-1028.1

Story, L., & Butts, J. B. (2010). Compelling teaching with the four Cs: Caring, comedy, creativity, and challenging. *Journal of Nursing Education, 49*(5), 291–294. 10.3928/01484834-20100115-08

Touchie, C., & Cate, O. (2016). The promise, perils, problems and progress of competency-based medical education. *Medial Education, 50*, 93–100. Http://dx.doi.org/10.1111/medu.12839

Tucker, C. A. (2020). Succession planning for academic nursing. *Journal of Professional Nursing, 36*(5): 334–342. 10.1016/j.profnurs.2020.02.002

Tyler, R. W. (1949). *Basic principles of curriculum and instruction.* Chicago, IL: University of Chicago Press.

Vaccaria, A., Figueiredo, F. G., & Porto, D. S. Implementation of a lesson plan model in the nursing laboratory: Strengthening learning. *Revista Gaucha de Enfermagem, 41*, 1–5. 10.1590/1983-1447.2020.20190174

Vinales, J. J. (2015). The mentor as a role model and the importance of belongingness. *British Journal of Nursing, 24*(10), 532–535.:10.12968/bjon.2015.24.10.532

Vroom, V. (1964). *Work and motivation.* New York, NY: Wiley.

Walker, S. (2003). Active learning strategies to promote critical thinking. *Journal of Athletic Training, 38*(3), 263–267.

Watson, G., & Glaser, E. M. (1964). *Watson–Glaser critical thinking appraisal manual.* New York, NY: Harcourt, Brace & World.

Wittmann-Price, R. A., & Fasolka, B. (2010). Objectives and outcomes: The fundamental difference. *Nursing Education Perspective, 31*(4), 233–236.:10.1043/1536-5026-31.4.233

Wittmann-Price, R. A., & Godshall, M. (2009). Strategies to promote deep learning in clinical nursing courses. *Nurse Educator, 34*(5), 214–216.

Wong, C. K., & Driscoll, M. (2008). A modified jigsaw method: An active learning strategy to develop the cognitive and affective domains through curricular review. *Journal of Physical Therapy Education, 21*(3), 15–23.

Wong, S. H. V., & Kowitlawakul, Y. (2020). Exploring perceptions and barriers in Developing critical thinking and clinical reasoning of nursing students: A qualitative study. *Nurse Education Today, 95,* N.PAG-N.PAG. 10.1016/j.nedt.2020.104600

Yeo, C. M. (2014). Concept mapping: A strategy to improve critical thinking. *Singapore Nursing Journal, 41*(3), 2–7.

Yeom, Y., Miller, M. A., & Delp, R. (2018). Constructing a teaching philosophy: Aligning beliefs, theories, and practice. *Teaching & Learning in Nursing, 13*(3), 131–134. Http://dx.doi.org.proxy1.lib.tju.edu/10.1016/j.teln.2018.01.004

Yildirim, S. N., Karaca, A., & Cangur, S. (2020). Factors affecting health-promoting behaviors in nursing students: A structural equation modeling approach. *Nurse Education in Practice, 48,* N.PAG-N.PAG. 10.1016/j.nepr.2020.102880

Yilmaz, R. (2020). Enhancing community of inquiry and reflective thinking skills of undergraduates through using learning analytics-based process feedback. *Journal of Computer Assisted Learning, 36*(6), 909–921. 10.1111/jcal.12449

Yonge, O., Lee, H., & Luhanga, F. (2006). Closing and not just ending a course. *Nurse Educator, 31*(4), 151–153.

Yoon, J. (2004). *Development of an instrument for the measurement of critical thinking disposition in nursing* (master's thesis). The Catholic University of Education, Seoul, Korea.

Younas, A. (2018). Practical tips for novice nurse educators. *Nursing, 48*(2), 21–22. Http://dx.doi.org.proxy1.lib.tju.edu/10.1097/01.NURSE.0000529815.29031.52

Zsohar, H., & Smith, J. A. (2006). Faculty issues. Top ten list of don'ts in classroom teaching. *Nurse Educator, 31*(4), 144–146.

Teaching and Learning Strategies

Karen K. Gittings

> *Those who know, do. Those that understand, teach.*
> —Aristotle

▶ **LEARNING OUTCOMES**

This chapter also addresses the Certified Nurse Educator Exam and the Certified Nurse Educator Novice Exam Content Area 1: Facilitate Learning

- Differentiate between teaching strategies and learning activities
- Contrast passive and active learning
- Identify key points for effective PowerPoint presentations
- Identify advantages and disadvantages of various passive learning strategies
- Describe advantages and disadvantages of various active learning strategies
- Discuss flipping the classroom and associated challenges
- Appraise the principles for good practice in online education
- Discuss how virtual simulation can be used as an alternative to face-to-face clinicals

INTRODUCTION

The teaching–learning process involves the planning and implementation of experiences that are designed to lead to the achievement of student learning outcomes. These learning experiences can be thought of in terms of teaching strategies and learning activities. Although these terms are sometimes used interchangeably, the difference is in their focus.

- Teaching strategies, also referred to as methods or techniques, are teacher-centered activities. These strategies are used by faculty when teaching.
- Learning activities focus more on the learner. Faculty design strategies that enhance learner involvement and participation (Scheckel, 2012).

In postsecondary education, the majority of today's students are aged 17–37 years. Labelled as generation Y or millennials, these students are used to working in teams, with a desire to be coached or mentored. They have grown up with technology and are comfortable communicating through multiple methods. Although learner-centered instruction is increasingly recommended for all learners, this is particularly relevant for teaching generation Y students. Learning activities encourage student involvement and place more of the responsibility on the learner for the acquisition of knowledge (Battersby, 2017).

 ## PASSIVE AND ACTIVE LEARNING

Learning activities can be further categorized as passive or active. With passive learning, learners take in information through their senses to be recalled at a later date; passive learning most commonly occurs through classroom lectures. This mode of learning is still used commonly in today's classrooms in nursing and healthcare education. With active learning, learners are more engaged and are encouraged to participate in the acquisition of knowledge. Active learning can lead to improved retention and better understanding (Battersby, 2017).

▶ PASSIVE LEARNING ADVANTAGES

- Faculty are able to present large amounts of information.
- Faculty have greater control over the learning environment.
- Learners often prefer this method because of their previous experience.
- Important concepts are identified for learners.
- Learners may feel less anxious with a method familiar to them (Scheckel, 2012).

▶ PASSIVE LEARNING DISADVANTAGES

- Leaves little time for questions or discussion.
- Faculty may not know whether learners understand the information presented.
- Requires little effort from learners.
- May limit retention of knowledge and understanding.
- Does not facilitate application of concepts or use of higher-level thinking (Scheckel, 2012).
- Students of today are less satisfied with passive learning methods (Battersby, 2017).
- Learners are less motivated to participate.
- Learners are less likely to achieve learning outcomes (Youngwanichsetha et al., 2019).

◎ **Critical Thinking Question**
  Role modeling is a passive-teaching strategy that can be used to influence the attitude of learners. What other active-learning strategy is effective for learning in the affective domain?

▶ ACTIVE LEARNING ADVANTAGES

- Increased attentiveness in the learning environment (Vetter & Latimer, 2017).
- Improved retention of content.
- Deeper understanding of the information.
- Reinforces ideas.
- Improves test scores (Battersby, 2017).

- Improved critical-thinking and problem-solving skills (Aljezawi & Albashtawy, 2015; Youngwanichsetha, 2019).
- Encourages reflection, exploration, creativity, and collaboration (Johnson & Barrett, 2017).

▶ ACTIVE LEARNING DISADVANTAGES

- Learners may be resistant to change.
- Learners may view these strategies as requiring extra work.
- Faculty may be resistant to change from their patterns of teaching and learning.
- Faculty may be concerned about student evaluations, especially if they are nontenured (Scheckel, 2012).

● LECTURE

Lecture, which is a type of passive learning, is still most commonly used in today's classroom. Nurse educators have to cover large amounts of content within their courses (Nowak et al., 2016). Lecturing allows the educator to control the pace and flow of the class so that instructional goals for each specific class time can be achieved. Despite using lecture as a primary teaching strategy, most educators supplement with visual slides or audio files. Microsoft's PowerPoint is a very popular tool that has replaced the transparencies of the past. Instead of learners hurriedly trying to write notes and keep up, the challenge today is to not provide every note, which would lessen learner engagement (Nowak et al., 2016). There are many other learning strategies that can be employed in the classroom to increase learner participation in their own knowledge acquisition.

EVIDENCE-BASED TEACHING PRACTICE

In a study conducted by Mahon et al. (2018), the researchers set out to determine if audience response systems (ARSs) offer any advantage over traditional classroom questioning (CQ) techniques. With questions that pertained to psychological safety, 90% of students identified that they liked the anonymity of the ARS. In other findings, 85.7% of respondents thought that ARS assisted learning, 71.4% found the ARS fun to use, and 85.7% thought the ARS would make it easier to respond to questions. The authors concluded that ARSs provide psychological security and enhance student interaction.

● POWERPOINT

PowerPoint has been described as a multimedia presentation of a speech or lecture (Grech, 2018). Many educators use PowerPoint presentations to supplement lectures in the classroom, but few have received any guidance on how to use PowerPoint effectively.

It is not uncommon that in an attempt to convey large amounts of information, faculty include too much detail on their PowerPoints. Learners can become quickly bored, particularly when slides are busy and the educator proceeds to read directly from the slides (Nowak et al., 2016). Because PowerPoint is likely here to stay, it is important that educators learn how to develop presentations that are effective for student learning.

▶ KEYS TO EFFECTIVE PRESENTATIONS

- Choose simple slide designs.
- Blue or green backgrounds with high contrast colors are most attractive.
- Font should contrast with the background and be easily readable (larger than 30).
- Choose easily readable font styles (Arial, Verdana, Lucida Console).
- Use bullets for key points—no more than six bullets per slide and six to eight words per bullet.
- Include title/topic, author, credentials, and date on the first slide.
- Include concisely written objectives early in the presentation.
- Limit one idea per slide if possible.
- Include graphics to facilitate understanding (no more than one per slide) in APA format.
- Use multiple strategies to engage the learners (websites, videos, discussions, and polls).
- Slides should serve as an outline only.
- Plan on covering 20–30 slides per 30-minute time frame.
- Never read directly from slides.
- Allow white space for note-taking (Nowak et al., 2016).
- Graphics and verbal presentation are more effective than words on a slide.
- Text and pictures are more effective than text alone.
- Identify key points as slide titles.
- The less information on the slide, the clearer the focus on the relevant message (Grech, 2018).

TEACHING GEM "A presentation is not a showcase for a speaker's IT skills (Grech, 2018, p. 37)." In PowerPoints, keep transitions smooth and avoid special effects that detract from the message (Grech).

Learning is optimized when visual and auditory methods are utilized simultaneously; thus, PowerPoint can be effective for conveying information if not overused (Grech, 2018). PowerPoint is additionally only as effective as the educator presenting; the presenter must stay cognizant of how the audience (learners) is responding and adapt accordingly. Other active learning strategies should be incorporated to keep the learners engaged in the classroom. Tables 2.1 and 2.2 provide examples of passive and active learning strategies.

Table 2.1 Passive Learning Strategies

Strategy	Description	Advantages	Disadvantages
Lecture	Educator presents the content. May include audio or visual aids and/or handouts	▪ Clarifies complex information for the learner ▪ Efficient for covering large amounts of information (Rowles, 2012) ▪ An inspiring teacher can engage learners and keep their attention ▪ Can be made more engaging by breaking up the lecture with other activities (Hagler & Morris, 2015) ▪ Highlights main ideas and summarizes data ▪ Effective for cognitive learning (Fitzgerald & Keyes, 2019) ▪ Educator serves as role model for critical thinking and problem-solving ▪ Opportunity for learners to develop listening skills (DeYoung, 2015) ▪ Recorded lectures can be viewed when convenient and watched multiple times (Furnes et al., 2018)	▪ Minimal learner engagement ▪ Initial lengthy faculty preparation (Rowles, 2012) ▪ Learners are unlikely to retain information when they are not actively engaged (Hagler & Morris, 2015) ▪ Mostly ineffective with affective and psychomotor learning ▪ All learners are taught the same despite differing abilities and limitations (Fitzgerald & Keyes, 2019) ▪ Focuses more on the teaching of facts and less on analytical thinking ▪ Effective for primarily auditory, linguistic learners ▪ Loss of attention occurs over time (DeYoung, 2015)
Demonstration	Educator shows the learner how to perform a specific skill	▪ Facilitates understanding (Rowles, 2012) ▪ Effective for visual learners (Hagler & Morris, 2015)	▪ Learners may get bored (Rowles, 2012) ▪ Limited to small groups so that all can observe (Fitzgerald & Keyes, 2019)

(continued)

Table 2.1 Passive Learning Strategies (*continued*)

Strategy	Description	Advantages	Disadvantages
Reading	It is the learner's responsibility to read assigned chapters that relate to course content	▪ Provides an opportunity to understand, interpret, and apply information ▪ Strategies exist to improve reading comprehension (Hagler & Morris, 2015)	▪ May be difficult to learn through this method ▪ Often difficult for learners to complete all of the assigned readings (Hagler & Morris, 2015)
Role modeling	Educators model behaviors and influence/teach by example; differs from mentoring	▪ Effective for affective learning ▪ Influences attitudes of learners ▪ Potential to instill socially desired behaviors (Fitzgerald & Keyes, 2019) ▪ Effective for promoting those professional attributes that are difficult to teach (e.g., integrity) ▪ Fosters the development of professionalism ▪ Cultivates the formation of a professional identity ▪ Assists to identify career choices (e.g., areas of specialization) (Passi & Johnson, 2016)	▪ Requires a positive relationship between the educator and learner ▪ May result in unacceptable behaviors if the role model has a negative influence (Fitzgerald & Keyes, 2019) ▪ Learners may have difficulty judging positive vs negative role modeling ▪ Learners may be conflicted when negative role modeling is observed in contrast to what is taught in the formal curriculum (Passi & Johnson, 2016)

Table 2.2 Active Learning Strategies (*continued*)

Strategy	Description	Advantages	Disadvantages
Algorithms	Step-by-step process for problem-solving	■ Assists learners in identifying the most relevant information ■ Generally easy to use and access ■ Guide for decision-making ■ Commonly used in healthcare (Lee et al., 2019)	■ Time-consuming for faculty to develop ■ Steps must be easy to understand ■ Learners need instruction in use (Rowles, 2012)
Audience response systems (ARS)/clickers	Electronic polling system that provides instant results	■ Instant feedback available ■ May be used for attendance or to gauge learner understanding of the material ■ Engages the student behaviorally, emotionally, and cognitively ■ Anonymous polling creates a safe learning environment ■ Generally enjoyable for the learner ■ Some systems allow statistical analysis of responses ■ Web-based systems allow use of smart devices ■ Increases two-way communication in the classroom (Mahon et al., 2018)	■ Some cost involved if clickers are used ■ Instructors need to learn the technology ■ May be time-consuming and a limitation on the amount of content delivered ■ May be distracting (Mahon et al., 2018)
Case study/case report	Application of nursing content and theory to analyze real-life situations	■ Retrospective look at a clinical case ■ Often highlights the diagnosis, treatment, and complications of an infrequent or unusual case (Morris, 2015) ■ Promotes critical thinking ■ Helps learners make the connection between didactic and practice events ■ Learners can practice problem-solving ■ When done in class, improves communication, collaboration, and creativity ■ Learners can construct their own knowledge (Youngwanichsetha et al., 2019)	■ Time-consuming for faculty to develop ■ Complex cases may be difficult to write ■ Cases must be detailed, structured, and organized to be effective (Morris, 2015)

(*continued*)

Table 2.2 Active Learning Strategies (*continued*)

Strategy	Description	Advantages	Disadvantages
Clinical conferences/ online conferences	Small-group discussions that occur pre-, mid-, or post-clinical experiences	▪ Assists learners to connect theory to practice ▪ Promotes clinical decision-making and critical thinking ▪ Increases learner confidence (Stokes & Kost, 2012)	▪ More effective if planned in advance (Stokes & Kost, 2012)
Collaborative/ cooperative learning	Learners work on assignments in teams	▪ Encourages teamwork ▪ Learners master knowledge by constructing content (Battersby, 2017) ▪ Promotes learner satisfaction, participation, and academic achievement (Peacock & Grande, 2016) ▪ Increases retention and promotes deeper learning ▪ Learners also learn group skills (Hagler & Morris, 2015) ▪ Strengthens communication skills (DeYoung, 2015)	▪ Learners are often resistant to group work ▪ Some learners may not participate to group standards ▪ Potential scheduling conflicts (Rowles, 2012) ▪ Educators must plan and create a highly structured group environment (Hagler & Morris, 2015)
Debate	A logical argument and defense of a position aimed at demonstrating the truth or falsity of the matter	▪ Promotes critical thinking ▪ Facilitates higher-order learning (analysis, synthesis, and evaluation) (Rao, 2019) ▪ Improves verbal communication ▪ Team building (Battersby, 2017) ▪ May be used to promote thinking about ethical or controversial issues (Hagler & Morris, 2015)	▪ Requires extensive knowledge of the subject matter ▪ Lengthy learner preparation time ▪ May increase learner anxiety ▪ Increases time committed to group work (Rowles, 2012)
Debriefing	Faculty assist learners to reflect on clinical experiences; often used with simulation	▪ May be done synchronously or asynchronously ▪ Empowers learners ▪ Facilitates the development of critical thinking skills and knowledge transfer ▪ Opportunity to review actions and clinical decisions and discuss ways to improve (Gerdes, 2018) ▪ May be planned (most common) or spontaneous (informal) (Werry, 2016)	▪ Faculty need training to provide effective debriefing ▪ Faculty may lack confidence in the debriefing process ▪ Some debriefing models are complex (Werry, 2016) ▪ Challenging to organize and enact with large course enrollments (Gerdes, 2018)

(*continued*)

Table 2.2 Active Learning Strategies (*continued*)

Strategy	Description	Advantages	Disadvantages
Flipped classroom	Learners complete learning activities prior to coming to class so that active learning can occur in the classroom; swaps lecture for active learning time	▪ More focused learning can occur in the classroom ▪ Facilitates collaboration and team work ▪ Higher learning occurs ▪ Dynamic classes often lead to greater student satisfaction (Luchetti, 2018)	▪ Learners are accountable for pre-work, which if extensive, may lead to discontent ▪ Requires a change in mindset of the learners and faculty ▪ Initially, may require more preparation time for faculty ▪ Faculty may require more technological support (Sharma, 2015)
Games	Learners compete against self, a game, peers, or a computer	▪ Fun for learners ▪ Creates real-life situations for learning ▪ Effective for kinesthetic/tactile learners ▪ In scaffolding, games begin with easily completed tasks, which are then built upon with more challenging tasks ▪ Develops skills in communication, problem-solving, and decision-making ▪ Improves retention (Day-Black, 2015) ▪ Engages learners even when the content is repetitive or dry (Fitzgerald & Keyes, 2019) ▪ Increases interaction among learners (DeYoung, 2015)	▪ Increased faculty time investment for creation of games ▪ Costs may be associated (Steinhardt, 2020) ▪ May take a significant amount of time from class ▪ Faculty may lose control of the classroom ▪ Difficult to evaluate individual learning (Rowles, 2012) ▪ Competition may deter some learners ▪ May require additional, adaptable space ▪ Potentially creates a noisy environment (Fitzgerald & Keyes, 2019)
Grand rounds	Educator discusses patient problems and nursing care	▪ Facilitates exchange of ideas among faculty, learners, and nursing staff (Stokes & Kost, 2012) ▪ Encourages critical thinking and problem-solving ▪ Collaboration with the health care team is enhanced ▪ Improves communication (Woodley, 2015)	▪ Requires planning ▪ Patient permission should be obtained (Stokes & Kost, 2012)

(*continued*)

Table 2.2 Active Learning Strategies (*continued*)

Strategy	Description	Advantages	Disadvantages
Group discussions/ seminars	Students and educator meet to discuss specific topics and share ideas	▪ Peer sharing occurs ▪ Problems can be discussed and solved as a group ▪ Creates an environment of teamwork and cooperation ▪ Increases learner motivation ▪ Facilitates skills in interpersonal communication and public speaking (Grover, 2018) ▪ Group participants are better able to clarify their own thoughts and beliefs when faced with the ideas of others (Hagler & Morris, 2015) ▪ Promotes deeper understanding and longer retention of information ▪ Promotes positive interpersonal relationships ▪ Effective for learning in the affective and cognitive domains (Fitzgerald & Keyes, 2019) ▪ Attitudes can be changed (DeYoung, 2015)	▪ Learners must be prepared with knowledge of the topic ▪ Some learners may be reluctant to speak and participate ▪ Difficult to evaluate student learning in those not participating (Grover, 2018) ▪ Learners may not be able to decipher the important points to remember (Hagler & Morris, 2015) ▪ More time-consuming to transmit information ▪ Most effective with small-size groups (Fitzgerald & Keyes, 2019)
Group projects	Cooperative project in which learners work together to achieve a common goal	▪ Increases long-term retention ▪ Encourages critical thinking and problem-solving ▪ Requires negotiation and collaboration ▪ Decreases the amount of work required of any individual learner ▪ Learners experience conflict resolution, compromise, and trust building (Ward-Smith, et al., 2010)	▪ The work may be divided unevenly, resulting in a few people doing all the work ▪ Learners may only learn the portion that they worked on ▪ Conflict may occur ▪ Scheduling time to work together may be a challenge (Ward-Smith et al., 2010)

(*continued*)

Table 2.2 Active Learning Strategies (*continued*)

Strategy	Description	Advantages	Disadvantages
Humor	The use of comical situations or comments to highlight important points and enhance learning	■ Increases learner interest in the topic ■ Helps to alleviate stress and anxiety ■ May improve retention ■ Educators may seem more relatable and approachable ■ Learners are more willing to ask questions (Azadbakht, 2019) ■ Enhances learner–educator rapport ■ Increases group cohesion by providing a sense of belonging ■ Increases inclusiveness by reducing the unequal role status between educator and learner (Mesquita, 2015)	■ May be inappropriate ■ May be demeaning if used inappropriately ■ May interfere with the learner educator relationship ■ Learners may find it distracting (Azadbakht, 2019)
Imagery	Forming a mental picture or rehearsing in one's mind before taking action	■ Enhances learning of psychomotor skills ■ Helps learners to better understand the steps of procedures ■ Assists in mental preparation before a procedure ■ Builds confidence ■ Identifies potential issues and/or solutions ■ Effective adjunct to physical practice (Anton et al., 2017)	■ Should not be the sole method of training (Anton et al., 2017) ■ Requires more time than just practice of skills ■ Faculty need to fully understand the strategy before educating learners in its use ■ Stress may interfere with effective use (Rowles, 2012)
Jigsaw	Group learning in which each member of the group is given a packet of information to learn and share with the rest of the group so that all benefit	■ Learners work together for success ■ Each group member is accountable for his or her portion ■ Builds comprehension ■ Encourages cooperation ■ Improves listening and communication skills (Bhandari et al., 2017)	■ Time-consuming for faculty to develop ■ Learners may complain that it is difficult for group members to meet outside the classroom ■ Learners may experience anxiety because of reliance on other students' contributions (Phillips & Fusco, 2015)

(continued)

Table 2.2 Active Learning Strategies (*continued*)

Strategy	Description	Advantages	Disadvantages
Just-In-Time Teaching	Learners complete questions/ exercises prior to class, which the educator then uses to direct instruction toward gaps in learning or areas of confusion	▪ Connects out-of-class with in-class learning ▪ Classroom instruction is tailored to the needs of the class ▪ May be combined with other strategies (e.g., flipping the classroom) (Clark, 2016)	▪ If written poorly, questions may be ineffective in identifying gaps in knowledge ▪ Learners may not find the questions/ exercises useful for learning (Clark, 2016)
Learning circles	Learners get together to discuss a focused topic in order to learn from each other; usually peer based with a facilitator	▪ Promotes equality ▪ Promotes open discussions (Walker et al., 2010)	▪ Takes time to plan and arrange ▪ Learners must be self-directed (Walker et al., 2010)
Learning contracts	Written contract between an individual learner and teacher specifying what needs to be accomplished to meet course outcomes	▪ Effective for adult learners ▪ Builds on prior knowledge and experiences ▪ Learners can work at their own pace (Rowles, 2012) ▪ May be used to clarify expectations for learners not meeting course requirements ▪ Often used for practicum courses or precepted clinical experiences (Hagler & Morris, 2015)	▪ Learners must be independent, self-motivated, and self-disciplined ▪ Time-consuming if faculty have a large number of learners with individualized contracts ▪ Learners may need instruction on developing contracts (Rowles, 2012)
Literature analogies/ newspaper analysis	Literature is used to clarify nursing concepts and to identify similarities and differences Newspapers are used to identify significant events during the week, both positive and negative	▪ Learners can relate unfamiliar concepts with those that are more familiar (Rowles, 2012) ▪ Enables dialogue and communication ▪ Provides an opportunity to discuss lived experiences and emotions (Alves et al., 2017)	▪ Difficult and time-consuming for faculty to locate relevant literature ▪ Learners may be unable to see the relationships (Rowles, 2012)

(continued)

Table 2.2 Active Learning Strategies (*continued*)

Strategy	Description	Advantages	Disadvantages
Mind mapping/ concept maps	Concepts and sub-concepts are diagrammed to visually demonstrate relationships. Although mind mapping and concept maps are often referred to interchangeably, they differ in some respects. Concept maps are linear and word-based. Mind mapping is a nonlinear approach that uses pictorial forms (Zipp et al., 2015)	▪ Effective for visual learners ▪ Graphically demonstrates relationships ▪ Hierarchical process to cross-link concepts and ideas ▪ Effective in recall of short- and long-term facts ▪ Improves understanding of complex information ▪ Encourages analytical thinking (Zipp et al., 2015)	▪ May initially be time-consuming until learners are practiced in organizing the concepts ▪ Skilled technique that requires practice (Zipp et al., 2015) ▪ Faculty may be unfamiliar with this strategy and also require instruction in its use (Clark & Spence, 2016)
One-to-one instruction/ tutoring	Face-to-face interaction designed to meet the needs of the learner; may be formal or informal	▪ Experience is unique to the learner ▪ Retention is improved when information is given in small amounts ▪ Content and pace of instruction are adapted to the learner's needs ▪ Effective for learning in the cognitive, affective, and psychomotor domains ▪ Provides immediate feedback for the learner (Fitzgerald & Keyes, 2019)	▪ Labor intensive ▪ Time-consuming for the educator ▪ Isolates the learner (Fitzgerald & Keyes, 2019)

(*continued*)

Table 2.2 Active Learning Strategies (*continued*)

Strategy	Description	Advantages	Disadvantages
Podcasts/vodcasts/ enhanced podcasts	Audio or video that is available over the Internet; may be played with multimedia devices, for example, PowerPoints with voice-over narration, pictures, images, and short videos	▪ May be used to record lectures ▪ Provides an opportunity for learners to relisten to course information outside the classroom ▪ May be used for inclement weather, faculty illness, or with virtual learning during community crises (e.g., pandemics) ▪ May be utilized to review confusing or complex concepts from lecture (Rae & O'Malley, 2017) ▪ May be used for teaching psychomotor skills prior to class/lab time, thus saving time for hands-on (Greenberger & Dispensa, 2015)	▪ Requires some faculty training ▪ Requires smartphone or other mobile device if used in mobile format ▪ Access to high-speed Internet required ▪ Learners may be more inclined to miss class (Rae & O'Malley, 2017) ▪ Additional resources/ experts may be needed to create quality products (Greenberger & Dispensa, 2015)
Portfolio/electronic portfolios	Electronic or printed documents that are evidence of learning; may be used to demonstrate best work or growth	▪ Encourages learners to self-reflect ▪ Documents progress of learner's work ▪ Effective with independent, self-directed learners ▪ Electronic portfolios are easy to store and update (Ryan, 2018)	▪ May become overly large if guidelines for inclusion are not provided ▪ Learners need guidance on what to include ▪ Time-consuming for faculty to review ▪ ePortfolios may be challenging for learners who have difficulty with technology (Ryan, 2018) ▪ Many ePortfolio platforms require a subscription ▪ Institutions may lack sufficient instructional technology (IT) support ▪ Access to the ePortfolio may end after graduation or a designated period of time (Collins & Crawley, 2016)

(*continued*)

Table 2.2 Active Learning Strategies (*continued*)

Strategy	Description	Advantages	Disadvantages
Poster	Electronic or printed document that may include text, graphs, or pictures to represent a concept	▪ Permits learners to be creative ▪ Complex ideas can be conveyed in a concise format ▪ Effective for dissemination of scholarly work or sharing of information in a short period of time ▪ Can be graded by faculty easily and quickly (Astroth & Hain, 2019)	▪ Supplies may be costly ▪ May be frustrating for some learners who lack creativity ▪ Planning is required for transport, display, and storage if in printed form (Astroth & Hain, 2019)
Problem-based learning	A curriculum approach in which clinical problems and professional issues are used to organize the content	▪ Develops critical thinking and clinical decision-making ▪ Effective with teams and group work ▪ Promotes cooperation and team building ▪ Can be used with interdisciplinary groups ▪ Learners develop a deeper understanding ▪ Prior learning is applied to real-life problems (Decelle, 2016) ▪ Increases learner autonomy ▪ Enhances comprehension and knowledge retention (Santra & Mani, 2017)	▪ Extensive time commitment for faculty to learn to develop problems ▪ Unfamiliar to most learners; requires extended orientation to learner expectations ▪ Difficult to use in larger classes (Rowles, 2012) ▪ Learners may find this methodology to be stressful and time consuming (Mrunalini & Chandekar, 2015)
Questioning/ Socratic questioning	Queries about content designed to elicit a response; questioning to explore complex ideas or analyze concepts	▪ Can be planned or used spontaneously ▪ Promotes clinical decision-making with high-level questions ▪ Encourages discussion and multiple points of view ▪ Strengthens test-taking abilities (Rowles, 2012) ▪ Can be used to review content (DeYoung, 2015) ▪ Inspires self-confidence and self-direction ▪ Initiates collective thinking ▪ Creates a shared responsibility for learning ▪ Provides learners with insight into their learning/performance relative to others (Mahon et al., 2018)	▪ Learners must understand the content ▪ Faculty must be prepared to deliver questions that require more than a statement of the facts ▪ May take a significant amount of class time in order to give learners sufficient time to formulate an answer ▪ Learners may refrain from answering for fear of being wrong or being seen as a 'know-it-all' (Mahon et al., 2018)

(*continued*)

Table 2.2 Active Learning Strategies (*continued*)

Strategy	Description	Advantages	Disadvantages
Reflection/ journaling/blogs	Electronic or written record of personal experiences related to specific content	▪ Learners are better able to connect classroom learning with clinical experiences ▪ Facilitates exploration of one's beliefs and emotions ▪ Learners gain valuable insight to improve their practice ▪ Faculty have better insight into student learning (Mahon & O'Neill, 2020) ▪ Effective for learning in the cognitive and affective domains ▪ Facilitates critical thinking ▪ Promotes self-directed learning (Naicker & van Rensburg, 2018)	▪ Learners may view this as busywork if the objectives are not clear ▪ May restrict thinking if assignment is overly structured ▪ Biases may result in errors of reflection ▪ Learners may minimize the assignment and invest little time ▪ Time-consuming for faculty to read and provide feedback (Mahon & O'Neill, 2020) ▪ Faculty must be skilled in reflective practice in order to provide guidance and support (Naicker & van Rensburg, 2018)
Return demonstration	This requires the learner to repeat a skill that was previously demonstrated	▪ Increases retention ▪ Facilitates understanding ▪ Novices are able to model expert technique (Rowles, 2012) ▪ Effective for the kinesthetic learner (Hagler & Morris, 2015) ▪ Confidence and competence are increased through repetition and frequent feedback (Fitzgerald & Keyes, 2019)	▪ Learners master skills at different speeds ▪ Learners may get bored with waiting ▪ Requires supervision, supplies, and space ▪ Costs associated (Rowles, 2012) ▪ Takes a considerable amount of time for learners to practice and educators to monitor ▪ Groups must be kept small to allow for practice and close supervision (Fitzgerald & Keyes, 2019)

(*continued*)

Table 2.2 Active Learning Strategies (*continued*)

Strategy	Description	Advantages	Disadvantages
Role play	Enactment of a specific role, usually unscripted, whereby others are observing and analyzing the demonstration	■ Learning occurs through observation and discussion ■ Promotes understanding of human behaviors ■ Effective for interpersonal and communication skills training ■ Useful for practicing less common or more challenging situations ■ Peer role play is easy to implement ■ Improves decision-making ■ Effective for processing skills and learning in the affective domain (Furnes et al., 2018) ■ Provides opportunity to explore attitudes and beliefs (Fitzgerald & Keyes, 2019)	■ Learners may not want to participate ■ Time investment needed for faculty to develop scenarios ■ May take a significant amount of class time (Rowles, 2012) ■ May reinforce stereotypical behavior (Moyer & Wittmann-Price, 2008) ■ May appear unrealistic if overly dramatic (Fitzgerald & Keyes, 2019)
Self-learning packet/module/ reusable learning objects (RLO)	Content is presented in sections that permit the learner to progress forward if he or she has demonstrated mastery, often through pre-tests/ post-tests	■ Students have more control over their learning ■ Self-directed and paced ■ Flexible (Curtis et al., 2016) ■ May be used to introduce new content or reinforce/ clarify existing content ■ May be used for learner prework when flipping the classroom (Hagler & Morris, 2015)	■ Learners may procrastinate ■ Time-consuming to prepare ■ Learners may not be sufficiently motivated (Rowles, 2012)
Service learning	A form of experiential learning that occurs outside the traditional classroom	■ Facilitates application of knowledge to the real world ■ Encourages civic involvement ■ Promotes problem-solving (Hagler & Morris, 2015) ■ Incorporates reflective practice (Preheim & Foss, 2015) ■ Promotes improved cultural competency, awareness of social determinants of health, and understanding of health disparities (Bryant-Moore, 2018)	■ Requires extensive planning to ensure that learning outcomes can be met ■ Time-consuming for the faculty to plan and develop experiences and monitor for effectiveness (Hagler & Morris, 2015)

(continued)

Table 2.2 Active Learning Strategies (*continued*)

Strategy	Description	Advantages	Disadvantages
Simulation	A situation that is designed to mimic real-life clinical experiences	■ Learners can practice in a safe environment ■ Learners can experience situations seldom encountered ■ Immediate feedback is provided ■ Increases learner confidence ■ Increases critical thinking ■ Improves clinical judgment and problem-solving skills (Karacay & Kaya, 2020) ■ Encourages teamwork ■ Effective for cognitive, psychomotor, and affective learning (Aebersold, 2018) ■ Acceptable, useful adjunct for clinical instruction ■ Provides an opportunity to develop/practice skills without putting the patient at risk ■ Useful for remediation (van Vuuren et al., 2018)	■ Faculty must develop or search for scenarios ■ Learning outcomes need to be clear for each simulation ■ Faculty adoption may be limited by time constraints in planning simulations, lack of experience with the technology, and insufficient resources/support ■ Equipment is expensive to purchase and maintain ■ Requires physical space and technical support (van Vuuren, 2018)
Social writing tools/wikis	A single document developed by a group that can be edited by each member	■ Promotes collaboration among group members ■ Thinking and writing skills are further developed (Halstead & Billings, 2012) ■ Facilitates group work without needing face-to-face meetings ■ Individual learner contributions can be seen using the history function (DeYoung, 2015)	■ An open wiki would be accessible by the public (Sopczyk, 2019) ■ Learners may be reluctant to critique or edit the work of others ■ Learners who procrastinate impact the work of the group (DeYoung, 2015)
Standardized patient (SP)	Live actors portray patients in a realistic clinical simulation	■ Effective for improving communication and/or physical-assessment skills ■ Learners can experience a situation not experienced in the clinical environment ■ Increases confidence (Aebersold, 2018) ■ Learners receive written and oral feedback (Oermann & Gaberson, 2019)	■ Must be realistic for knowledge to transfer to real life ■ Actors must be trained and scripts provided for each simulation ■ May be costly (Aebersold, 2018)

(*continued*)

Table 2.2 Active Learning Strategies (*continued*)

Strategy	Description	Advantages	Disadvantages
Storytelling/ dialogue/ narrative pedagogy	A conversation between at least two people in which relevant stories are shared	■ Encourages reflection and analysis ■ Reinforces affective learning (Ironside, 2015) ■ Improves recall through evoked emotions and sensory associations ■ Facilitates translation of theory to practice ■ Provides an opportunity to role model good practice (Hardie et al., 2020)	■ Faculty must keep stories relevant and realistic ■ Stories may lead to peer sharing, which can become lengthy and cause learners to lose focus (Rowles, 2012)
Team-based learning	Learners work on assignments in groups, taking accountability for the quality of their own work and that of the group	■ Can be used in larger classes ■ Enhances team building ■ Introduces peer assessment and accountability ■ Improves depth of knowledge and problem-solving skills ■ Increases in-class participation and student engagement ■ Improves communication and collaboration ■ Facilitates development of leadership skills (Roh et al., 2015)	■ Learners and faculty need time to learn this strategy ■ May be challenging for groups to schedule time to work on assignments outside of class time ■ Conflict may interfere with effective group functioning (Rowles, 2012) ■ Learner reactions may be mixed ■ Learners may see this strategy as adding to their workload (Roh et al., 2015)
Think–pair–share	A type of cooperative learning whereby the educator asks a question, allows time for the learners to think, pairs up learners for discussion, and then requests that the collaborative response be shared with the class	■ Increases learner engagement ■ Improves understanding of difficult content ■ Encourages collaboration ■ Enhances interpersonal and small-group skills (Fitzgerald, 2013)	■ Requires learners to come to class prepared ■ Learners may initially be resistant to the additional work required (D. Fitzgerald, 2013)
Top 10 list	Learners prioritize topics from their reading in a list format	■ Helps learner to organize, prioritize, and compare their results with others (Beitz & Snarponis, 2006)	■ Learners will probably prioritize differently (Beitz & Snarponis, 2006)

(*continued*)

Table 2.2 Active Learning Strategies (*continued*)

Strategy	Description	Advantages	Disadvantages
Unfolding case studies	Learners follow a patient through a series of events and, using the data provided, make decisions related to the patient's care; usually integrated into individual lessons	■ Develops critical thinking and clinical decision-making ■ Assists in making connections between theory and practice through the use of realistic clinical cases ■ Effective with teams and group work ■ Can be used with interdisciplinary groups ■ Increases learner responsibility for learning ■ Promotes collaborative learning (Chan et al., 2016)	■ Extensive time commitment needed for faculty to develop realistic, challenging cases ■ Difficult to use in larger classes (Chan et al., 2016)
Vignettes	Hypothetical situation that simulates real-life experiences; often presented in short video clips	■ Used to explore attitudes, beliefs, and perceptions ■ Effective for cognitive, affective, and psychomotor learning ■ Demonstrates the nurse-patient relationship ■ Facilitates discussion and problem-solving ■ Improves knowledge retention and comprehension ■ Facilitates the transfer of theory to practice ■ May be viewed multiple times if available online or through an LMS (Wirihana et al., 2017)	■ Learners may be reluctant to share personal feelings ■ Cannot entirely replicate real-life ■ Accessibility may be a challenge for some students who lack broadband connection ■ Requires compatible computer hardware/ software for use outside the classroom ■ IT support may be insufficient for integration (Wirihana et al., 2017)

(*continued*)

Table 2.2 Active Learning Strategies (*continued*)

Strategy	Description	Advantages	Disadvantages
Virtual reality/ worlds/clinical experiences	Computer-based, three-dimensional technology that creates virtual clinical environments or practicums, for example, Second Life	▪ Provides distance/online clinical experiences ▪ Can also be used as classrooms and meeting spaces ▪ Learners gain practice skills, demonstrate professional behaviors, and learn teamwork and collaboration ▪ Useful when clinical sites are limited as in rural areas or with virtual learning during community crises (e.g., pandemics) ▪ Facilitates improved personal reflection ▪ Fosters development of communication and decision-making skills (Mitchell, 2020) ▪ Learners can gain experience with culturally diverse patients (DeYoung, 2015)	▪ Expensive ▪ Faculty and learners need to be oriented to use (O'Connor, 2019)
Warm-up/start-up exercises	Activities used to check reading assignments at the beginning of class; may count toward grade	▪ Encourages learners to read before class	▪ Takes class time
Webinars	Internet-based web conference that attendees join via telephone or computer	▪ Effective for distance teaching or meetings ▪ Allows discussion and interaction (Sopczyk, 2019)	▪ Requires technological expertise ▪ Background noise can become a problem (Sopczyk, 2019)
Writing/research paper	The act of conveying ideas or knowledge through the written word in the form of scholarly papers, journals, etc	▪ Promotes critical thinking ▪ Students learn to organize their ideas ▪ Enhances communication skills (Rowles, 2012)	▪ Grading can be subjective ▪ Time-consuming for both learners and faculty ▪ Does not lend itself well to use in large classes

(*continued*)

Table 2.2 Active Learning Strategies (*continued*)

Strategy	Description	Advantages	Disadvantages
YouTube/DVDs	Films or video clips used to enhance content	▪ Appeals to millennials ▪ Faculty can create their own YouTube channels to share video clips at no cost ▪ Discussions can enhance learning and encourage critical thinking ▪ Effective for demonstration of psychomotor skills ▪ Deepens understanding through visualization ▪ Usually inexpensive (Mustafa et al., 2020)	▪ May be time-consuming for faculty to locate relevant videos ▪ Faculty must review all required videos for accuracy and appropriateness for all learners ▪ No quality control or regulations exist ▪ Longer films or clips may take up a significant amount of class time (Mustafa et al., 2020) ▪ Passive unless the educator is involved (DeYoung, 2015)

● FLIPPED CLASSROOMS

The flipped or inverted classroom has generated much interest in recent years because it is a learner-centered approach with the potential to keep learners actively engaged in the learning process. In flipping the classroom, learners are required to review content and complete prework before coming to class. In the classroom, active learning strategies are used to assist learners in developing higher-order thinking and problem-solving skills (Betihavas et al., 2016).

Although many nurse educators continue to use the traditional lecture as the primary mode of transmission of information, it is well recognized that for learners to retain and apply the information, they must be actively engaged in their learning. Nursing students, in particular, must learn how to think critically, solve problems, and apply theory to practice. The recognition of the importance of student-centered learning has led to the increased use of active learning strategies, including flipped classrooms (Betihavas et al., 2016).

● TEACHING GEM Team-based learning and unfolding case studies are two strategies that lend themselves well to use in the flipped classroom. Learners are divided into small groups (four to six) to work through unfolding case studies. After the group has had time to work together, the full class can come back together to further discuss the case. This enhances team building and clinical decision-making.

Most research into the effectiveness of flipped classrooms has been done in the disciplines of pharmacology and medicine. In a systematic review by Betihavas and colleagues (2016), five studies of flipped classrooms used in nursing education showed evidence of mixed results on academic performance and student satisfaction. Several challenges in implementing flipped classrooms were identified.

▶ STUDENT CHALLENGES

- Difficulty in adjusting
- Unable to see the value
- Increased preparation time
- Dissatisfaction with group work (Betihavas et al., 2016)

▶ FACULTY CHALLENGES

- Inexperience
- Increased preparation time (Betihavas et al., 2016)

Despite a limited number of studies in using flipped classrooms in nursing education, most studies in the health disciplines support the use of this learner-centered approach to prepare learners for practice. Although learners may be less satisfied with this approach, likely related to increased workload, several studies have reported improved academic performance. Flipped classrooms increase the opportunity for students to learn higher-level thinking, which can facilitate their transition to practice (Betihavas et al., 2016).

 ## VIRTUAL LEARNING

Virtual learning is a learning approach that incorporates information technology to support teaching and learning off-site (Leigh et al., 2020). Following the onset of the COVID-19 pandemic in the spring of 2020, schools were suddenly thrust into a position of moving from face-to-face learning to virtual. In a short period of time, nursing faculty were moving lectures online and figuring out ways to continue clinical learning, as practice sites closed their doors to students. Although many faculty utilized teaching strategies and learning activities that have been in the literature for years, for many, it was the first time enacting them in their courses. Faculty around the world were challenged to change their practices in a short period of time, all while ensuring that learners met their student learning outcomes and were well prepared for practice in a stressed healthcare system and an ever-changing world. Fortunately, many learning activities could continue with slight adaptations to the online world.

ONLINE EDUCATION

Online education has been viewed in the past as a non-traditional, self-directed method of instruction. Learners are required to be motivated, autonomous, and ready to learn in order to achieve success in this environment (Decelle, 2016). Educators are required to have knowledge in content, pedagogy, and technology. Although it is expected that educators will be experts in their area of instruction and have a working knowledge of pedagogy, skill and comfort level with technology is most variable. Technology must be appropriately incorporated so that teaching strategies are student-centered, collaborative, and engaging (Calloway-Graham, 2016).

Multiple digital platforms exist for use with online learning. Most learning management systems (LMSs) have some online classroom component (e.g., Blackboard Collaborate). These online classrooms can be used for synchronous classes, meetings, tutoring, or office hours. Zoom is another platform that gained popularity in 2020 for use with classes, teleconferences, and meetings. Microsoft Teams is yet another platform available for use (Leigh et al., 2020). Although some of these platforms have free subscriptions, many require an upgraded subscription for a larger number of users or extended time.

▶ ASYNCHRONOUS VS. SYNCHRONOUS TECHNOLOGY

In using online platforms for learning, faculty can choose to use either synchronous or asynchronous. There are advantages and disadvantages to both. Most faculty choose to use what is most familiar and comfortable to them, especially when time is of the essence. The challenge is to engage learners in problem-solving and collaboration (Decelle, 2016).

▶ ASYNCHRONOUS ADVANTAGES

- More time for learners to prepare responses to discussions
- Learners do not interrupt each other when responding
- Learners can access course documents and other resources before responding (Decelle, 2016)

▶ ASYNCHRONOUS DISADVANTAGES

- Lacks direct contact and communication
- Places some limits on discussions (Decelle, 2016)

▶ SYNCHRONOUS ADVANTAGES

- Increases communication
- Faculty and students may be able to assist each other in troubleshooting technical issues (Decelle, 2016)

▶ SYNCHRONOUS DISADVANTAGES

- Technological issues may occur with "live" discussions
- Less convenient since students will need to be online at a specified time
- Faculty and students may talk over each other

There are seven principles of good practice that should be considered when integrating online learning into coursework. These principles are applicable when using both asynchronous and synchronous technology. Utilizing these guidelines is important in achieving teaching effectiveness that will benefit the learner in the online environment.

- Contact between faculty and students is extremely important
- Mutual exchange should be developed among learners
- Active learning strategies should still be encouraged in the online setting
- Feedback should be timely, whether for assignments, or in response to questions
- Time on task is important for providing quality instruction
- Expectations should remain high
- Respect student diversity and ways of learning (Chickering & Ehrmann, 1996, as cited in Calloway-Graham et al., 2016, p. 289)

In addition to the principles identified above, educators must also consider the geographical area in which students are located. Many rural areas continue to have limited access to internet and wifi. Connectivity for online exams and extended synchronous class times should be considered. The key to online education, at least during a pandemic when faculty and students alike are forced into virtual learning, is patience, understanding, and flexibility.

EVIDENCE-BASED TEACHING PRACTICE

Sedden and Clark (2016) reviewed 40 peer-reviewed, scholarly journal articles published between 2006 and 2015 to examine students' perspectives on motivation in the classroom. Researchers found students respond best to instructors who are themselves motivated. The student-instructor relationship and the instructor's teaching and social ability were identified as being important. Instructors who were open-minded, knowledgeable, and enthusiastic were better received. Students reported feeling more motivated in an organized, positive setting where they were free to ask questions and share their views.

 ## ONLINE CLINICAL

Alternatives to face-to-face clinicals became a challenge with the pandemic of 2020. Many schools turned to the use of virtual simulation. Some programs develop their own virtual simulations by recording scenarios in their simulation labs, while other programs purchase commercial products (e.g., Second Life, vSim, or Shadow Health). Commercial products contain pre-built cases and activities that can be used in a variety of courses. Studies have demonstrated that simulation is effective for the acquisition of knowledge, psychomotor skills, self-efficacy, satisfaction, confidence, and critical thinking skills. In a landmark study conducted by the National Council of State Boards of Nursing (NCSBN), it was found that students who had up to 50% of their clinical hours replaced with simulation had no difference in NCLEX pass rates or end of program outcomes when compared to the control group who had 10% or less simulation hours (Aebersold, 2018). Although many studies have been done on the effectiveness of simulation, there is limited evidence to date on the effectiveness of virtual simulation.

Teaching strategies and learning activities continue to grow and evolve. Although there will likely always be a place for lecture in nursing education, educators are increasingly motivated to include active learning strategies to engage students in their learning. If the pandemic of 2020 can be said to have one positive, it may be that educators were forced out of their comfort zone to explore and incorporate strategies they might never have otherwise considered. Faculty across the world have responded by changing and adapting to provide their students with the best education possible under difficult circumstances.

 CASE STUDIES

CASE STUDY 2.1

A new nurse educator was hired to teach in the undergraduate Bachelor of Science in Nursing (BSN) program. The primary course that the nurse educator is teaching this semester is Health Assessment. After the first exam, the nurse educator's mentor finds the new educator upset and discouraged. The new nurse educator shares that the students did poorly on their first exam, and they are complaining that they do not know what to study. The new nurse educator says that they have spent countless hours creating new PowerPoints that include extensive pictures, embedded videos, and animations.

As the mentor, what suggestions can you provide to focus the instruction and PowerPoint on key concepts needed for learning?

CASE STUDY 2.2

instructor new nurse educator in the undergraduate, BSN program assigned to teach the pediatrics course. The new nurse educator has attended multiple conferences and webinars to learn more about teaching and learning strategies. The new nurse educator is particularly excited about incorporating simulation into the new course. The new nurse educator shares that they plan to extensively use simulation in the laboratory as well as virtual simulation since clinical sites are very difficult to find in the specialty.

As the nurse educator mentor, what advice would you provide about incorporating simulation? What does the evidence show?

1. A nurse educator is interested in using a learning strategy that is effective for affective learning and will allow learners to self-reflect on the experience. A colleague suggests that she considers incorporating:

    A. Storytelling
    B. Case studies
    C. Games
    D. YouTube videos

2. Nursing faculty are planning a two-day orientation for new students admitted to the nursing program. Since the majority of the students are Millennials, faculty are looking for an activity that is engaging and an effective learning tool for this group of students. In discussing ideas, faculty decide that the least effective choice would be to have students:

    A. Work in teams using a Jeopardy-style game
    B. Participate in a short simulation using the high-fidelity manikin
    C. Complete an electronic self-learning module
    D. Work as a group to develop a poster

3. A novice nurse educator is preparing PowerPoint slides to be used with her lectures in a Health Assessment course. What statement by the novice educator should the mentor question?

    A. "I am going to use a medium blue background with black print for contrast"
    B. "My font size is 30, and I checked to see that it was readable from the back of the room"
    C. "I am going to embed some polls to keep the students engaged"
    D. "I am trying to use multiple graphics on each slide rather than words"

4. One of the outcomes in a Fundamentals of Nursing course is for new nursing students to develop and improve their communication skills. The best way to learn these skills is by having students:

    A. Watch vignettes of nurses communicating with patients
    B. Participate in a simulation/debriefing with a standardized patient
    C. Role model professional communication in the classroom setting
    D. Journal about situations observed in the laboratory/clinical setting

1. A) Storytelling

Storytelling provides an opportunity for faculty to role model good practice and behaviors. Learners are able to reflect and later recall their learning through sensory association. Case studies are more effective for cognitive learning and the development of critical thinking. Games are effective for the kinesthetic/tactile learner. YouTube videos are effective for teaching psychomotor skills.

2. C) Complete an electronic self-learning module

Most millennials are comfortable working in teams; they enjoy the interaction and communication. A self-learning module would be a less engaging activity, whereas the game, simulation, and group poster would all serve to promote team learning.

3. D) "I am trying to use multiple graphics on each slide rather than words"

Graphics are effective but should generally be limited to only one per slide. Extensive use of graphics makes it more difficult for identification of key points. A blue or green background with a contrasting font color and a size of 30 or greater is most effective. Embedded polls, videos, etc., keep the learner engaged, but care should be taken to not overuse.

4. B) Participate in a simulation/debriefing with a standardized patient

Practicing with standardized patients is an effective way of improving communication and learner confidence. Vignettes, role modeling, and journaling all allow the learner to observe behaviors and communication skills, but they do not provide an opportunity for practice. Only the simulation experience provides the educator with the opportunity to evaluate the learning that has occurred and provide additional opportunities for ongoing improvement.

5. A nursing faculty member is discussing with her mentor ways in which to engage students following the sudden change from face-to-face to online learning. Which method of teaching and learning would best meet her objective of student engagement?

    A. Develop a voice-over PowerPoint that students can view on their own time
    B. Post modules and PowerPoints for students to review asynchronously
    C. Require reading assignments followed by synchronous Zoom sessions for questions
    D. Develop PowerPoints with polling and discussion questions for synchronous use

6. A nurse educator is teaching a clinical decision-making course at the end of the nursing curriculum. In order to determine gaps in learner knowledge in preparing for the class, what method would be most useful to the educator in identifying areas in which students need more practice?

    A. Just-in-time teaching
    B. Start-up exercises
    C. Top 10 list
    D. Group discussion

7. A nurse educator is discussing the advantages of adding a portfolio assignment to the nursing curriculum. A colleague would question which of the following statements?

    A. "Portfolios provide an opportunity for students to self-reflect on their work"
    B. "Learners are able to document the progress that they have made in their knowledge development"
    C. "Portfolios require students to be self-directed so that little guidance is required"
    D. "Electronic portfolios may require a subscription for continued access"

8. A novice nurse educator is telling their mentor about a new virtual simulation product that they would like to incorporate in their course as a replacement for clinical hours. What statement would indicate that the educator has a clear understanding of simulation?

    A. "Scenarios for simulation can be written in a short period of time and used repeatedly"
    B. "Virtual simulation can be used to replace up to 50% of clinical hours"
    C. "The clinical educators can be quickly taught to debrief the simulations"
    D. "The virtual simulations can be assigned and require little time from faculty"

(See answers next page.)

5. D) Develop PowerPoints with polling and discussion questions for synchronous use

Lecture with PowerPoints that incorporate activities that engage the student are most effective for learning. Polling and discussions are designed to involve the students. Voice-over PowerPoints, modules, and reading assignments require students to be self-directed, but they are less effective at engaging them.

6. B) Start-up exercises

Using just-in-time teaching, students complete exercises prior to class that the educator then uses to tailor the classroom instruction to meet learner needs. Start-up exercises also provide insight into knowledge gaps, but because they are done at the beginning of class, information cannot be used until subsequent classes. The top 10 list and group discussions allow learners to self-identify their needs but are ineffective if students are unable to identify their areas of weakness.

7. C) "Portfolios require students to be self-directed so that little guidance is required"

Portfolios require students to be more independent in their work, but guidance is still required to avoid overly large documents and inclusion of items that have little benefit in showcasing the learner's knowledge development. Portfolios are effective in facilitating self-reflection and documentation of educational progress. In selecting a platform for an ePortfolio, care must be taken to determine cost and accessibility after graduation.

8. B) "Virtual simulation can be used to replace up to 50% of clinical hours"

Prior research has found that up to 50% of clinical time can be replaced with simulation with no effect on NCLEX-RN pass rates or student learning outcomes. To date, there is limited research on the effect of virtual simulation in the replacement of clinical hours. Simulation scenarios take skill and time in writing them. Debriefing is extremely important to the learning that occurs with simulation; those who are debriefing should receive thorough training. Learners also require debriefing and feedback following virtual simulations.

9. A seasoned faculty member overhears some adjunct faculty discussing online teaching. Which statement would indicate that they have a clear understanding of good practice in online learning?

   A. "Expectations in an online course are always lower than face-to-face"

   B. "All online learners are the same and should be treated as such"

   C. "It is so important that faculty maintain contact with their students in this setting"

   D. "Less active learning strategies are needed online because students must be self-directed"

10. A new faculty member completed a continuing education module on service learning, and she would now like to incorporate this into her course. What statement indicates that she may need some clarification about service learning?

   A. "Service learning provides a wonderful opportunity for students to learn about health disparities"

   B. "Successful service learning opportunities take an extensive amount of planning and organization"

   C. "It is important to match service learning sites to student learning outcomes"

   D. "If students are required to identify their own locations, faculty workload is lessened"

(See answers next page.)

9. C) "It is so important that faculty maintain contact with their students in this setting"

Since online learning typically lacks face-to-face contact on a regular basis, it is important that contact be maintained so that students feel supported in their learning. Contact may be in the form of announcements, emails, synchronous class dates, or virtual office hours. Students will have variable levels of comfort with technology, so some students may require more support than others. High expectations and strategies that engage the student are as important in online learning as face-to-face.

10. D) "If students are required to identify their own locations, faculty workload is lessened"

Service learning is not the same as volunteering. Care must be taken to identify sites in which learning can occur and outcomes achieved. Nurse educators must be fully involved in identifying sites and planning learning activities for a successful service-learning experience. Students have the opportunity to develop a greater knowledge of cultural competency and determinants of health.

REFERENCES

Aebersold, M. (2018). Simulation-based learning: No longer a novelty in undergraduate education. *Online Journal of Issues in Nursing*, 23(2), 1–17. 10.3912/OJIN.Vol23No02PPT39

Aljezawi, M., & Albashtawy, M. (2015). Quiz game teaching format versus didactic lectures. *British Journal of Nursing*, 24(2), 86–92. 10.12968/bjon.2015.24.2.86

Alves, R. M., Alves, J. B., de Menezes, M. H. D., & Moraes, A. (2017). Strategies for teaching learning in the hospital nursing school of an integrated curriculum. *Journal of Nursing UFPE On Line*, 11(11), 4289–4297. 10.5205/reuol.23542-49901-1-ED.1111201703

Anton, N. E., Bean, E. A., Hammonds, S. C., & Stefanidis, D. (2017). Application of mental skills training in surgery: A review of its effectiveness and proposed next step. *Journal of Laparoendoscopic & Advanced Surgical Techniques*, 27(5), 459–469. 10.1089/lap.2016.0656

Astroth, K. S., & Hain, D. (2019). Disseminating scholarly work through nursing presentations. *Nephrology Nursing Journal*, 46(5), 545–549.

Azadbakht, E. (2019). Humor in library instruction: A narrative review with implications for the health sciences. *Journal of the Medical Library Association*, 107(3), 304–313. dx.doi.org/10.5195/jmla.2019.608

Battersby, L. (2017). Education strategies that best engage Generation Y students. *The Canadian Journal of Dental Hygiene*, 51(3), 118–125.

Beitz, J., & Snarponis, J. (2006). Strategies for online teaching and learning. *Nurse Educator*, 31(1), 20–24.

Betihavas, V., Bridgman, H., Kornhaber, R., & Cross, M. (2016). The evidence for flipping out: A systematic review of the flipped classroom in nursing education. *Nurse Education Today*, 38, 15–21.

Bhandari, B., Mehta, B., Mavai, M., Singh, Y. R., & Singhal, A. (2017). Jigsaw method: An innovative way of cooperative learning in physiology. *Indian Journal of Physiology and Pharmacology*, 61(3), 315–321.

Bryant-Moore, K., Bachelder, A., Rainey, L., Hayman, K., Bessette, A., & Williams, C. (2018). *Journal of Transcultural Nursing*, 29(5), 473–479. 10.1177/1043659617753043

Calloway-Graham, D., Sorenson, C. J., Roark, J., & Lucero, J. (2016). Technology-enhanced practice courses and collaborative learning in distance education. *Journal of Technology in Human Services*, 34(3), 285–299. http://dx.doi.org/10.1080/15228835.2016.1219898

Carifa, L., & Goodin, H. J. (2011). Using games to provide interactive perioperative education. *AORN Journal*, 94(4), 370–376. doi:10.1016/j.aorn.2011.01.018

Chan, A. W. K., Chair, S. Y., Sit, J. W. H., Wong, E. M. L., Lee, D. T. F., & Fung, O. W. M. (2016). Case-based web learning versus face-to-face learning: A mixed-method study on university nursing students. *The Journal of Nursing Research*, 24(1), 31–39. 10.1097/jnr.0000000000000.104

Clark, K. R. (2016). Just-in-time teaching. *Radiologic Technology*, 87(4), 465–467.

Clark, K. R., & Spence, B. (2016). Using concepts maps in radiologic science education. *Radiologic Technology*, 88(1), 107–110.

Collins, E., & Crawley, J. (2016). Introducing ePortfolios into nursing schools. *Kai Tiaki Nursing New Zealand*, 22(5), 34–35.

Connors, H. B., & Tally, K. (2015). Integrating technology in education. In M. H. Oermann (Ed.), *Teaching in nursing and role of the educator* (pp. 61–81). New York, NY: Springer Publishing.

Curtis, K., Wiseman, T., Kennedy, B., Kourouche, S., & Goldsmith, H. (2016). Implementation and evaluation of a ward-based elearning program for trauma patient management. *Journal of Trauma Nursing*, 23(1), 28–35. 10.1097/JTN.0000000000000177

Day-Black, C., Merrill, E. B., Konzelman, L., Williams, T. T., & Hart, N. (2015). Gamification: An innovative teaching-learning strategy for the digital nursing students in a community health nursing course. *The Association of Black Nursing Faculty*, 26(4), 90–94.

Decelle, G. (2016). Andragogy: A fundamental principle of online education for nursing. *Journal of Best Practices in Health Professions Diversity*, 9(2), 1263–1273.

Della Ratta, C. B. (2015). Flipping the classroom with team-based learning in undergraduate nursing education. *Nurse Educator*, 40(2), 71–74.

DeYoung, S. (2015). *Teaching strategies for nurse educators* (3rd ed.). Pearson.

Dusaj, T. K. (2013). Pump up your PowerPoint® presentations. *American Nurse Today*, 8(7), 43–46.

Fatmi, M., Hartling, L., Hillier, T., Campbell, S., & Oswald, A. E. (2013). The effectiveness of team-based learning on learning outcomes in health professions education: BEME guide no. 30. *Medical Teacher*, 35, e1608–e1624. doi:10.3109/0142159X.2013.849802

Fitzgerald, D. (2013). Employing think-pair-share in associate degree nursing. *Teaching and Learning in Nursing*, 8(3), 88–90.

Fitzgerald, K., & Keyes, K. (2014–2019). Instructional Teaching methods and settings. In S. B. Bastable (Ed.), *Nurse as educator: Principles of teaching and learning for nursing practice* (4th 5th ed., pp. 469–515). Jones & Bartlett.

Friesth, B. M. (2012). Teaching and learning at a distance. In D. M. Billings & J. A. Halstead (Eds.), *Teaching in nursing: A guide for faculty (pp. 386–400)*. St. Louis, MO: Elsevier Saunders.

Furnes, M., Kvaal, K. S., & Hoye, S. (2018). Communication in mental health nursing – Bachelor students' appraisal of a blended learning training programme – An exploratory study. *BioMed Central Nursing*, 17(20), 1–10. https://doi.org/10.1186/s12912-018-0288-9

Gerdes, M. (2018). Teaching-learning strategy for promoting student success: Asynchronous post-exam reflections. *Nursing Science Quarterly*, 31(4), 335–339. 10.1177/0894318418792876

Grech, V. (2018). The application of the Mayer multimedia learning theory to medical PowerPoint slide show presentations. *Journal of Visual Communication in Medicine*, 41(1), 36–41. https://doi.org/10.1080/17453054.2017.1408400

Greenberger, H. B., & Dispensa, M. (2015). Usage and perceived value of video podcasts by professional physical therapist students in learning orthopedic special tests. *Journal of Physical Therapy Education*, 29(3), 46–57.

Grover, S., Sood, N., & Chaudhary, A. (2018). Student perception of peer teaching and learning in pathology: A qualitative analysis of modified seminars, fishbowls, and interactive classroom activities. *Indian Journal of Pathology and Microbiology*, 61(4), 537–544. https://www.ijpmonline.org/text.asp?2018/61/4/537/242971

Hagler, D., & Morris, B. (2015). Teaching methods. In M. H. Oermann (Ed.), *Teaching in nursing and role of the educator* (pp. 35–59). Springer Publishing.

Hainsworth, D., & Keyes, K. (2014). Instructional materials. In S. B. Bastable (Ed.), *Nurse as educator: Principles of teaching and learning for nursing practice* (4th ed., pp. 518–558). Burlington, MA: Jones & Bartlett.

Halstead, J. A., & Billings, D. M. (2012). Teaching and learning in online learning communities. In D. M. Billings & J. A. Halstead (Eds.), *Teaching in nursing: A guide for faculty* (pp. 401–421). St. Louis, MO: Elsevier Saunders.

Hardie, P., Darley, A., Carroll, L., Redmond, C., Campbell, A., & Jarvis, S. (2020). Nursing & midwifery students' experience of immersive virtual reality storytelling: An evaluative study. *BioMed Central Nursing*, 19(78), 1–12. https://doi.org/10.1186/s12912-020-00471-5

Hayne, A. N., & McDaniel, G. S. (2013). Presentation rubric: Improving faculty professional presentations. *Nursing Forum*, 48(4), 289–294.

Innes, G., & Main, M. (2013). Improving learning with personal response systems. *Nursing Times*, 109(13), 20–22.

Ironside, P. M. (2015). Narrative pedagogy: Transforming nursing education through 15 years of research in nursing education. *Nursing Education Perspectives*, 36(2), 83–88. 10.5480/13-1102

Jefferies, P. R., & Clochesy, J. M. (2012). Clinical simulations: An experiential, student-centered pedagogical approach. In D. M. Billings & J. A. Halstead (Eds.), *Teaching in nursing: A guide for faculty* (pp. 352–368). St. Louis, MO: Elsevier Saunders.

Jefferies, P. R., Dreifuerst, K. T., Aschenbrenner, D. S., Adamson, K. A., & Schram, A. P. (2015). Clinical simulations in nursing education: Overview, essentials, and the evidence. In M. H. Oermann (Ed.), *Teaching in nursing and role of the educator* (pp. 83–101). New York, NY: Springer Publishing.

Johnson, H. A., & Barrett, L. C. (2017). Your teaching strategy matters: How engagement impacts application in health information literacy instruction. *Journal of the Medical Library Association*, 105(1), 44–48. dx.doi.org/10.5195/jmla.2017.8

Karacay, P., & Kaya H. (2020). Effects of a simulation education program on faculty members' and students' learning outcomes. *International Journal of Caring Sciences*, 13(1), 555–562. 10.7748/ns.25.49.35

Lee, J. H., Ju, H. O., & Lee, Y. J. (2019). Effects of an algorithm-based education program on nursing care for children with epilepsy by hospital nurses. *Child Health Nursing Research*, 25(3), 324–332. https://doi.org/10.4094/chnr.2019.25.3.324

Leigh, J., Vasilica, C., Dron, R., Gawthorpe, D., Burns, E., Kennedy, S., Kennedy, R., Warburton, T., & Croughan, C. (2020). Redefining undergraduate nurse teaching during the coronavirus pandemic: Use of digital technologies. *British Journal of Nursing*, 28(10), 566–569. 10.12968/bjon.2020.29.10.566

Lim, F. A. (2012). Wake up to better PowerPoint presentations. *Nursing*, 42(2), 46–48.

Luchetti, A. L. G., Ezequiel, O., de Oliveira, I. N., Moreira-Almeida, A., & Luchetti, G. (2018). Using traditional or flipped classrooms to teach "geriatrics and gerontology"? Investigating the impact of active learning on medical students' competences. *Medical Teacher*, 40(12), 1248–1256. 10.1080/0142159X.2018.1426837

Mahon, P., Lyng, C., Crotty, Y., & Farren, M. (2018). Transforming classroom questioning using emerging technology. *British Journal of Nursing*, 27(7), 389–394. 10.12968/bjon.2018.27.7.389

Mahon, P., & O'Neill, M. (2020). Through the looking glass: The rabbit hole of reflective practice. *British Journal of Nursing*, 29(13), 777–783. 10.12968/bjon.2020.29.13.777

Mareno, N., Bremner, M., & Emerson, C. (2010). The use of audience response systems in nursing education: Best practices guidelines. *International Journal of Nursing Education Scholarship*, 7(1), 1–17. doi:10.2202/1548-923X.2049

Mesquita, I., Coutinho, P., De Martin-Silva, L., Parente, B., Faria, M., & Afonso, J. (2015). The value of indirect teaching strategies in enhancing student-coaches learning engagement. *Journal of Sports Science and Medicine*, 14, 657–668.

Mitchell, A. (2020). Pandemic inspires innovative use of virtual simulation to teach practical skills. *British Journal of Nursing*, 29(20), 1214.

Morris, C. (2015). Writing a wound care case study. *Wounds UK*, 11(1), 61–64.

Moyer, B. A., & Wittmann-Price, R. A. (2008). *Nursing education: Foundations for practice excellence*. Philadelphia, PA: F. A. Davis.

Mrunalini, V. S., & Chandekar, P. A. (2015). Perception and opinion of problem based learning (PBL) among student nurses. *International Journal of Nursing Education*, 7(3), 1–7. 10.5958/0974-9357.2015.00131.2

Mustafa, A. G., Taha, N. R., Alshboul, O. A., Alsalem, M., & Malki, M. I. (2020). Using YouTube to learn anatomy: Perspectives of Jordanian medical students. *BioMed Research International*, 2020(5), 1–8. https://doi.org/10.1155/2020/6861416

Naicker, K., & van Rensburg, G. H. (2018). Facilitation of reflective learning in nursing: Reflective teaching practices of educators. *Africa Journal of Nursing and Midwifery*, 20(2), 1–15. https://doi.org/10.25159/2520-5293/3386

Nowak, M. K., Speakman, E., & Sayers, P. (2016). Evaluating PowerPoint presentations: A retrospective study examining barriers and strategies. *Nursing Education Perspectives*, 37(1), 28–31. 10.5480/14-1418

O'Connor, S. (2019). Virtual reality and avatars in health care. *Clinical Nursing Research*, 28(5), 523–528. 10.1177/1054773819845824

Oermann, M. H., & Gaberson, K. B. (2014–2019). *Evaluation and testing in nursing education* (6th ed.). New York, NY: Springer Publishing.

Passi, V., & Johnson, N. (2016). The impact of positive doctor role modeling. *Medical Teacher*, 38(11), 1139–1145. http://dx.doi.org/10.3109/0142159X.2016.1170780

Peacock, J. G., & Grande, J. P. (2016). An online app platform enhances collaboration medical student group learning and classroom management. *Medical Teacher*, 38(2), 174–180. https://doi.org/10.3109/0142159X.2015.1020290

Phillips, J., & Fusco, J. (2015). Using the jigsaw technique to teach clinical controversy in a clinical skills course. *American Journal of Pharmaceutical Education*, 79(6), 1–7. https://doi.org/10.5688/ajpe79690

Preheim, G., & Foss, K. (2015). Partnerships with clinical settings: Roles and responsibilities of nurse educators. In M. H. Oermann (Ed.), *Teaching in nursing and role of the educator* (pp. 163–190). New York, NY: Springer Publishing.

Rae, M. G., & O'Malley, D. (2017). Do prerecorded lecture VODcasts affect lecture attendance of first-year pre-clinical graduate entry to medicine students? *Medical Teacher*, 39(3), 250–254. http://dx.doi.org/10.1080/0142159X.2017.1270436

Rao, B. J. (2019). Innovative teaching pedagogy in nursing education. *International Journal of Nursing Education*, 11(4), 176–180. 10.5958/0974-9357.2019.00114.4

Roh, Y. S., Lee, S. J., & Choi, D. (2015). Learner perception, expected competence, and satisfaction of team-based learning in Korean nursing students. *Nursing Education Perspectives*, 36(2), 118–120. 10.5480/13-1200

Rowles, C. J. (2012). Strategies to promote critical thinking and active learning. In D. M. Billings & J. A. Halstead (Eds.), *Teaching in nursing: A guide for faculty* (pp. 258–284). Elsevier Saunders.

Ryan, J. A. (2018). Which resources are most helpful to support development of an ePortfolio? *British Journal of Nursing*, 27(5), 266–271.

Santra, P., & Mani, S. (2017). Comparative assessment of problem-based learning and traditional teaching to acquire knowledge on ventilator associated pneumonia. *International Journal of Nursing Education*, 9(4), 101–106. 10.5958/0974-9357.2017.00104.0

Scheckel, M. (2012). Selecting learning experiences to achieve curriculum outcomes. In D. M. Billings & J. A. Halstead (Eds.), *Teaching in nursing: A guide for faculty* (pp. 170–187). St. Louis, MO: Elsevier Saunders.

Sedden, M. L., & Clark, K. R. (2016). Motivating students in the 21st century. *Radiologic Technology*, 87(6), 609–616.

Sharma, N., Lau, C. S., Doherty, I., & Harbutt, D. (2015). How we flipped the medical classroom. *Medical Teacher*, 37(4), 327–330. 10.3109/0142159X.2014.923821

Sopczyk, D. L. (2014–2019). Technology in education. In S. B. Bastable (Ed.), *Nurse as educator: Principles of teaching and learning for nursing practice* (4th 5th ed., pp. 559–600). Burlington, MA: Jones & Bartlett.

Steinhardt, S. J., Kelly, W. N., Clark, J. E., & Hill, A. M. (2020). An artistic active-learning approach to teaching a substance use disorder elective course. *American Journal of Pharmaceutical Education*, 84(4), 498–503. https://doi.org/10.5688/ajpe7634

Stokes, L. G., & Kost, G. C. (2012). Teaching in the clinical setting. In D. M. Billings & J. A. Halstead (Eds.), *Teaching in nursing: A guide for faculty* (pp. 311–334). St. Louis, MO: Elsevier.

Saunders Van Vuuren, V. J., Seekoe, E., & Goon, D. T. (2018). *The perceptions of nurse educators regarding the use of high fidelity simulation in nursing education*. Africa Journal of Nursing and Midwifery, 20(1), 1–20. https://doi.org/10.25159/2520-5293/1685

Vetter, M. J., & Latimer, B. (2017). Tactics for teaching evidence-based practice: Enhancing active learning strategies with a large class of graduate EBP research in nursing students. *Worldviews on Evidence-Based Nursing*, 14(5), 419–421. https://doi.org/10.1111/wvn.12227

Walker, R., Henderson, A., Cooke, M., & Creedy, D. (2010). Impact of a learning circle intervention across academic and service contexts on developing a learning culture. *Nurse Educator Today*, 31(4), 378–382. doi:10.1016/j.nedt.2010.07.010

Ward-Smith, P., Peterson, J., & Schmer, C. (2010). Students' perceptions of group projects. *Nurse Educator, 35*(2), 79–82. doi:10.1097/NNE.0b013e3181ced87e

Werry, J. (2016). Informal debriefing: Underutilization in critical care settings. *The Canadian Journal of Critical Care Nursing, 27*(4), 22–26.

Wirihana, L., Craft, J., Christensen, M., & Bakon, S. (2017). A nursing education perspective on the integration of video learning: A review of the literature. *Singapore Nursing Journal, 44*(1), 24–32.

Woodley, L. K. (2015). Clinical teaching in nursing. In M. H. Oermann (Ed.), *Teaching in nursing and role of the educator* (pp. 141–161). New York, NY: Springer Publishing.

Wright, J. M., Heathcote, K., & Wibberley, C. (2014). Fact or fiction: Exploring the use of real stories in place of vignettes in interviews with informal carers. *Nurse Researcher, 21*(4), 39–43.

Youngwanichsetha, S., Chatchawet, W., Kritcharoen, S., Kala, S., & Thitimapong, B. (2019). Field trip for case study: Action research to improve teaching and learning in midwifery course. *International Journal of Nursing Education, 11*(2), 83–86. 10.5958/0974-9357.2019.00046.1

Yuan, H. B., Williams, B. A., & Fang, J. B. (2011). The contribution of high-fidelity simulation to nursing students' confidence and competence: A systematic review. *International Nursing Review, 59*, 26–33.

Zipp, G. P., Maher, C., & D'Antoni, A. (2015). Mind mapping: Teaching and learning strategy for physical therapy curricula. *Journal of Physical Therapy Education, 29*(1), 43–48.

Zwirn, E. E., & Muehlenkord, A. (2012). Creating interactive learning environments using media and digital media. In D. M. Billings & J. A. Halstead (Eds.), *Teaching in nursing: A guide for faculty* (pp. 369–385). St. Louis, MO: Elsevier Saunders.

Educational Technology

3

Frances H. Cornelius and Linda Wilson

The great aim of education is not knowledge but action.
—Herbert Spencer (1820–1903)

▶ LEARNING OUTCOMES

This chapter also addresses the Certified Nurse Educator Exam and the Certified Nurse Educator Novice exam Content Area 1: Facilitate Learning

- Analyze the nurse educator's role with respect to the use of educational technology to support learning
- Examine the importance of the appropriate integration of technology in a meaningful and relevant manner to support learning
- Describe how to devise strategies to integrate technology in a learning activity

● INTRODUCTION

Different types of digital courseware or technology tools are available to educators. The goal is to maximize learning and not simply to use the latest cool tool. Learning should be action-oriented, promoting active learning and engagement with the content, faculty, and other learners. Technology should be relevant and interactive to the coursework at hand, that is, supporting learning. So, when selecting teaching technology, it is important to start at the end. What do you want the outcome to be? What do you want the learners to understand/master? Then select the tool that will help you get there.

As technology progresses, academic nurse educators must keep up with technological advancement. Although this may be challenging at times, as an academic nurse educator, it is important to be open-minded, eager to learn, and willing to look outside of nursing for innovative ideas to enhance the quality of nursing education. Professional and special-interest organizations offer opportunities to stay current and to network. Some organizations include:

- Educause (www.educause.edu)—this nonprofit association's mission is to advance higher education by promoting the intelligent use of information technology.
- National Education Association (NEA; www2.nea.org/he/techno.html)—this organization was founded in 1857 with the goal to "both elevate the character and advance the interests of teaching, promoting the cause of education in the United States" (NEA, 2020, p. 1). The NEA higher education website offers a forum to discuss the role of technology in education as well as an opportunity to learn about new trends.

- Online Learning Consortium (OLC, onlinelearningconsortium.org)—OLC is a collaborative community of higher education leaders and innovators, dedicated to advancing quality digital teaching and learning experiences designed to reach and engage the modern learner—anyone, anywhere, anytime.
- Society for Applied Learning Technologies (SALT; www.salt.org)—SALT is a society oriented toward professionals whose work requires knowledge and communication in the field of instructional technology.
- United States Distance Learning Association (USDLA; https://usdla.org) is a nonprofit distance learning association focused upon supporting distance learning research, development, and practice across the complete arena of education, training, and communications.

Additional resources include Innovate (www.innovateonline.info) or EmergingEdTech (www.emergingedtech.com), which provide the faculty an opportunity to stay current with new technologies and innovations.

TECHNOLOGY IN THE LEARNING ENVIRONMENT

The learning environment has morphed into an arena where learners are no longer passive recipients of information. Learning has become an interactive and social experience, resulting in richer, more meaningful experiences for learners and faculty alike (Educause, 2019). Whether in the traditional face-to-face classroom, the clinical setting, or a virtual/hybrid environment, new technologies, Web 2.0 tools and Web 3.0 functionality provide many opportunities to enhance learning far beyond the traditional "ivory towers." As renowned educational thought leader Sealy Brown predicted:

> One would also expect a form of spiral learning to evolve, initially rooted in one community but then branching out to encompass expanding interests and skills. The spiral would weave a tapestry between activities in the niche communities of interest and the core curriculum, with both serving to ground and complement the other. This new learning scape would be supported by an understanding of the interplay between the social and cognitive basis of learning, and enabled by the networked age of the 21st century. Such an educational experience would undoubtedly build a strong foundation for life-long learning in a world of accelerating change (2006, p. 29).

Technology enables the delivery of educational content to learners across a variety of settings, with the ability to accommodate diverse learning needs. This technology capabilities and flexibility can be leveraged to deliver teaching and assessment that is convenient, interactive, and engaging for learners (Button, Harrington, & Belan, 2014; O'Connor & Andrews, 2015; O'Connor, Hubner, Shaw, Blake, & Ball, 2017).

There are many opportunities to incorporate new technologies into learning. For example, as a result of emerging technologies, all courses can be "web-enhanced" and can support any curriculum no matter if it is traditional Face2Face, hybrid, or fully online. As the global COVID pandemic has highlighted, embedding teaching/learning technologies provide opportunities to be facile when radical curricular pivots are required. The Internet, video streaming, podcasting, and Web 2.0 tools can help to enhance any classroom activity, providing a mechanism for enhancing learning, student engagement, and continuing the discussion beyond the classroom. Some popular Web 2.0 tools include:

- Wikis—A wiki is a collection of web pages that may be edited by anyone.
- Blogs—Journal entries that are presented in reverse chronological order.
- Social networking—Websites that build relationships and connections/networks, strengthening learning communities.
- Twitter—A "microblog" that allows users to send short text messages, not exceeding 140 characters in length, to a personalized homepage.
- Podcasting or video podcasting—A method of distributing multimedia content (lectures, discussions, etc.) via the Internet for playback on mobile devices and personal computers. This can be accomplished using simple syndication (RSS) feeds that are freely available on the Internet.
- Social bookmarking or tagging—An online service that allows resources to be categorized using user-defined keywords or tags. Principally, social bookmarking allows users to assemble and annotate (tag) preferred web links/resources, to share with others. This creates a vast repository of shared resources, organized in a meaningful manner.
- Gaming—Often referred to as serious gaming, the use of games for educational purposes is growing exponentially. There are many free tools available that can be utilized, such as Baamboozle (www.baamboozle.com), Quizlet (quizlet.com), or Socrative (www.socrative.com). Gaming can provide opportunities for authentic learning and can generate a "tremendous amount of transactional data that can reveal insights not only about student success or failure but also about student teamwork and collaboration preferences, learning styles, and a variety of other learning issues" (Epper, Derryberry, & Jackson, 2012, p. 2).

While these technologies can provide considerable support in developing higher-level thinking among learners, the focus should not be on the technology because the "technology by itself does not yield the greatest impact on learning; it does so when it is embedded in a scaffolding of support for learners and instructors" (Educause, 2020, p. 13). The goal of educational technology is to improve engagement and learning, but it must be aligned with the curriculum in order to be effective (Zirawaga, Olusanya, & Maduku, 2017). For example, Twitter or FlipGrid (flipgrid.com could be used to continue the class discussion on a given topic beyond the classroom, but it must be linked with a specific student learning outcome.

TEACHING GEM   Blogging is a great method to use when a portion of learners are on service-learning trips; this will keep the learning community at home in touch with the travels and experiences of the others.

Metacognition—the practice of thinking about and reflecting on your learning—has been shown to benefit comprehension and retention. As a tool for students or professional colleagues to compare thoughts about a topic, Twitter can be a viable platform for metacognition, forcing users to be brief and to the point—an important skill in thinking clearly and communicating effectively (Educause Learning Initiative, 2016, p. 2).

Similarly, Flipgrid can require learners not only to be succinct but also to develop verbal communication skills. Tools such as ThingLink (www.thinglink.com) or Coggle (https://coggle.it/) can be used to help students make important connections between concepts and previously learned material, supporting metacognitive skill development (Astriani, Susilo, Suwono, Lukiati & Purnomo, 2020).

Another way to use technology to support metacognition is to change HOW the technology is used. For example, reframing PowerPoint presentations using the PechaKucha (www.pechakucha.com) approach supports student learning by requiring them to synthesize content into brief presentations consisting of 20 slides and 20 seconds of commentary per slide. Just as with Twitter, the Pechakucha approach would force students to be brief and to the point, guiding students in a learning process that embeds repetition and practice, provides students with an opportunity to practice time management and organization, and demonstrate their learning creatively (Hayashi & Holland, 2017; Ave, Beasley & Brogan, 2020).

◎ **Critical Thinking Question**

Can you use metacognition to decrease the number of words on each PowerPoint slide by 10%?

EVIDENCE-BASED TEACHING PRACTICE

Ricker and Richert (2021) studied metacognition in children 6 to 10 years old using 15 different digital games. The games were rated for interactivity, level-of-control, feedback, and adaptivity, and results demonstrated that exposure to games high in interactive features was positively associated with children's metacognitive awareness and exposure to games that were less interactive did not affect metacognitive awareness.

Recently, there has been considerable discussion regarding the next generation of the web—Web 3.0—and particularly what this next step in the evolution of the Internet will offer education. A variety of predictions regarding anticipated functionalities of Web 3.0 are available. Web 3.0 is described as the "intelligent web or semantic web with technologies like big data, linked data, cloud computing, 3D visualization, augmented reality and more" (p. 8), further scaffolding the transition from passive to active learning (Dominic, Francis, & Pilomenraj, 2014). Early in 2007, Google's chief executive officer, Eric Schmidt, predicted that Web 3.0 would transform things in a big way (Yun, 2007; Rudman & Bruwer, 2016). There has been significant transformation while the full potential has not yet been fully realized. Specifically, for educators, Web 3.0 functionality can now assist in the areas of course development, record keeping, learner support, and assessment through very robust learning analytics (Prinsloo & Slade, 2017; Rienties, Cross & Zdrahal, 2017). In addition, students will benefit from learning personalization and knowledge construction powered by the Semantic Web (Morris, 2011; Watson, Watson, & Reigeluth, 2015; Amith, Fujimoto, Mauldin, & Tao, 2020).

Web 3.0 will be characterized by the following:

- A series of combined applications that are very small will be "pieced" together and will run using data stored in the cloud.
- These applications will be very fast, will run on any device (mobile phone, computer, etc.), and will be highly customizable.
- Applications will be distributed "virally" from person to person via text, e-mail, and so on.

The core software technology in Web 3.0 is artificial intelligence (AI). Online test security has been significantly enhanced through AI, lightening the load for 'live' proctors. It is anticipated that AI proctoring will be secure and self-sufficient not long in the future (Ismail, Osmanaj & Jaradat, August 2019).

The tools and functionalities offered by Web 3.0 create a more flexible and open approach to teaching/learning and a more personalized learning experience (Singh & Lal, 2012; Watson, Watson & Reigeluth, 2015). This customization will permit users (educators and learners alike) to forge new linkages between components/features, transforming content to build new knowledge, further enriching the learning experience.

These tools include:

- Intelligent Search Engines and Intelligent Tutoring Systems—providing direct, highly personalized, and customized information searching, instruction, and/or feedback to learners.
- 3-D Wikis, 3-D Online Games, and 3-D Encyclopedias—providing increased interaction with content through 3-D representation of content and the capability for 360° camera rotation, allowing the user to examine content from multiple perspectives or vantage points.
- Semantic Digital Libraries, Semantic Blogs, and Semantic Forums and Community Portals—connecting content and making distinctions/connections among words, symbols, and concepts resulting in richer and deeper learning experiences.
- Virtual Worlds—providing "an interactive simulated environment accessed by multiple users through an online interface" and available in a "wide variety of forms, including 3-D re-creations of museum and gallery spaces, computer programming tutorials, virtual libraries, and meeting spaces for online university courses" (Creative Commons, n.d., pp. 1, 11).
- Microblogging—"Microblogging is the practice of posting small pieces of digital content—which could be text, pictures, links, short videos, or other media—on the Internet" (Educause Learning Initiative, 2016, p. 1).
- Virtual Laboratories/Education Laboratories—similar to the virtual worlds described earlier, virtual laboratories will provide a realistic 3-D laboratory experience for the learners.

▶ SHIFT FROM PASSIVE TO ACTIVE LEARNING

Student engagement is critical to learning and is "positively related to academic outcomes" and "has a compensatory effect on first-year grades and persistence to the second year of college at the same institution" (Kuh, Cruce, Shoup, Kinzie, & Gonyea, 2008, p. 555). Furthermore, students who have opportunities to engage in level-appropriate academic challenges, participate actively in collaborative learning, encounter enriching educational experiences, and have frequent interaction with faculty are more likely to be successful and persist (Canney, 2015; Robinson & Hullinger, 2008; Riggs & Linder, 2016). National Survey of Student Engagement reported that "when students are both challenged and provided the appropriate amount of support, they are motivated to reach their potential" and are "more likely to engage in a variety of effective educational practices," which include reflection, quantitative reasoning, collaborative learning, discussions with diverse others, and student–faculty interactions (National Survey of Student Engagement, 2015, p. 3). The good news is that generally there is consensus among educators that student engagement is essential; however, Kuh (2009) stresses that these efforts must be individualized, pointing out that some educators

> sometimes adopt a hegemonic, one-size-fits-all way of thinking. Student engagement is too important, as well as too complicated, for the educational community to allow this to happen. For example, as with other college experiences, engagement tends to have conditional effects, with students with certain characteristics benefiting from some types of activities more so than other students. (p. 15)

Active learning supports student engagement in that it involves all the senses. Integrating technologies that provide a "hands-on" learning experiences build learner confidence in their ability to apply what they have learned (Snow, 2019).

EVIDENCE-BASED TEACHING PRACTICE

Snow (2019) reports benefits of a 1.5-hour hands-on learning experience added to a masters-level graduate nursing program in which learners "applied various creative thinking tools to actual problems they were experiencing in practice. Results indicate participants perceived they can learn to be more creative, can role model methods to inspire creativity, and can use education to empower staff to use creative thinking techniques to solve problems in practice" (p. 309).

Strategies to engage students in active learning include opportunities for students to interact with content, instructors, and other learners. Teaching/learning technologies have expanded capabilities to support this interaction. For example, an audience-response system (ARS) can be used to engage the learner in the classroom and in online environments and has demonstrated positive impact on learning (Kay & LeSage, 2009; Hunsu, Adescope & Bayly, 2016; Hung, 2017). These can be actually distinct "stand-alone" devices distributed to the participants, or these can be set up to invite participants to respond to questions using a mobile phone or laptop connected to the Internet, an approach often referred to as "Bring Your Own Device" (BYOD).

- One method for incorporating this technology is to create some preclass questions that the learners can respond to using the clicker technology, and then, following the lecture, the same questions are presented as postclass questions to see whether there is an increase in correct responses, thereby demonstrating learner comprehension of the content presented (Toothaker, 2018).
- Another method is to pose questions to which there may be differing opinions. Learners can respond anonymously, and "the stage is set to support and deepen engagement and articulation as students try to mount arguments for their position" (Brown, 2006, p. 29).

In another example, students can be asked to create content using a variety of freely available tools and resources that not only permit student "authoring" of content but also support collaborative learning. These include tools like PlayPosit (www.playposit.com), Screencastomatic (screencast-o-matic.com), Trello (trello.com), and Padlet (padlet.com). Students can use these tools to create reports, group presentations, and more.

▶ OPEN EDUCATIONAL RESOURCES

The United Nations Educational, Scientific and Cultural Organization (UNESCO) defines Open Educational Resources (OER) as "teaching, learning and research materials in any medium – digital or otherwise – that reside in the public domain or have been released under an open license that permits no-cost access, use, adaptation and redistribution by others with no or limited restrictions" (UNESCO, 2019).

OERs save money for students and faculty alike. As technology and access continually evolve, these resources continue to grow. In addition, OER allows instructors flexibility in assembling content to create a more personalized, engaging learning experience for learners. Some commonly used OERs that offer extensive resources content and tools include:

- College Open Textbooks (collegeopentextbooks.org)
- Merlot (www.merlot.org)
- MIT Open Courseware (ocw.mit.edu)
- OER Commons (www.oercommons.org)
- Open Course Library (opencourselibrary.org)
- Open Education Consortium (www.oeconsortium.org)
- Open Learning Initiative (oli.cmu.edu)
- Openstax (openstax.org)

▶ EMERGING TRENDS

A challenge faced by nurse educators is to consider and implement novel approaches to teaching students. The advancement of nursing education and practice "depends on the continual improvement of our work; improvement occurs when innovative ideas are introduced and tested. Nurse educators must be encouraged to explore new and alternative methods for teaching, learning, and practice" (Giddens, 2015). This means that the nurse educator must be aware of emerging trends and be proactive in efforts to examine and test new emerging technology.

For example, Educause's 2019 Horizon Report identifies the following important developments in educational technology for higher education and estimates when these technologies will be widely adopted (Alexander et al., 2019):

One Year or Less:

- Mobile Learning: "Mobile learning is no longer focused directly on apps but instead on connectivity and convenience, with the expectation that learning experiences will include mobile-friendly content, multidevice syncing, and anywhere/anytime access" (p. 21).
- Analytics Technologies: "Analytics technologies are a key element of student success initiatives across institutions and a driving force behind the collaborative, targeted

strategic planning and decision-making of higher education leaders" supporting not only the organization but providing critical information of student learning that is timely and facilitates early faculty intervention to support student success (p. 23).

Two to Three Years:

- Mixed Reality (MR): "This hybrid space integrates digital technologies into the physical world and creates virtual simulations of physical spaces, blurring the differentiation between worlds. Augmented reality layers information over physical spaces and objects, such as labels and other supplementary data over museum displays." A key characteristic of MR is its interactivity, enhancing opportunities for learning and assessment, allowing learners to "construct new understanding based on experiences with virtual objects that bring underlying data to life" (p. 25).
- Artificial Intelligence (AI): AI applications associated with teaching and learning are expected to grow significantly due to AI's ability to "reduce workloads and assist with analysis of large and complex data" as well as "reducing college costs and allowing students to personalize their learning experiences to best meet their needs" (p. 27).

Four to Five Years:

- Blockchain: This technology may have broad application in higher education as a secure measure to monitor adaptive learning and award micro credentials. Currently, "colleges and universities are investigating ways in which the technology could be used for areas including transcripts, smart contracts, and identity management" (p. 29).
- Virtual Assistants: "As the capability of interacting through natural conversation increases, educational uses for learners of all languages multiply. Virtual assistants are expected to be used for research, tutoring, writing, and editing. Similarly, virtual tutors and virtual facilitators will soon be able to generate customizable and conversational learning experiences currently found in a variety of adaptive learning platforms. Investments in the education sector of AI demonstrate the potential for robust growth for virtual assistant solutions for learners" (pp. 31–32).

EVIDENCE-BASED TEACHING PRACTICE

Tar-Ching, Loney, Elias, Ali, and Adam (2016) studied audience response system's (ARS's) ability to obtain student consensus on presented issues in a modified three-stage Delphi process. The modified Delphi process included (a) agreeing on the topic(s) of interest for which consensus is sought, (b) identifying key stakeholders whose opinions are required, and (c) assembling the stakeholders for a one-day event. The ARS provided immediate feedback and students could consider the group view before moving forward in the process. This study resulted in expediting the Delphi method by decreasing the time needed to arrive at consensus.

▶ SUPPORTING FACULTY DEVELOPMENT

To support academic nurse educators with the use of technology, a university can implement a variety of professional development opportunities to faculty as well as build an infrastructure that supports and rewards creativity and innovation in education (Giddens, 2015; White, Pillay & Huang, 2016). It is important to be facile and timely in the supports provided, an essential characteristic highlighted during the COVID pandemic but will remain a valuable organizational competency in years to come.

- Provide access to new learning technologies.
- Encourage faculty to explore new and alternative methods for teaching, learning, and practice (Snow, 2016; Gidden, 2019).
- Offer faculty training to support the integration of new technologies into teaching.
- Establish web-based resource centers, such as Drexel University's Virtual Nursing Faculty Resource Center (Hasson, Cornelius, & Suplee, 2008).
  - The purpose of this type of resource center is to provide web-based support.
  - "This resource center can serve as a 'one-stop shopping' area for all faculty to access not only resources but also tutorials to support 'just-in-time' training needs" (Hasson et al., 2008, p. 23).
- Provide library liaisons and instructional designers to work with teaching faculty to "develop courses and/or class assignments, interactive teaching models, learning objects, and tutorials that introduce information literacy concepts, resources, and tools" (Donald, 2009, p. 2).

INFORMATICS IN THE LEARNING ENVIRONMENT

The NLN (2008) "advocates for support of faculty development initiatives and innovative educational programs that address informatics preparation. This call for reform is relevant to all prelicensure and graduate nursing education programs as the informatics revolution will impact all of nursing practice" (p. 1; see Exhibit 3.1).

Exhibit 3.1 Faculty Development

For Nurse Educators
- Participate in faculty development programs to achieve competency in informatics
- Designate an informatics champion in every school of nursing to (a) help faculty distinguish between using instructional technologies to teach versus using informatics to guide, document, analyze, and inform nursing practice, and (b) translate state-of-the-art practices in technology and informatics that need to be integrated into the curriculum
- Incorporate informatics in the curriculum
- Identify clinical informatics exemplars, those drawn from clinical agencies and the community or from other nursing education programs, to serve as examples for the integration of informatics into the curriculum
- Achieve competency through participation in faculty development programs
- Partner with clinicians and informatics specialists at clinical agencies to help faculty and learners develop competence in informatics

(*continued*)

Exhibit 3.1 Faculty Development (*continued*)

- Collaborate with clinical agencies to ensure that learners have hands-on experience with informatics tools
- Collaborate with clinical agencies to demonstrate transformations in clinical practice produced by informatics
- Establish criteria to evaluate informatics goals for faculty

For Deans/Directors/Chairs
- Provide leadership for necessary information technology (IT) infrastructure that will ensure education that prepares graduates for 21st-century practice roles and responsibilities
- Allocate sufficient resources to support IT initiatives
- Ensure that all faculty members have competence in computer literacy, information literacy, and informatics
- Provide opportunities for faculty development in informatics
- Urge clinical agencies to provide hands-on informatics experiences for learners
- Encourage nurse-managed clinics to incorporate clinical informatics exemplars that have transformed nursing practice to provide safe, quality care
- Advocate that all learners graduate with up-to-date knowledge and skills in each of the three critical areas: computer literacy, information literacy, and informatics
- Establish criteria to evaluate outcomes related to achieving informatics goals

For the NLN
- Disseminate this position statement widely
- Seek external funding and allocate internal resources to convene a think tank to reach a consensus on definitions of informatics, competencies for faculty and learners, and program outcomes that include informatics
- Participate actively in organizations that focus on education in nursing informatics to ensure that recommendations from those organizations are congruent with the NLN's positions on the curriculum
- Use the Educational Technology and Information Management Advisory Council (ETIMAC) and its task groups to (a) develop programs for faculty, showcasing exemplar programs and (b) disseminate outcomes from the think tank
- Encourage and facilitate accrediting bodies, regulatory agencies, and certifying bodies to reach a consensus on definitions related to informatics and minimal informatics competencies for practice in the 21st century (NLN, 2001, 2006)

Key driving forces in this process include:
- Reports and recommendations from the Institute of Medicine (IOM)
- Creation of the Office of the National Coordinator of Health Information Technology and its federal mandates
- The Technology Informatics Guiding Educational Reform (TIGER) Initiative
- The Robert Wood Johnson Foundation–funded Quality and Safety Education for Nurses (QSEN) Initiative (NLN, 2008)

▶ THE TIGER INITIATIVE

The Technology Informatics Guiding Education Reform (TIGER) Initiative is a global interprofessional community that focuses on education reform, interprofessional community development, and global workforce development. TIGER offers "tools and resources for learners to advance their skills and for educators to develop valuable curricula. By providing the necessary resources to integrate technology and informatics into education, clinical practice, and research, the TIGER initiative helps prepare the next generation of global healthcare professionals to improve patient care" (Healthcare Information and Management Systems Society, Inc. (HIMSS), 2020). TIGER recommendations for schools of nursing include:

- Adopt informatics competencies for all levels of nursing education (undergraduate/graduate) and practice (generalist/specialist).
- Encourage faculty to participate in development programs in informatics.
- Develop a task force or committee at each school to examine the integration of informatics throughout the curriculum.
- Encourage the Health Services Resources Administration's (HRSA) Division of Nursing to continue and expand its support for informatics specialty programs and faculty development.
- Measure changes from baseline in informatics knowledge among nursing educators and learners and among the full range of clinicians seeking continuing education.
- Collaborate with industry and service partners to support faculty creativity in the design, acceptance, and adoption of informatics technology.
- "Develop strategies to recruit, retain, and educate current and future nurses in the areas of informatics education, practice, and research" (NLN, 2008, p. 3).

▶ INFORMATICS COMPETENCIES

Specific informatics competencies include, but are not limited to, computer literacy or computer skills, information literacy or the ability to retrieve information, and general informatics skills. These skills include the ability to use informatics strategies and system applications to manage data and information and the ability to process the data retrieved (Saba & Calderone, 2010; Saba & McCormick, 2006: Kupferschmid, Creech, Lesley, & Schoville, 2020). Informatics competencies for nurses are typically organized according to three proficiency levels:

1. Beginner, entry, or user level
2. Intermediate or modifier level
3. Advanced or innovator level of competency (Saba & Calderone, 2010; Saba & McCormick, 2006)

    Informatics requires competency in three areas:

1. Technical competency
2. Utility competency
3. Leadership competency (Kaminski, 2007)

    In 2008, the NLN issued a statement with recommendations for schools of nursing to prepare learners for practice in the dynamic health care arena. These recommendations are listed in Exhibit 3.2.

Exhibit 3.2 Recommendations for Nursing Educational Units

Technical competencies	Technical competencies are related to the actual psychomotor use of computers and other technological equipment. Specific nursing informatics competencies include the ability to use selected applications in a comfortable and knowledgeable way. It is important for nurses to feel confident in their use of computers and software in the practice setting, and especially at the bedside, to be able to attend to the client while using these devices
Utility competencies	Utility competencies are the process of using computers and other technological equipment within nursing practice, education, research, and administration. Specific nursing informatics competencies include the process of applying evidence-based practice, critical thinking, and accountability to the use of selected applications in a comfortable and knowledgeable way
Leadership competencies	Leadership competencies are related to the ethical and management issues of using computers and other technological equipment within nursing practice, education, research, and administration. Specific nursing informatics competencies include the process of applying accountability, client privacy and confidentiality, and quality assurance in documentation to the use of selected applications in a comfortable and knowledgeable way

Rapidly advancing computer information technology mandates that the nurse educator not only acquire skills associated with teaching/learning technologies but also attain and maintain competencies related to the technology nursing graduates will be required to utilize in the workplace. These include lifelong learning skills, computer and information literacy, informatics, and technology competency (Button, Harrington, & Belan, 2014; Rajalahti, Heinonen, & Saranto, 2014; Martin, Budhrani, Kumar & Ritzhaupt, 2019).

MOBILE LEARNING

The mobile device has emerged as a ubiquitous and powerful tool that can support learning in the mobile environment, and as mentioned earlier, mobile learning will have a dominant role in the educational arena moving forward. According to Alexander et al. (2019) the driving factor for mobile learning is the ownership of mobile devices, particularly the smartphone, with 95% of undergraduate students owning smartphones. As mobile device ownership and usage have increased, mobile learning is no longer just focused on asynchronous interaction, content creation, and reference. More emphasis is emerging on content that is responsive instead of adaptive and on creating microlearning experiences that can sync across multiple devices and give learners the flexibility to learn on the device of their choice.

Key trends include:

- Smartphone ownership by 84% of all adults in the United States in 2020. A higher percentage of younger adults own smartphones—96% of those aged 18–29 and 92% of those aged 30–49 (PEW Research Center, 2019).

■ Ownership of tablets/e-readers among American adults rose from 45% to 52% between 2015 and 2020 (PEW Research Center, 2019).

■ Postsecondary learners value technology—particularly mobile technology—in education (Derryberry, 2011; Martin, Budhrani, Kumar & Ritzhaupt, 2019).

These devices have become smaller and faster and have the capacity to contain a vast library of resources to support learning. The advent of "cloud" computing has further expanded these capabilities. There are a large variety of mobile devices that share several common characteristics:

■ Highly portable (smartphone, reader, iPad, etc.)
■ Internet capable
■ Able to display rich content (images/videos)
■ Delivery of "chunks" of information; just-in-time information
■ Highly customizable (productivity tools, resources, references, decision support tools, etc.)
■ Storage capacity (data)
■ Autonomous ("stand-alone" devices)
■ Mobility of devices supports contextual learning through use of Quick Response codes and the Global Positioning System

Mobile devices can be used to support learning in any setting and with a variety of activities. For example:

■ Classroom: The electronic resources on these devices can be used in activities such as
  ● Gaming activities (e.g., Jeopardy) to review class content and stimulate learners in the classroom
  ● Modeling strategies to bring new evidence into practice
■ Lab/clinical: The electronic resources on these devices may be used to
  ● Reference step-by-step instructions for a nursing procedure, such as nasogastric tube insertion or tracheostomy care
  ● Model point-of-care/point-of-need information access such as drug compatibility/ interactions

E-BOOKS

E-books have become a growth industry. By 2011, more e-books were sold than traditional books (Minzesheimer, 2012). E-book sales revenue in the United States from 2008 to 2014 rose from $63.9 million to $3.5 billion (Statista, Inc., 2016a, 2016b). Industry experts maintain that this trend will persist and is forecasted to reach $8.7 billion in 2018. The growth is also impacting higher education as well but not at such speed. Surprisingly, despite the lower cost and convenience, e-book purchases by college-age learners increased modestly from 12% in October 2010 to 26% in 2012 (Greenfield, 2013; NACS OnCampus Research, 2011, 2013). Currently, the use of e-books in higher education remains stable, offering learners options between print vs. electronic seems to be the way to go, however, given the emerging trends identified by Educause, it is likely that e-books will be gaining popularity over print for a variety of reasons.

- Ease of access and use
- Additional features and functionalities not available in the "hard copy" format
- Portability
- Cost
- Environmental factors (paperless, minimal environmental footprint)
- Interactivity (with the content)

E-books offer the following important features that support and enrich the learning experience. These include:

- Embedded links
- Note-taking capability
- Social interactivity with peers and faculty
- Video, audio enhancements to content
- Bookmarking and highlighting content (Dixon, 2020)

Another important aspect is that e-books can easily accommodate different learning styles by providing electronic reader functionalities as well as enhanced visual images or videos for the visual learner. Some people, especially millennials, simply prefer learning materials in electronic format. In addition, the use of e-books provides improved accessibility for those students who require accommodations and meets the requirements for compliance with Section 504 of the Rehabilitation Act of 1973 and Title III of the Americans with Disabilities Act. (More information about generational learner differences can be found in Chapter 9).

● CASE STUDIES

CASE STUDY 3.1

A new academic nurse educator is assigned to teach two sections of a medical–surgical nursing course. One of the sections of the course will have traditional, 4-year undergraduate nursing learners, whereas the other section will have accelerated undergraduate nursing learners.

While planning the course and the use of technology, what types of technology could you use if you were teaching this course? Would you use the same types of technology for both sections of the course? Would you use different types of technology for each section?

CASE STUDY 3.2

A nurse educator is clinically teaching a group of nursing learners on a medical–surgical unit within a busy urban hospital. The nurse educator wants to make the most of the learning opportunities for the learners and thus plans to fully integrate mobile technology into the day's experience.

Discuss how the nurse educator can leverage the "teachable moments" encountered at the bedside with the learners.

1. The novice nurse educator states: "I do believe I need informational competency so I can use technology more efficiently and have a vision for the use of it in the class. I must also learn how to manage the students' use of information technology." The best response from the nurse educator mentor is:

   A. "Understanding the technical functionality is not a priority"
   B. "Developing new possible uses for information technology should not occur until you have taught the course several times"
   C. "Do not try to lead information technology changes until you are more experienced"
   D. "Managing students' use of informational technology is not a priority"

2. The nurse educator understands the impact of serious gaming when they state: "Serious gaming ...

   A. needs to be done independently to be effective"
   B. provides opportunities for research"
   C. has more effect on socialization than anything else"
   D. provides a method to assess learning"

3. A nursing student needs better understanding about using the educational institution's officially issued mobile device when the student tries to use it for:

   A. Gaming activities
   B. Patient documentation
   C. Medication reference
   D. Reference books

4. A nurse educator provides presence to her online learners by posting small pieces of text, pictures, links, short videos, and other media. The students rate the interactions highly on the course evaluation. The method being used is:

   A. Semantic blog
   B. Virtual memos
   C. Microblogging
   D. Micromemos

5. A nurse educator uses an e-book for a course because they understand that an important feature is:

   A. Embedded links
   B. Individualism
   C. Book pages
   D. Annotated index

1. D) "Managing students' use of informational technology is not a priority"
The nurse educator does not have to function on a managerial level. The nurse educator must have technical, utility and leadership informatics competencies. The educator must understand the functionality of the technology, needs to know the utilization and possibilities of technology, and must demonstrate vision for technology use.

2. D) "Serious gaming provides a method to assess learning"
Serious gaming provides a method to assess learning by providing an evaluative piece. It does not have to be completed independently, and is usually not used for research purposes or socialization.

3. B) Patient documentation
A mobile device be utilized to support learning through gaming activities, medication reference, and reference books. A mobile device is usually not used for patient information that is identified due to Health Insurance Portability and Accountability Act of 1996 (HIPAA) violations.

4. C) Microblogging
The practice of posting small pieces of digital content—which could be text, pictures, links, short videos, or other media—on the Internet is called microblogging.

5. A) Embedded links
Embedded links are an important feature that e-books offer. Both e-books and paper books offer individualism for study and referencing, pages, and annotated indexes.

6. A nurse educator includes an electronic concept map in her assignment section worth three percent (3%) of the final course grade. A student's grade is 20 points off out of a possible 100 points on the rubric for missing a link between the medications and the interventions. The student's final course percentage for the assignment would be calculated as:

   A. 3.0%
   B. 2.8%
   C. 2.4%
   D. 2.0%

7. The nurse educator understands that by developing a wiki to facilitate course content may:

   A. Assist recording journal entries that are presented in reverse chronological order
   B. Help develop community sites that build relationships and connections/networks
   C. Provide space for a collection of web pages that may be edited only by those invited
   D. Establish a method of distributing videos and web content

8. The Technology Informatics Guiding Educational Reform (TIGER) initiative assisted nurse educators to:

   A. Gain informatics competencies for clinical practicums
   B. Promote informatics competencies for all levels of nursing education
   C. Enhance informatics competencies for skills laboratory
   D. Assist with informatics competencies for electronic medical records

9. The nurse educator is teaching students to use social bookmarking so they can:

   A. Tag a website so that you can easily return later
   B. Share websites with others who are interested
   C. Distribute multimedia content moong peers
   D. Record short video and audio clips for education

10. The nurse educator uses Twitter to get small bits of information across to students. The nurse educator if effectively using a(n):

    A. Social networking site
    B. Wiki
    C. E-book format
    D. Microblog

(See answers next page.)

6. C) 2.4%
Eighty percent (80%) or points is 2.4% of a total of three percent (3%).

7. C) Provide space for a collection of web pages that may be edited only by those invited
A wiki is a collection of web pages that may be edited only by those invited. A wiki is not an open community site, a place to record ongoing documents, or a distribution platform.

8. B) Promote informatics competencies for all levels of nursing education
The TIGER initiative focused on the development of informatics competencies for all levels of nursing education—for students and nursing faculty alike.

9. A) Tag a website so that you can easily return later
social bookmarking is a way to tag or 'save' a website to make it easier to return to it later. Social bookmarking is not generally used for sharing, distribution, or recording.

10. D) Microblog
Twitter is an example of a microblog and is not an actual full-size social network. It is not in an e-book format or a wiki.

REFERENCES

Amith, M., Fujimoto, K., Mauldin, R., & Tao, C. (2020). Friend of a Friend with Benefits ontology (FOAF+): extending a social network ontology for public health. BMC Medical Informatics & Decision Making, Supplement 10, 20: 1-14.10.1186/s12911-020-01287-8

Alexander, B., Ashford-Rowe, K., Barajas-Murphy, N., Dobbin, G., Knott, J., McCormack, M., Pomerantz, J., Seithamer, R., & Weber, N. (2019). EDUCAUSE Horizon Report 2019 Higher Education Edition, https://library.educause.edu/-/media/files/library/2019/4/2019horizonreport.pdf?la=en&hash=C8E8D444AF372E705FA1BF9D4FF0DD4CC6F0FDD1

Anderson, M. (2015). Technology device ownership: 2015, Pew Research Center Internet, Science & Tech. R http://www.pewinternet.org/2015/10/29/technology-device-ownership-2015

Astriani, D., Susilo, H., Suwono, H., Lukiati, B. & Purnomo, A. (2020). Mind Mapping in Learning Models: A Tool to Improve Student Metacognitive Skills. *International Journal of Emerging Technologies in Learning (iJET)*. 15 (6), pp. 4–17. Kassel, Germany: International Journal of Emerging Technology in Learning.

Ave, J.S., Beasley, D. & Brogan, A. (2020). A Comparative Investigation of Student Learning through PechaKucha Presentations in Online Higher Education. *Innov High Educ* 45, 373–386, https://doi.org/10.1007/s10755-020-09507-9

Brown, J. S. (2006). *New learning environments for the 21st century*. Forum for the Future of Higher Education's 2005 Aspen Symposium. http://www.johnseelybrown.com/newlearning.pdf

Button, D., Harrington, A., & Belan, I. (2014). E-learning and information communication technology (ICT) in nursing education: A review of the literature. *Nurse Education Today, 34*(10), 1311–1323.

Byrne, M. M. (2016). Presentation innovations: Using Pecha Kucha in nursing education. *Teaching and Learning in Nursing*, 11, 20–22. https://doi.org/10.1016/j.teln.2015.10.002

Canney, C. (2015). *Elements that affect student engagement in online graduate courses* (Thesis). Available from ProQuest Dissertations & Theses Global (1682465830). (Order No. 3702588)

Creative Commons. (n.d.). What is a virtual world? Retrieved from http://www/virtualworldsreview.com/info/whatis.shtml

Derryberry, A. (2011, April 26). Dispatch from the digital frontier: Insights from and about Generation Z. *Learning Solutions Magazine*, 1. http://www.learningsolutionsmag.com/articles/672/dispatch-from-the-digital-frontier-insights-from-and-about-generation-z

Dixon, N. (2020). ETEXTBOOKS: What's Their Future and How Can Libraries Prepare? Computers in Libraries 40(7), 14–17.

Dominic, M., Francis, S., & Pilomenraj, A. (2014). E-learning in web 3.0. *International Journal of Modern Education and Computer Science, 2*(2), 8–14. 10.5815/ijmecs.2014.02.02

Donald, J. W. (2009). Using technology to support faculty and enhance coursework in academic institutions. *Texas Library Journal, 85*(4), 129–131.

Educause. (2020). 2020 EDUCAUSE Horizon Report: Teaching and Learning Edition Retrieved from https://library.educause.edu/-/media/files/library/2020/3/2020_horizon_report_pdf

Educause Learning Initiative. (2016a). 7 Things you should know about... Twitter. www. educause.edu/ir/library/pdf/ELI7027.pdf

Educause Learning Initiative. (2016b). 7 Things you should know about... Microblogging. http://net.educause.edu/ir/library/pdf/ELI7051.pdf

Epper, R. M., Derryberry, A., & Jackson, S. (2012). *Game-based learning: Developing an institutional strategy (Research Bulletin)*. Louisville, CO: EDUCAUSE Center for Applied Research. http://www.educause.edu/ecar

Greenfield, J. (2013). Students still not taking to e-textbooks, new data show. *Digital Publishing News for the 21st Century*. http://www.digitalbookworld.com/2013/students-still-not-taking-to-e-textbooks-new-data-show

Hasson, C., Cornelius, F., & Suplee, P. D. (2008). A technology driven nursing faculty resource center. *Nurse Educator, 23*(1), 22–25.

Hunsu, N. J., Adesope, O. & Bayly, D. J. (2016). A meta-analysis of the effects of audience response systems (clicker-based technologies) on cognition and affect, Computers & Education, Volume 94, 02-119, ISSN 0360-1315, https://doi.org/10.1016/j.compedu.2015.11.013.

Hung, H. T. (2017). Clickers in the flipped classroom: bring your own device (BYOD) to promote student learning, *Interactive Learning Environments*, 25:8, 983–995

Ismail, R. Osmanaj, V. & Jaradat, A. (August 2019). Moving towards e-university: Modelling the online proctored exams, Conference Proceedings, Oxford Conference Series, AICMSE-AICSSH 2019, ISBN 978-913016-08-1

Kaminski, J. (2007). Nursing informatics competencies: Self-assessment. http://www.nursing-informatics.com/niassess/index.html

Kay, R. H., & LeSage, A. (2009). Examining the benefits and challenges of using audience response systems: A review of the literature. *Computers & Education, 53*(3), 819–827. 10.1016/j.compedu.2009.05.001

Kuh, G. D. (2009). The national survey of student engagement: Conceptual and empirical foundations. *New Directions for Institutional Research, 141*, 5–20. http://onlinelibrary.wiley.com/doi/10.1002/ir.283/abstract

Kuh, G. D., Cruce, T. M., Shoup, R., Kinzie, J., & Gonyea, R. M. (2008). Unmasking the effects of student engagement on first-year college grades and persistence. *Journal of Higher Education, 79*(5), 540–563. http://muse.jhu.edu/article/248905

Kupferschmid, B., Creech, C., Lesley, M., & Schoville, R. (2020). Understanding support for a nursing informatics leadership pipeline: An ANI emerging leader project. *CIN: Computers, Informatics, Nursing, 38*(11), 543–596.

Martin, F., Budhrani, K., Kumar, S., & Ritzhaupt, A. (2019). Award-winning faculty online teaching practices: Roles and competencies. Online Learning, 23(1),184-205. 10.24059/olj.v23i1.1329

Minzesheimer, B. (2012, January). E-books sales surge after holidays. *USA Today*. http://www.usatoday.com/life/books/news/story/2012-01-09/ebooks-sales-surge/52458672/1

Morris, R. D. (2011). Web 3.0: Implications for Online Learning. *TechTrends* 55, 42–46. https://doi.org/10.1007/s11528-011-0469-9

NACS OnCampus Research 2011. (2011). Update: Electronic book and eReader device report March 2011. http://www.nacs.org/LinkClick.aspx?fileticket=uIf2NoXApKQ%3D&tabid=2471&mid=3210

NACS OnCampus Research 2013. (2013). Student watch: Behaviour and trends of student consumers. http://www.nacs.org/email/html/OnCampusResearch/SPR-080-03-12_Client%20Newsletter.pdf

National Education Association. (2020). Higher education faculty and staff. www2.nea.org/he/techno.html

National League for Nursing. (2001). *Position statement: Lifelong learning for nursing faculty.* Washington, DC: NLN Press. http://www.nln.org/docs/default-source/about/archived-position-statements/lifelong-learning-for-nursing-faculty-pdf.pdf?sfvrsn=8

National League for Nursing. (2006). Position statement: Mentoring of nurse faculty. *Nursing Education Perspectives, 27*(2), 110–113.

National League for Nursing. (2008). Position statement: Preparing the next generation of nurses to practice in a technology-rich environment: An informatics agenda. Washington, DC: NLN Press. http://www.nln.org/docs/default-source/professional-development-programs/preparing-the-next-generation-of-nurses.pdf?sfvrsn=6

National League for Nursing. (2021). Certified Nurse Educator (CNE) 2021 candidate handbook. http://www.nln.org/docs/default-source/default-document-library/cne-handbook-2021_revised_07-01-2021.pdf?sfvrsn=2

National League for Nursing. (2021). Certified Nurse Educator Novice (CNEn) 2021 candidate handbook. http://www.nln.org/Certification-for-Nurse-Educators/cne-n/cne-n-handbook

National Survey of Student Engagement. (2015). *Engagement insights: Survey findings on the quality of undergraduate education: Annual results 2015.* Bloomington: Indiana University Center for Postsecondary Research.

O'Connor, S & Andrews, T. (2015). Mobile technology and its use in clinical nursing education: a literature review. Jouranl of Nursing Education,(54) 3 137–144, 10.3928/01484834-20150218-01

O'Connor, S., Hubner, U., Shaw, T., Blake, R. & Ball, M. (2017). Time for TIGER to ROAR! Technology informatics guiding education reform, Nurse Education Today, 58, 78-81,ISSN 0260-6917, https://doi.org/10.1016/j.nedt.2017.07.014.

Pew Research Center (2019). Mobile fact sheet.https://www.pewresearch.org/internet/fact-sheet/mobile/

Prinsloo, P. & Slade, S. (2017). An elephant in the learning analytics room: The obligation to act. In Proceedings of the Seventh International Learning Analytics & Knowledge Conference (LAK '17). Association for Computing Machinery, New York, NY, USA, 46–55. https://doi.org/10.1145/3027385.3027406

Rajalahti, E., Heinonen, J., & Saranto, K. (2014). Developing nurse educators' computer skills towards proficiency in nursing informatics. *Informatics for Health & Social Care, 39*(1), 47–66.

Ricker, A. A. & Richert, R. A. (2021). Digital gaming and metacognition in middle childhood. Computers in Human Behavior, 115, N.PAG-N.PAG. 10.1016/j.chb.2020.106593

Rienties, B., Cross, S. & Zdrahal, Z. (2017). Implementing a learning analytics intervention and evaluation framework: What works? In B. Kei Daniel (ed.), Big Data and Learning Analytics in Higher Education, Springer International Publishing Switzerland. 10.1007/978-3-319-06520-5_10

Robinson, C. C., & Hullinger, H. (2008). New benchmarks in higher education: Student engagement in online learning. *Journal of Education for Business, 84*(2), 101–108.

Rudman, R. & Bruwer, R. (2016). Defining Web 3.0: Opportunities and challenges. *Electronic Library, 34*(1), 132–154. 10.1108/EL-08-2014-0140

Saba, V. K., & Calderone, T. L. (2010). What nurse educators need to know about the TIGER initiative. *Nurse Educator, 35*(2), 56–60.

Saba, V. K., & McCormick, K. A. (2006). *Essentials of nursing informatics* (4th ed.). McGraw-Hill.

Singh, R., & Lal, M. (2012). Web 3.0 in education & research. *BVICAM's International Journal of Information Technology, 3*(2). http://www.bvicam.ac.in/bijit/Downloads/pdf/issue6/02.pdf

Snow, F. (2019). Creativity and innovation: An essential competency for the nurse leader, Nursing Administration Quarterly, (43)4, 306–312.

Statista, Inc. (2016a). Trade e-book sales revenue in United States from 2008–2014 (in million U.S. dollars). http://www.statista.com/statistics/278235/e-book-sales-revenue-in-the-us

Statista, Inc. (2016b). Revenue from e-book sales in the United States from 2008 to 2018 (in billion U.S. dollars). http://www.statista.com/statistics/190800/ebook-sales-revenue-forecast-for-the-us-market

Tar-Ching, A., Loney, T. J., Elias, A., Ali, S., & Adam, B. (2016). Use of an audience response system to maximise response rates and expedite a modified Delphi process for consensus on occupational health. *Journal of Occupational Medicine & Toxicology, 11,* 1–6. 10.1186/s12995-016-0098-5

Technology Informatics Guiding Education Reform. (2016). The TIGER initiative: Evidence and informatics transforming nursing: 3-year action steps toward a 10-year vision. http://www.aacn.nche.edu/education-resources/TIGER.pdf

Toothaker, R. (2018). Millennial's perspective of clicker technology in a nursing classroom: A Mixed methods research study. Nurse Education Today, 62, 80-84. 10.1016/j.nedt.2017.12.027

United Nations Educational, Scientific, and Cultural Organization (UNESCO) (2019). Open educational resources (OER) https://en.unesco.org/themes/building-knowledge-societies/oer

Watson, W. R., Watson, S. L. & Reigeluth, C. M. (2015). Education 3.0: breaking the mold with technology, Interactive Learning Environments, 23: 3, 332–343, 10.1080/10494820.2013.764322

White, K. R., Pillay, R. & Huang, X. (2016). Nurse leaders and the innovation competence gap, *Nursing Outlook,* 64, 255–261.

Yun, C. (2007). Eric Schmidt, Web 2.0 vs. Web 3.0. http://youtu.be/T0QJmmdw3b0

Zirawaga, V. S., Olusanya, A. I. & Maduku, T. (2017). Gaming in education: Using games as a support tool to teach history. *Journal of Education and Practice,* v8 n15 p.55–64.

Online Learning

4

Frances H. Cornelius and Linda Wilson

Education is not the filling of a pail, but the lighting of a fire.
—William Butler Yeats

▶ LEARNING OUTCOMES

This chapter also addresses the Certified Nurse Educator Exam and the Certified Nurse Educator Novice exam Content Area 1: Facilitate Learning

- Analyze nurse educator's role in an online learning environment to support learning
- Examine the importance of the appropriate integration of technology in a meaningful and relevant manner to support online learning
- Describe how to devise strategies to integrate technology in an online learning activity

⬤ INTRODUCTION

As described in Chapter 3, there has been a significant transformation of the learning environment primarily because of the wide array of technological advancements currently available. This transformation has served as a catalyst in the shift away from traditional teaching paradigms. Learners are no longer passive recipients of information; the learning that takes place is deeper. As discussed in the previous chapter, new technologies and Web 2.0 tools provide many opportunities to engage students in active learning. The online learning environment is growing exponentially. Industry experts believe that this trend is likely to continue, citing the following facts:

- In the United States, the number of learners taking at least one online course increased from 5.6 million in the fall of 2009 to 6.1 million in the fall of 2010, an increase of approximately 560,000 learners (Allen & Seaman, 2011; Terantino & Agbehonou, 2012).
- Thirty-one percent of all higher education learners were taking at least one course online (Allen & Seaman, 2011), and then the pandemic (COVID-19) proliferated in the United States and remote learning instantly became the mode for almost all learners.
- The future of learning modalities may be forever changed and include variations of remote online and face-to-face (F2F) learning environments.

ONLINE TEACHING VERSUS TRADITIONAL CLASSROOM TEACHING

Although there are some important differences, there are many similarities between online teaching and traditional classroom teaching. Both traditional and online courses use lectures, class discussions, readings and assignments, group activities, projects, and other activities. The difference lies in how these activities are delivered in the online environment. For example, a class lecture (a stalwart standard in education) in the online learning environment can be delivered in the following ways:

- Written text
- PowerPoint slides
- Audio only
- Voice-over PowerPoint slides
- Video
- Podcast
- Live (using a synchronous meeting room)

Strategies/techniques to deliver content in an online course are similar to those of the traditional F2F classroom. However, with the use of available technologies, these activities can be enhanced with rich media and high levels of interaction and feedback. Some strategies include:

- Problem-based learning
- Self-directed learning
- Just-in-time learning
- Case-based learning
- Self-assessment
- Feedback
- Journals and portfolios
- Instructor feedback

In an online teaching environment, course content for learners can be presented or enhanced through the use of the following:

- Outside reading
- Links to websites
- Visual materials
- Audio and video recordings
- Links or folders that contain your own personal lectures, notes, and papers

The ability to have access to so many different materials is an advantage for nurse educators engaged in remote education because the opportunities for enriching the learning experience are limitless. Table 4.1 provides some examples of how traditional classroom activities can be transitioned into online learning activities.

Table 4.1 Comparison of Traditional F2F and Online Classroom Activities

Activity	Online activity	Comments
Class lecture—traditional with faculty at the podium	Asynchronous, prerecorded lectures that can be viewed independently by learners at any time Opportunity for faculty to tweak or rerecord improvements Opportunity for learners to go back as many times as they want to listen to the prerecorded lecture	Accomplishes the same goal, but an online activity provides more learner control; more easily viewed again for review and clarification. Learners can view lectures in their own time. Lectures can be saved in different formats so that they are portable (mp3 and mp4 files). Learners can email questions to presenters or post them to a discussion forum
Class discussion	Synchronous class discussion using virtual meeting rooms such as WebCT, Adobe Connect, Eluminate, or Zoom	A virtual meeting room provides a venue for dynamic, interactive class meetings. This is a great option for individual, group, or outside speaker presentations and Q&A sessions Encourages introverted learners to actively participate in discussions Benefit is that discussions are in "real time" so that the faculty can get a sense of how the learners think "on their feet" and can articulate thoughts and ideas clearly Use of webcam allows learners to see the instructor, which can make visual learners more comfortable
	Discussion board (text-based, asynchronous)	Great venue for learners to have discussions about various topics, readings, and assignments One benefit is the asynchronous mode allows learners to participate at their convenience, around their schedule Learners have a good opportunity to reflect and formulate a more powerful response to questions and have time to bring in the literature to support their position
	Voice discussion board (audio-based, asynchronous)	Provides opportunity to actually hear verbal comments from learners and instructors as well as the tone/verbal inflections of the speaker Helps the auditory learner grasp important concepts

(continued)

Table 4.1 Comparison of Traditional F2F and Online Classroom Activities

Activity	Online activity	Comments
Class debate	Discussion board/voice discussion board	A debate on a discussion board can be asynchronous to allow learners to respond at their convenience and have more time to reflect on their answers so as to respond in a more substantive way
	Live debate in synchronous class meeting rooms	Benefit is that synchronous debate allows the faculty to get a sense of the learner's ability to construct a persuasive argument and articulate thoughts and ideas clearly
Group work—small breakout groups during class to respond to questions	Synchronous class meeting using breakout rooms	This is a great way to manage group activities in online courses. Groups can work together in the synchronous classroom. Faculty can move from room to room to assist as needed Benefit of using these small-group activities during synchronous class meetings is that it is an effective way the faculty can provide the structure to help build learner connections with the learning community
Group projects— learner teams work on projects outside the class	Group projects— using dedicated synchronous learner meeting rooms, wikis, and group discussion boards	This is another great idea. The learners can meet outside of "class" in the learner meeting rooms to work on a project during a time that is convenient for the members of small groups
Group presentations in class	Group presentations in a synchronous classroom	There really isn't much difference between the group presentations in class versus the one in a synchronous class meeting room. Learners can use PowerPoint slides, handouts, etc., in both settings. Learners can be viewed through a webcam in a synchronous classroom so that other learners can see their expressions, etc
Tests/quizzes— traditional F2F	Online quizzes and tests using Blackboard and additional test security options (i.e., Remote Proctor, ProctorU) or live proctors	Live proctors can assist with test security and ensure that the learner is actually the one taking the examination If quizzes are taken online, it is important to time them and randomize the questions If desired, the online quizzes can be set up to provide immediate feedback to the learner. If the test is "high stakes," it is a good idea to give learners only the score until after the test is closed. If correct answers are given prior to closing of the test, the learners will share the correct answers
Similar to the traditional F2F classroom, questions can be discussed in depth to drill down into deeper understanding regarding the rationale for why a particular answer was correct. The discussion can be engaging to get them to think critically about what the question demands truly, and why the correct answer is the "best" answer		

Table 4.1 Comparison of Traditional F2F and Online Classroom Activities

Activity	Online activity	Comments
Case study— presentations with questions about the case	Case studies posted on discussion board, learners respond to questions through discussion board (asynchronous)	This can be accomplished by either a lone learner or multiple learners in breakout groups to compile a case study or build upon each other ideas Case studies presented in this way provide the learners time to look up information in reference books/articles so that they can build their understanding at their own pace
	Synchronous class meetings in which learners present case studies and engage in real-time in-depth discussion	Benefit is that synchronous presentation allows the faculty to get a sense of the learners' understanding as well as their ability to think "on their feet" and articulate thoughts and ideas clearly

In an online course, lectures are already completed before the learners get to class. Therefore, an instructor spends more time engaged in discussions, feedback, and supervising activities/assignments. Keep in mind that in the online course, the instructor can put many more activities and assignments into each unit, and consequently, there is more to discuss and supervise. In addition, frequent constructive and meaningful feedback ensure that students remain engaged and on task (Bonnel & Boehm, 2011; Shim & Lee, 2020).

The benefits of online learning are well documented in the literature. The online learning environment increases the student's control over the content, as well as the time and place learning occurs—creating a more individualized, learner-centered experience. The online learning environment also provides more opportunities for students to be more engaged and to interact with faculty, peers, and content (Robinson & Hullinger, 2008). Furthermore, it can help students gain knowledge and skills more quickly than traditional instructor-led methods (Cook, 2007; Ilkay & Zeynep, 2014; McGarry, Theobald, Lewis, & Coyer, 2015; Shim & Lee, 2020).

Courses can be fully online, hybrid, or web facilitated, depending on how much of the course is delivered online. In general, courses that deliver less than 20% of content online are considered web facilitated. A **web-facilitated** course usually delivers course materials, such as the syllabus, assignments, or readings, via an online course management system. Courses that provide a substantial amount of the content online (between 29% and 79%) are considered to be **blended** or **hybrid**. This type of course frequently uses online discussions in place of F2F meetings. A course that provides 80% or more content online or has no F2F meetings is considered to be an online course, although for the most part, many academic institutions offer online courses that are 100% online (Sener, 2015). Online courses can be delivered using a variety of software applications and benefit from academic collaboration (McGillian, 2020). Some of these include:

- **Learning management systems** (LMS): An LMS may be a commercial product or an open-source system. It is defined as an "information system that administers instructor-led and e-learning courses and keeps track of student progress" (Learning management system, n.d.). There are four major LMS platforms currently in use. These include Blackboard (www.blackboard.com) Canvas (www.instructure.com), Desire2Learn (www.d2l.com) and Moodle (moodle.org).

- **Content management system** (CMS): "An application (more likely web-based), that provides capabilities for multiple users with different permission levels to manage (all or a section of) content, data or information of a website project, or Internet/intranet application. Managing content refers to creating, editing, archiving, publishing, collaborating on, reporting, distributing website content, data and information" (Kohan, 2010). Examples of a CMS are:

  - Crownpeak DXM (www.crownpeak.com)
  - WordPress (wordpress.org)
  - Wix (www.wix.com)
  - Drupal (drupal.org)
  - Joomla! (www.joomla.org)
  - MS Sharepoint (www.microsoft.com)
  - ExpressionEngine (ellislab.com/expressionengine)
  - TextPattern (textpattern.com)

- Ackehurst and Polvere (2020) studied the use of a new content management system to organize journals for accessibility and use. After 3 years, the maintenance effort decreased for users, and the topic structure changed to increase accessibility assisting the professionals who need the information.

EVIDENCE-BASED TEACHING PRACTICE

Price, Whitlatch, Jane, Burdi, and Peacock (2016) discuss improvement in online teaching by providing faculty with an online teaching workshop. Results were positive from this pilot study, which used faculty ($N = 11$) and RN to BSN student ($N = 6$) focus groups.

BENCHMARKS AND QUALITY MEASURES FOR ONLINE TEACHING

The Institute for Higher Education Policy (IHEP) has identified 24 benchmarks as essential to ensuring excellence in Internet-based distance learning. These benchmarks include seven areas of quality measures presently used on college and university campuses nationwide (Phipps & Merisotis, 2000). These benchmark areas are:

1. Institutional support
2. Course development
3. Teaching/learning
4. Course structure
5. Student support
6. Faculty support
7. Evaluation and assessment

For a complete list of the 24 benchmarks, refer to Table 4.2.

Table 4.2 Benchmarks That Are Essential for Quality Internet-Based Distance Education

Educational organization support	The educational organization has a technological system that has protections build in to maintain student and faculty privacy. The technology is effective, and there are back-ups in case of system failure
Course Use of Technology	The course is designed at the appropriate level of the students, and the course student learning outcomes are clear. The technology needs for the course are understood by students and assist the students to reach the course goals
Using Technology in the Teaching/Learning Process	Students feel connected in the course through peer and faculty responses. They use a variety of online methods to learn, and those methods are explained to them adequately
Course Development	Before students enroll in an online course, they understand the expectations and resources needed to be successful
Technical Support	Students are able to access the technology department when needed, and they have their questions answered well and in a timely manner
Faculty Professional Development	Faculty professional development in online teaching is ongoing and accessible
Course Evaluation	Online courses should be evaluated for effectiveness. Were the students able to complete the SLOs? Was there rigor in the courses? Were students satisfied, and would they recommend taking another online course?

Source: Adapted from Phipps and Merisotis (2000).

The Online Learning Consortium (OLC) (formerly Sloan Consortium) identified five Pillars for Quality Online Education. These include: (1) learning effectiveness, (2) student satisfaction, (3) faculty satisfaction, (4) cost-effectiveness, and (5) access. The 2002 *Sloan Consortium Report to the Nation* states that "Sloan-C's five pillars are a framework for measuring and improving an online program within any institution," noting that most organizations evaluate the quality of online education considering only "learning effectiveness," however, "learning effectiveness has greater meaning when it is combined within a framework that encompasses all five pillars" (Lorenzo & Moore, 2002, p. 3).

The OLC and IHEP have had a lasting impact on efforts to ensure quality online education and are still utilized today. Esfijani (2018) conducted an in-depth, meta-synthesis of online education quality standards and benchmarks and noted that the "quality pillars outlined by the OLC and the quality benchmarks developed by the IHEP are the most well-known and oft-cited approaches and have been employed in different educational cultures with no modifications" (p. 69).

In addition to the 24 benchmarks identified by the IHEP (Phipps & Merisotis, 2000), there are many other quality resources/measures available to help the nurse educator ensure quality online course delivery. Quality Matters™ (QM) is an organization that provides quality assurance regarding the course design. The QM approach is designed to be a collegial, faculty-centered, peer-review process to evaluate the design of online and blended courses through the use of eight general standards and 43 specific standards (Table 4.3; QM, 2016). The full rubric provides a point value for each standard to aid in scoring for peer review. Additional information can be obtained at the QM website (www.qualitymatters.org).

Table 4.3 Quality Matters™ Standards From the QM *Higher Education Rubric*, Sixth Edition

Course overview and introduction	1.1 Instructions make clear how to get started and where to find various course components
	1.2 Learners are introduced to the purpose and structure of the course
	1.3 Communication expectations for online discussions, email, and other forms of interactions are clearly stated
	1.4 Course and/or institutional policies with which the student is expected to comply are clearly stated, or a link to current policies is provided
	1.5 Minimum technology requirements are clearly stated, and information on how to obtain the technologies is provided
	1.6 Computer skills and digital information literacy skills expected of the learner are clearly stated
	1.7 Expectations for prerequisite knowledge in the discipline and competencies are clearly stated
	1.8 The self-introduction by the instructor is appropriate and available online
	1.9 Learners are asked to introduce themselves to the class
Learning objectives (competencies)	2.1 The course learning objectives, or course/program competencies, describe outcomes that are measurable
	2.2 The module/unit-level learning objectives or competencies describe outcomes that are measurable and consistent with the course-level objectives or competencies
	2.3 Learning objectives or competencies are stated clearly, written from the learner's perspective, and are prominently located in the course
	2.4 The relationship between learning objectives or competencies and learning activities is clearly stated
	2.5 The learning objectives or competencies are suited to the level of the course
Assessment and measurement	3.1 The assessments measure the achievement of the stated learning objectives or competencies
	3.2 The course grading policy is stated clearly at the beginning of the course
	3.3 Specific and descriptive criteria are provided for the evaluation of learners' work, and their connection to the course grading policy is clearly explained
	3.4 The assessments used are sequenced, varied, and suited to the level of the course
	3.5 The course provides learners with multiple opportunities to track their learning progress with timely feedback
Instructional materials	4.1 The instructional materials contribute to the achievement of the stated objectives or competencies
	4.2 The relationship between the use of instructional materials in the course and completing learning activities is clearly explained
	4.3 The course models the academic integrity expected of learners by providing both source references and permissions for the use of instructional materials
	4.4 The instructional materials represent up-to-date theory and practice in the discipline
	4.5 A variety of instructional materials is used in the course

Learning Activities and Learner interaction	5.1 The learning activities promote the achievement of the stated learning objectives or competencies 5.2 Learning activities provide opportunities for interaction that support active learning 5.3 The instructor's plan for interacting with learners during the course is clearly stated 5.4 The requirements for learner interaction are clearly stated
Course technology	6.1 The tools used in the course support the learning objectives or competencies 6.2 Course tools promote learner engagement and active learning 6.3 A variety of technology is used in the course 6.4 The course provides learners with information on protecting their data and privacy
Learner support	7.1 The course instructions articulate or link to a clear description of the technical support offered and how to obtain it 7.2 Course instructions articulate or link to the institution's accessibility policies and services 7.3 Course instructions articulate or link to the institution's academic support services and resources can help learners succeed in the course 7.4 Course instructions articulate or link to the institution's student services and resources can help learners succeed
Accessibility and Usability	8.1 Course navigation facilitates ease of use 8.2 The course design facilitates readability 8.3 The course provides accessible text and images in files, documents, LMS pages, and web pages to meet the needs of diverse learners 8.4 The course provides alternative means of access to multimedia content in formats that meet the needs of diverse learners 8.5 Course multimedia facilitates ease of use 8.6 Vendor accessibility statements are provided for all technologies required in the course

Note: The use of this 2018 Quality Matters™ rubric document is restricted to institutions that subscribe to the Quality Matters™ program and may not be copied or duplicated without written permission of MarylandOnline© 2018 MarylandOnline, Inc. www. qualitymatters.org. *Source:* QM (2018).

The following key points are to be kept in mind:

- Course organization style can drive instructional intensity for the learners and the instructor and can affect the quality of the learning experience.
- Course structure generally refers to the organization of the course content and logical flow of the content.
- Course structure is particularly important in an online course because, for the most part, learners are working independently going through the course content.
- Learner satisfaction with a course is closely related to how well the course is organized.
- A well-organized course is like a well-constructed house—all the pieces fit and work together.

The key benefit of good course structure is that it gives the learner a sense of how the learning process will unfold. Elements that provide the structure are as follows:

- Course schedule
- Course syllabus
- Overview of how the course content is organized
- Statement in the course introduction providing information to the learner regarding how the course is structured
- A "getting started" module

Course structure presents course content in a logical manner, permitting learners to focus on learning rather than spending time trying to find information within the course. Content can be distributed by the week or by modules. It is advisable to use the same format of presentation for each week/module.

Another key consideration is **alignment**. It is important that course and module/unit level learning objectives are aligned with course materials and learning activities and directly support the assessments for the course. When these elements are aligned, students are able to see how learning activities and materials connect with their assignments and, as a result, have a better learning experience. Conversely, this also helps the instructor see how course outcomes are being met and can more easily identify areas in which the course can be improved (Carnegie Mellon University, n.d.; Matuga, 2006; Shaltry, 2020). In addition, several studies have noted that students perform better in courses that are aligned (Jensen, McDaniel, Woodard, Kummer, 2014; Pape-Zambito & Mostrom, 2018).

Creating a quality online learning experience requires "more than simply uploading materials from a pre-existing face-to-face class onto a web-based course management system… course design must begin with a foundation of measurable competencies, essential outcomes, and evidence-based practice," accompanied with educational materials that "not only actively engage and resonate with the learner but also encourage him or her to seek mentorship and the support of his or her peers" (Hoffmann, Klein, & Rosenzweig, 2016, p. 4). This includes the use of multiple interactive and engaging learning activities that "accommodate the multiple learning styles, skills, and experiences of the adult learners" (p. 4).

ROLE OF NURSE EDUCATORS

In the online environment, more so than in the traditional classroom environment, it is essential that the nurse educator role shifts to a facilitator role rather than one of deliverer of content. Qualities of a successful online instructor include content knowledge, teaching commitment, communication ability, time management, flexibility, and tolerance for ambiguity (Bigatel, Ragan, Kennan, May, & Redmond, 2012; Hathaway, 2013; Varvel, 2007; Gay, 2016).

There are other perspectives regarding the essential competencies of online educators, and for the most part, all are in agreement. Some, such as Varvel's (2007), are more detailed, but all agree that the online educator must possess these competencies. Varvel (2007) identifies seven roles that comprise master online teacher competencies, and within each role, there are numerous specific criteria:

1. **Administrative Roles (Systems, Ethical, and Legal Issues)**: "The competent instructor has an understanding of and belief in the administrative system under which he or she is employed" (p. 8).
2. **Personal Roles (Personal Qualities and Characteristics)**: "The competent instructor possesses certain personal attributes that enhance his or her ability to instruct within any given educational paradigm" (p. 9).
3. **Technological Roles (Technology Knowledge and Abilities)**: "The competent instructor is knowledgeable about the technologies used in the virtual classroom and can make effective use of those technologies" (p. 11).
4. **Instructional Design Roles (Instructional Design Processes, Knowledge, and Abilities)**: "The competent instructor can judge the appropriateness and adequacy of materials and technology used in a course for the given audience, and can make materials and technology adjustments due to shifting audience needs and abilities" p. 14).
5. **Pedagogical Roles (Teaching Processes, Knowledge, and Abilities)**: "The competent instructor must be well versed and capable in the instruction of a high quality and effective educational experience for all participants" (p. 16).
6. **Assessment Roles (Assessing Student Learning and Abilities)**: "The competent instructor is aware of online assessment issues and can effectively assess students using a variety of techniques in the online classroom that are designed not just to determine student progress but to aid in student learning" (p. 24).
7. **Social Processes and Presence (Social Roles)**: "The competent instructor recognizes that a social aspect to education exists. The instructor will effectively incorporate that aspect into the teaching and learning process with the intent of creating a learning community" (p. 27).

Cook and Dupras (2004) point out that the educator should attend to the following principles when delivering online content:

- "Learners should be active contributors to the educational process
- Learning should closely relate to understanding and solving real-life problems
- Learners' current knowledge and experience need to be taken into account
- Learners should use self-direction in their learning
- Learners should be given opportunities and support for practice, accompanied by self-assessment and constructive feedback from teachers and peers
- Learners shoud be given opportunities to reflect on their practice" (p. 704)

Martin, Budhrani, Kumar, and Ritzhaupt (2019) identify five broad competencies for online instructors and identify specific skillsets within each competency (Exhibit 4.1). These competencies correspond with the 24 benchmarks for excellence in the IHEP discussed earlier in this chapter.

Exhibit 4.1 Competencies for Online Instruction

Technical Skills	▪ Use a learning management system (LMS) to design and deliver courses ▪ Email ▪ Navigate browser windows ▪ Upload and download files ▪ Create PDFs ▪ Develop audio/video materials (e.g., screencasts, videos) ▪ Record others and themselves with a microphone ▪ Record voice narration with PowerPoint ▪ Use free tools ▪ Use a webcam ▪ Provide online feedback ▪ Use collaborative technologies ▪ Create additional materials for students experiencing difficulties ▪ Write for media and the web to communicate in video and audio formats (i.e., technical writing) ▪ Communicate with a visual perspective
Willingness to learn	▪ Grow in pedagogy and technology skills ▪ Make the move to teaching online from teaching face-to-face ▪ See oneself as a learner ▪ Embrace oneself as a life-long learner ▪ Allot time to learn about online learning and how to teach online ▪ Have the desire to teach well, to help facilitate student learning, to be very engaged, and to be dedicated to students and the mission of the school ▪ Experiment with technologies ▪ Willingness to make mistakes and learn from mistakes ▪ Be exposed to new things ▪ Stay abreast with the latest research, theories, techniques on teaching online ▪ Participate in training
Knowledge of "how people learn"	▪ Understand how students learn in synchronous and asynchronous modes ▪ Develop a mix of activities for various learning styles (e.g., social vs. solitary, oral vs. visual) ▪ Evaluate courses according to learning style
Content Expertise	▪ Be an expert in the field ▪ Know the content or subject matter ▪ Understand content to be able to deliver it effectively for learners ▪ Translate content knowledge into "teaching"
Course Design	▪ Instructional design skills ▪ Knowledge of backward course design ▪ Knowledge of web accessibility regulations ▪ Write learning objectives ▪ Chunk content into manageable parts ▪ Develop lessons in a logical sequence ▪ Assess students formatively to ensure they make progress ▪ Create a community among online students ▪ Build social presence ▪ Create online environments that are safe and comfortable ▪ Instill rules for netiquette

Assess student learning	■ Design assessment for courses
	■ Provide timely, meaningful, and consistent feedback
	■ Evaluate and revise assessments in courses
	■ Provide individual and group feedback
	■ Use student data to guide the feedback process
	■ Provide information to students about their progress
	■ Provide feedback in written, audio, and video forms

Source: Martin, Budhrani, Kumar, & Ritzhaupt, 2019, p. 193.

◎ **Critical Thinking Question**

What teaching activities can be used to decrease the number of responses that nurse educators need to make to each learner on discussion boards?

Ragan (2012) identifies 10 principles of effective online teaching. The principles simply include; showing up on time, being proactive and communication, organizing the course, being flexible is a plan B is needed, providing timely feedback, communicating well, in other words, making sure the students understand the directions and intent of the communication, return assignments in an appropriate amount of time so students can learn from the comments, maintain course integrity, communicate in a secure system, and know the technology that is being used in the course.

Becoming skilled in online instruction is an iterative process. Jacobs (2015) offers some advice to the online instructor.

> The mechanics of preparing and teaching online courses is a constant learning process. There are new techniques developed every day to support instructors and students in online courses. This is what makes this particular aspect of academia exciting and challenging. The successful online instructor must be aware and comfortable with new innovative techniques designed to improve the operation of online courses. To benefit from these techniques, it is also important to understand the factors that affect student ability. One such factor would be the creation of a learning community fostered by a sense of social connectedness. It is equally important to understand the various factors that affect student satisfaction with an online course. The challenges can seem overwhelming at times. The key is to always maintain a sense of humor about the process (Jacobs, 2015, p. 6).

Evidence-Based Teaching Practice

Bravo-Agapito, Romero, and Pamplona (2021) completed a five-year investigation related to students learning completely online. The researchers used a multiple regression analysis to predict academic performance using the learning management platform Moodle. The variables studied were access (how many times the student used the platform), questions (interactions with faculty), task (completing assignments), and age. The results identified younger age as a negative predictor of students' performance.

COMMUNICATION

In an online learning environment, timely communication is essential. Fortunately, the instructor and learners can interact and communicate with each other, often in more substantive ways than traditionally afforded in the F2F classroom. Within the LMS, the instructor and learners can use built-in tools such as the following:

- Announcements (instructor only)—an easy way to disseminate course update information and remind learners of upcoming events and due dates
- Discussion board/voice board—can provide a centralized asynchronous message board to keep the lines of communication open among all class members
- Email/voicemail
- CMS/LMS instant messages
- Wikis and blogs—offer more robust authoring and collaborative capabilities, which can be effective in engaging students in active learning
- Synchronous class meeting rooms—virtual meeting rooms where attendees are present in "real time" although geographically dispersed (at remote locations)

Communication is essential when building a learning community within the online learning environment. The nurse educator must take a leadership role in "setting the stage" for expectations related to communication—either verbal or written—often referred to as netiquette. Ormrod (2011) identifies key features of learning communities in educational settings:

- All learners are active participants.
- Discussion and collaboration are common key elements.
- Diversity in learner interests and progress is expected and respected.
- Learners and teachers coordinate in helping one another learn; no one has exclusive responsibility for teaching others.
- Everyone is a potential resource for others; different individuals serve as resources for different topics and tasks.
- The teacher provides guidance and direction for activities, but learners also contribute.
- Constructive questioning and critiquing of one another's work is practiced.
- Process is emphasized as much as product.

Finally, the most important point regarding communication in the online learning environment is timeliness. Timely response to learners' questions or posts is absolutely essential.

Timely feedback contributes to student learning in that it helps reinforce new concepts that students are acquiring and helps prevent students from forming misconceptions. Generally, students will not incorporate feedback if it is not provided close to the time they have completed the assignment because the feedback loses relevance as the student has already "moved on" to the next assignment. Providing feedback in a timely manner allows students to better integrate what they have learned and incorporate your suggestions to improve their understanding (Spencer, 2017).

BENEFITS OF THE ONLINE LEARNING ENVIRONMENT

There are many benefits associated with the online learning environment. These include the following:

- Online courses can be packed with study material.
  - Instructors have limited contact hours each week in an on-campus class and, as a result, have to pick and choose their activities to fit the time.
  - In an online course, instructors are not bound by the limits of these contact hours and can provide additional materials, videos, demonstrations, discussions, and assignments that are not limited to 3 or 4 hours of "contact" with the course content each week.
  - However, instructors must consider ways to make the learning environment rich and not overload the course too much.
- Flexibility
  - The asynchronous nature of the majority of the course provides learners with great flexibility for participation
  - The time flexibility also applies to instructors
  - Classes can be conducted at any time of the day or night on any days of the week
- Opportunities for higher-level learning. Specifically, Web 2.0 tools:
  - Increase social engagement to enrich learning
  - Promote engagement and learning
  - Use of these technologies resulted in higher-order thinking, metacognitive awareness, teamwork/collaboration, improved affect toward school/learning, and ownership of learning (Chittleborough, Maybery, Patrick, & Reupert, 2009; Astriani, Susilo, Suwono, Lukiati & Purnomo, 2020).
- Increased opportunities for dialogue and questions.
  - Instructors can ask questions at any time during the course and have learners respond in a variety of ways, including discussion boards and emails
  - The online discussion may have deeper meaning, and learners have time to reflect on their responses
  - A typically "quiet" learner has an opportunity to participate fully
  - Learners can ask questions any time by email or by posting a question on a Q&A discussion forum
- Online course materials are reusable.
  - Instructors can reuse all or parts of their courses, including pithy comments and interesting discussions. (Although instructors might think that they are giving the same lecture from term to term in an on-campus course, they really are giving the same lecture in an online course, if they so choose.)
  - This gives instructors the opportunity to keep all the components that work well and modify the questionable ones.

COPYRIGHT LAW AND FAIR USE IN ONLINE LEARNING ENVIRONMENTS

The nurse educator who teaches in the online learning environment must have knowledge of copyright laws as these relate to academic use and the online learning environment. There are several laws that affect the use of materials for academic purposes. These include the following:

- The copyright laws
- Fair use
- The Technology, Education and Copyright Harmonization Act (TEACH Act) ("TEACH," 2006)

▶ COPYRIGHT LAWS

- "A form of protection provided by the laws of the United States to the authors of 'original works of authorship,' that are fixed in a tangible form of expression"
- Protects both published and unpublished works
- Protects exclusive rights of authors but authorizes others to do the following:

  - Reproduce the work in copies or phonorecords
  - Prepare derivative works based upon the work
  - Distribute copies or phonorecords of the work to the public by sale or other transfer of ownership, or by rental, lease, or lending
  - Perform the work publicly, in the case of literary, musical, dramatic, and choreographic works, pantomimes, and motion pictures and other audiovisual work
  - Display the work publicly, in the case of literary, musical, dramatic, and choreographic works, pantomimes, and pictorial, graphic, or sculptural works, including the individual images of a motion picture or other audiovisual work
  - Perform the work publicly (in the case of sound recordings) by means of a digital audio transmission" (U.S. Copyright Office, 2019, p. 2).

Refer to Exhibit 4.2 for more information regarding what materials are protected under the copyright laws and what materials are not.

TEACHING GEM Establish in the syllabus how often you will answer emails and questions, and if they will be answered on the weekends, so learners know what to expect regarding the nurse educator's response time.

Exhibit 4.2 Works Protected and Works Not Protected Under Copyright Laws

What Works Are Protected?

Copyright protects "original works of authorship" that are fixed in a tangible form of expression. The fixation need not be directly perceptible so long as it may be communicated with the aid of a machine or device. Copyrightable works include the following areas:

- Literary works
- Musical works, including any accompanying words
- Dramatic works, including any accompanying music
- Pantomimes and choreographic works
- Pictorial, graphic, and sculptural works
- Motion pictures and other audiovisual works
- Sound recordings
- Architectural works

These areas should be viewed broadly. For example, computer programs and most "compilations" may be registered as "literary works"; maps and architectural plans may be registered as "pictorial, graphic, and sculptural works."

What Is Not Protected by Copyright?

Several areas of material are generally not eligible for federal copyright protection. These include, among others:

- Ideas, procedures, methods, systems, processes, concepts, principles or discoveries
- Works that have not been fixed in a tangible form of expression (e.g., choreographic works that have not been notated or recorded, or improvisational speeches or performances that have not been written or recorded)
- Titles, names, short phrases, and slogans;
- Familiar symbols or designs
- Mere variations of typographic ornamentation, lettering or coloring
- Mere listings of ingredients or contents

Source: U.S. Copyright Office, 2019, p. 2.

▶ FAIR USE

"Section 107 under the copyright laws identifies four factors to be considered in determining whether or not a particular use is fair.

1. The purpose and character of the use, including whether such use is of commercial nature or is for non-profit educational purposes
2. The nature of the copyrighted work
3. The amount and substantiality of the portion used in relation to the copyrighted work as a whole
4. The effect of the use upon the potential market for, or value of, the copyrighted work" (United States Copyright Office, 2020)

If the concept of "fair use" is correctly applied, then it allows for the use of copyright-protected work without permission. However, it behooves the educator to be thoughtful in how materials are being used (Lamberson, 2020).

▶ THE TEACH ACT (TECHNOLOGY, EDUCATION AND COPYRIGHT HARMONIZATION ACT OF 2002)

- "Facilitates and enables the performance and display of copyrighted materials for distance education by accredited, non-profit educational institutions (and some government entities) that meet the TEACH Act's qualifying requirements.
- Its primary purpose is to balance the needs of distance learners and educators with the rights of copyright holders.
- The TEACH Act applies to distance education that includes the participation of any enrolled student, on or off campus" (Copyright Clearance Center, 2011, p. 1).

Crews (2010) provided a clear review and update regarding the TEACH Act and identified the following responsibilities of an instructor:

Exhibit 4.3 The TEACH Act: Description of Works Allowed and Excluded

Works explicitly allowed:

- Performances of nondramatic literary works
- Performances of nondramatic musical works
- Performances of any other work, including dramatic works and audiovisual works, but only in "reasonable and limited portions"
- Displays of any work "in an amount comparable to that which is typically displayed in the course of a live classroom session"

Works explicitly excluded:

- Works that are marketed "primarily for performance or display as part of mediated instructional activities transmitted via digital networks"
- Performances or displays given by means of copies "not lawfully made and acquired" under the U.S. Copyright ActU.S. Copyright Act, if the educational institution "knew or had reason to believe" that they were not lawfully made and acquired

Adapted from Crews (2010).

---

1. Select materials that are allowed by the TEACH Act (see Exhibit 4.3).
2. Instructor oversight: "An instructor seeking to use materials under the protection of the new statute must adhere to the following requirements:
   - The performance or display 'is made by, at the direction of, or under the actual supervision of an instructor.'
   - The materials are transmitted 'as an integral part of a class session offered as a regular part of the systematic mediated instructional activities' of the educational institution.
   - The copyrighted materials are 'directly related and of material assistance to the teaching content of the transmission.'
   - The requirements share a common objective: 'to assure that the instructor is ultimately in charge of the uses of copyrighted works and that the materials serve educational pursuits and are not for entertainment or any other purpose' (Crews, 2010, p. 5).

- The "use of the materials is integral to the course and under the instructor's supervision" (Crews, 2010, p. 5).
- Precludes "an instructor from including, in a digital transmission, copies of materials that are specifically marketed for and meant to be purchased by students outside of the classroom in the traditional teaching model" (Crews, 2010, p. 5). Specifically, instructors are prohibited from scanning textbook content for distribution to students—circumventing the required purchase of a textbook.

LEARNER ASSESSMENT IN THE ONLINE LEARNING ENVIRONMENT

Test security is always a concern in both the traditional and online classrooms. A concern expressed frequently by educators is that it is hard to monitor students in the online environment to ensure they are not cheating on tests. There are several techniques to use to prevent, or at least minimize, cheating.

- Proactive measures:
  - Education regarding academic integrity—some organizations provide mandatory training for all students to heighten awareness and understanding
  - Clear statements in student handbooks
- Low-tech measures:
  - Signature of integrity—required for all assignments and tests—is accompanied by a statement that attests to the originality of the document (Exhibit 4.4)
- High-tech measures:
  - Originality verification
    - Turnitin
    - iThenticate
    - WriteCheck
- Proctoring resources
  - ProctorU
  - Remote proctor

These tools and strategies can be effective deterrents, but it is important to note that it is not possible to prevent or detect all incidents of cheating. The most important proactive measure that an educator can take is to convey the expectation of academic integrity and endeavor to create a culture of ethics.

Exhibit 4.4 Intellectual Honesty Certification Statement

I certify that this assignment is presented as entirely my own intellectual work. Any words and/or ideas from other sources (e.g., printed publications, Internet sites, electronic media, other individuals, groups, or organizations) have been properly indicated using the appropriate scholarly citation style required by the department or college.

I have not submitted this assignment in its entirety to satisfy the requirements of any other course. Any parts of this assignment from other courses have been discussed thoroughly with the faculty member before this submission so that there is an understanding that I have used some of this work in a prior assignment.

Student's Signature: _____

Course Submitted: _____

Term: _____

Date: _____

Source: Gambescia (2010). Reprinted with permission.

CASE STUDIES

CASE STUDY 4.1

A nurse educator at a small midwestern hospital has just joined a regional consortium of health care systems that have formed the alliance to address mutual interests and share costs. One priority area that has been identified is that of ongoing staff education and in-service updates. The nurse educator has been asked to develop a series of online courses that can be distributed to all partner-organization employees, starting with one on the health insurance portability and accountability act. Describe an approach to the design and implementation of this online course. How will the course be structured? How will the content be delivered?

CASE STUDY 4.2

A nurse educator has taught a very popular course in the traditional F2F classroom. Within this course, she uses a variety of interactive classroom strategies designed to engage the students in active learning—including small-group work, debates, case studies, guest speakers, and student-led panel discussions. The dean wants this educator to take the course online. Discuss the strategies that would be used to transfer the course to the online learning environment while still maintaining these highly interactive learning activities.

1. A priority asset of online teaching includes:

   A. Student control over the content
   B. Lock-step module engagement
   C. An individualized, learner-centered learning experience
   D. More opportunities to interact with classmates

2. An online nurse educator provides a written transcript for a video that is including in the course. The nurse educator is incorporating which of the following quality design standards identified by QualityMatters™ (2016)?

   A. Course technology
   B. Accessibility
   C. Learner interaction
   D. Learner support

3. In an online course, which of the following will provide one-on-one interaction with the nurse educator:

   A. Asynchronous office hours
   B. Discussion board responses
   C. Synchronous office hours
   D. Class lecture with content quiz

4. A nurse educator is mapping the course student learning outcomes to the course content and assignments. The nurse educator understands that this is referred to as:

   A. Curriculum mapping
   B. Scaffolding
   C. Levelling
   D. Alignment

5. A nurse educator requests a recommendation to use a low-tech strategy to improve test integrity. A suggestion may be:

   A. Clear statement in student handbook
   B. Originality verification
   C. Education regarding academic integrity
   D. Collecting a signature of integrity

1. C) An individualized, learner-centered learning experience

Generally, online courses provide students with a more individualized, learner-centered learning experience and are often self-paced to a limited extent. Not all online learning courses are lock-step, and many have varying degrees of control or may not have peer interactions.

2. B) Accessibility

The online nurse educator must provide alternative formats to students in order to accommodate diverse learning needs of the student. Learner support, interactions, and technology needs are addressed by different online methods.

3. C) Synchronous office hours

Providing an opportunity for the student to meet with faculty synchronously, via a synchronous office hour virtual meeting, is a good strategy to increase 1:1 student/faculty interaction. Discussion board responses, asynchronous hours, and lectures will not provide one-to-one interactions.

4. D) Alignment

Alignment refers to how learning outcomes are linked with course materials and assessments. It is important to make sure the learning outcomes are met, and alignment ensures that this occurs.

5. A) Clear statement in student handbook

A low-tech strategy to ensure academic integrity would be to obtain a signature of integrity (that attests to the originality of the assignment submitted) from the student and require this for all assignments and tests. Originality verification, education, and collection of signatures take more effort.

6. A nurse educator who is designing an online course to be usable by all people to the greatest extent possible is employing which design?

   A. Usable
   B. Accessible
   C. Universal
   D. Versatile

7. The nurse educator wants to ensure that learners can complete course requirements with a reasonable amount of effort and achieve the course student learning outcomes. The nurse educator is ensuring:

   A. Efficiency and effectiveness
   B. Learnability and efficiency
   C. Consistency and effectiveness
   D. Usability and efficiency

8. A nurse educator would like to increase the cognitive presence in an online course. The best way to do this would be to:

   A. Develop an introduction discussion board
   B. Use a video to orientate students to the course
   C. Provide reflective questions after content
   D. Use warm-up exercises that add points to the grade

9. The nurse educator is providing alternative means of access to course materials in formats that meet the needs of diverse learners. This teaching method is called:

   A. Support
   B. Accessibility
   C. Interaction
   D. Engagement

10. The nurse educator developed a course that delivers less than 20% of the content online. The college registrar has correctly listed this course as:

    A. Blended
    B. Hybrid
    C. Dual
    D. Web-facilitated

(See answers next page.)

6. C) Universal

Universal design ensures that the course and course content is usable by all people regardless of their abilities. Usability, accessibility, and versatile designs do not reach as many people as universal.

7. A) Efficiency and effectiveness

Ensuring learners can perform requirements with a minimal amount of effort and achieve the course goals is called efficiency and effectiveness. Usability, learnability, and consistency are different attributes of a course.

8. C) Provide reflective questions after content

Using a reflective assignment about content assists the student to process the information. Using introductions and orientations assist with social presence. Warm-ups may assist with test taking.

9. B) Accessibility

Providing alternative means of access to course materials in formats that meet the needs of diverse learners is called providing accessibility to the learner.

10. D) Web-facilitated

Courses that deliver less than 20% of content online are considered Web-facilitated. Online just assists in making course material available to the learner.

REFERENCES

Ackehurst, M. & Polvere, R. (2020). Evolutional librarianship: From supermarket to smorgasbord. *Journal of Web Librarianship, 14*(3/4), 74–85. 10.1080/19322909.2020.1823299

Allen, I. E., & Seaman, J. (2011). Going the distance: Online education in the United States, 2011. *Babson Survey Research Group and Quahog Research Group, LLC.* http://www.onlinelearningsurvey.com/reports/goingthedistance.pdf

Astriani, D., Susilo, H., Suwono, H., Lukiati, B. & Purnomo, A. (2020). Mind mapping in learning models: A tool to improve student metacognitive skills. *International Journal of Emerging Technologies in Learning (iJET), 15*(6), 4–17.

Bigatel, P. M., Ragan, L. C., Kennan, S., May, J., & Redmond, B. F. (2012). The identification of competencies for online teaching success. *Journal of Asynchronous Learning Networks, 16*(1), 59–77.

Brinthaupt, T., Fisher, L., Gardner, J., Raffo, D., & Woodard, J. (2011). What the best online teachers should do. *Journal of Online Learning and Teaching, 7*(4). http://jolt.merlot.org/vol7no4/brinthaupt_1211.htm

Bravo-Agapito, J., Romero, S. J., & Pamplona, S. (2021). Early prediction of undergraduate Student's academic performance in completely online learning: A five-year study. *Computers in Human Behavior, 115.* 10.1016/j.chb.2020.106595

Bonnel, W., & Boehm, H. (2011). Improving feedback to students online: Teaching tips from experienced faculty. *Journal of Continuing Education in Nursing, 42*(11), 503–509.

Carnegie Mellon University. (n.d.). Why should assessments, learning objectives, and instructional strategies be aligned? http://www.cmu.edu/teaching/assessment/basics/alignment.html

Chittleborough, P., Maybery, D., Patrick, K., & Reupert, A. (2009). The importance of being human: Instructors' personal presence in distance programs. *International Journal of Teaching & Learning in Higher Education, 21*(1), 47–56. http://files.eric.ed.gov/fulltext/EJ896241.pdf

Cook, D. A. (2007). Web-based learning: Pros, cons and controversies. *Clinical Medicine, 7*(1), 37–42. http://www.clinmed.rcpjournal.org/content/7/1/37.full.pdf+html

Cook, D. A., & Dupras, D. M. (2004). A practical guide to developing effective web-based learning. *Journal of General Internal Medicine, 19*(6), 698–707. http://www.ncbi.nlm.nih.gov/pmc/articles/PMC1492389/pdf/jgi_30029.pdf

Copyright Clearance Center. (2011). The TEACH Act: New roles, rules and responsibilities for academic institutions. http://www.copyright.com/wp-content/uploads/2015/04/CR-Teach-Act.pdf

Crews, K. (2010). Copyright law and distance education: Overview of the TEACH Act. http://www.ala.org/advocacy/copyright/teachact/distanceeducation#newc

Esfijani, A. (2018). Measuring quality in online education: A meta-synthesis. *American Journal of Distance Education, 32*(1), 57–73. 10.1080/08923647.2018.1417658

Gambescia, S. (2010). *Intellectual honesty certification.* Philadelphia, PA: Drexel University College of Nursing and Health Professions. http://www.pages.drexel.edu/~cnhp/blackboard/ihcertification.html

Gay, G. H. E. (2016). An assessment of online instructor e-learning readiness before, during, and after course delivery. *Journal of Computers in Higher Education*, 28, 199–220. 10.1007/s12528-016-9115-z

Hathaway, K. L. (2013). An application of the seven principles of good practice to online courses. *Research in Higher Education Journal*, 22, 1–13. http://www.aabri.com/manuscripts/131676.pdf

Hoffmann, R. L., Klein, S. J., & Rosenzweig, M. Q. (2017). Creating quality online materials for specialty nurse practitioner content: Filling a need for the graduate nurse practitioner. *Journal of Cancer Education*, 32, 522–527. 10.1007/s13187-015-0980-3

Ilkay, A. O., & Zeynep, C. O. (2014). Impacts of e-learning in nursing education: In the light of recent studies. *World Academy of Science, Engineering and Technology International Journal of Social Behavioural, Education, Economic and Management Engineering*, 8(5), 1285–1287.

Jacobs, P. (2015). Suggestions for a smooth running online course. *Research in Higher Education Journal*, 29, 1–8.

Jensen, J. L., McDaniel, M. A., Woodard, S. M., & Kummer, T. A. (2014). Teaching to the test…or testing to teach: exams requiring higher order thinking skills encourage greater conceptual understanding. *Educational Psychology Review*, 26, 307–329. 10.1007/s10648-013-9248-9.

Kohan, B. (2010). What is a content management system (CMS)? Views about enterprise web application development research and reports. http://www.comentum.com/what-is-cms-content-management-system.html

Lamberson, N. (2020). Six copyright concepts your K-12 students should know. Library of Congress. https://blogs.loc.gov/copyright/category/copyright-in-education/

Learning management system. (n.d.). In *PC Mag.com encyclopedia*. http://www.pcmag.com/encyclopedia

Lorenzo, G. & Moore, J. (2002). The Sloan Consortium Report to the Nation: Five pillars of quality online education. https://www.understandingxyz.com/index_htm_files/SloanCReport-five%20pillars.pdf

Martin, F., Budhrani, K., Kumar, S., & Ritzhaupt, A. (2019). Award-winning faculty online teaching practices: Roles and competencies. *Online Learning*, 23(1), 184–205. 10.24059/olj.v23i1.1329

Matuga, J. M. (2006). The role of assessment and evaluation in context: Pedagogical alignment, constraints, and affordances in online courses. In D. Williams, M. Hricko & S. Howell (Eds.), *Online assessment, measurement and evaluation: Emerging practices* (pp. 316–330). Idea Group Publishing. 10.4018/978-1-59140-747-8.ch019

McCutcheon, K., Lohan, M., Traynor, M., & Martin, D. (2015). A systematic review evaluating the impact of online or blended learning vs. face-to-face learning of clinical skills in undergraduate nurse education. *Journal of Advanced Nursing*, 71(2), 255–270. 10.1111/jan.12509

McGarry, B. J., Theobald, K., Lewis, P. A., & Coyer, F. (2015). Flexible learning design in curriculum delivery promotes student engagement and develops metacognitive learners: An integrated review. *Nurse Education Today*, 35(9), 966. 10.1016/j.nedt.2015.06.009

McGillion, A. (2020). Collaboration —the key to success in transitioning to online learning. *Australian Nursing & Midwifery Journal*, 27(2), 47.

National League for Nursing. (2021). Certified Nurse Educator (CNE) 2021 candidate handbook. http://www.nln.org/docs/default-source/default-document-library/cne-handbook-2021_revised_07-01-2021.pdf?sfvrsn=2

National League for Nursing. (2021). Certified Nurse Educator Novice (CNEn) 2021 candidate handbook. http://www.nln.org/Certification-for-Nurse-Educators/cne-n/cne-n-handbook

Ormrod, J. E. (2011). *Human learning* (6th ed.). Prentice Hall.

Pape-Zambito, D. A. & Mostrom, A. M. (2018). Improving teaching through triadic course alignment. *Journal of Microbiology Biology Education, 19*, 1–6. 10.1128/jmbe.v19i3.1642.

Phipps, R., & Merisotis, J. (2000). *Quality on the line: Benchmarks for success in Internet-based distance education*. The Institute for Higher Education Policy. http://www.ihep.org/assets/files/publications/m-r/QualityOnTheLine.pdf

Quality Matters™. (2018). *Higher education rubric* (6th ed.). Author. https://www.qualitymatters.org/sites/default/files/PDFs/StandardsfromtheQMHigherEducationRubric.pdf

Quality Matters™. (2016). What is the QM Program? http://www.qmprogram.org

Ragan, L. (2012). 10 principles of effective online teaching: Best practices in distance education. *Magna Publications*. https://www.mnsu.edu/cetl/teachingwithtechnology/tech_resources_pdf/Ten%20Principles%20of%20Effective%20Online%20Teaching.pdf. Reprinted by permission of the author.

Rouamba, G. H. (2020). An online institute for teaching graduate students to design online courses: A design-based research study (Order No. 27737284). Available from ProQuest One Academic. (2382059220).

Robinson, C. C., & Hullinger, H. (2008). New benchmarks in higher education: Student engagement in online learning. *Journal of Education for Business, 84*(2), 101–108.

Sheffield, M. (2015). Exploring future teachers' awareness, competence, confidence, and attitudes regarding teaching online: incorporating blended/online experience into the teaching and learning in higher education course for graduate students. *Canadian Journal of Higher Education, 45*(3), 1–14.

Shim, T. E., & Lee, S. Y. (2020). College students' experience of emergency remote teaching due to COVID-19. *Children & Youth Services Review, 119*, N.PAG-N.PAG. 10.1016/j.childyouth.2020.105578

Smith, T. C. (2005). Fifty-one competencies for online instruction. *Journal of Educators Online, 2*(2), 1–18.

Spencer, B. (2017). The importance of timely and effective feedback, Satche. https://blog.teamsatchel.com/the-importance-of-timely-and-effective-feedback

TEACH Act—A Distance educator's update. (2006). *Distance Education Report, 10*(23), 5–8.

Terantino, J. M., & Agbehonou, E. (2012). Comparing faculty perceptions of an online development course: Addressing faculty needs for online teaching. *Online Journal of Distance Learning Administration, XIV*(II). http://www.westga.edu/~distance/ojdla/summer152/terantino_agbehonou152.html

U.S. Copyright Office. (2019). Copyright basics. https://www.copyright.gov/circs/circ01.pdf

U.S. Copyright Office. (2020). U.S. Copyright Office fair use index. https://www.copyright.gov/fair-use/

Varvel, V. E. (2007). Master online teacher competencies. *Online Journal of Distance Learning Administration, X*(I).http://www.westga.edu/~distance/ojdla/spring101/varvel101.htm

Skills Laboratory Learning

Carol Okupniak and Anita Fennessey

When you know better, you do better.
—Maya Angelou

► LEARNING OUTCOMES

This chapter also addresses the Certified Nurse Educator Exam and the Certified Nurse Educator Novice exam Content Area 1: Facilitate Learning

- Define skills laboratory learning
- Identify skills that can be practiced in a learning laboratory
- Develop practice and testing environment for fundamental and advanced nursing skills
- Understand how to rehearse clinical skills safely before learners take care of real patients
- Prepare and organize a skills laboratory
- Incorporate nursing research and evidence-based practice into clinical skills training
- Understand laboratory training in relation to clinical expectations of the nursing programs
- Evaluate learner competencies in the skills laboratory

INTRODUCTION

In the skills laboratory, nurse educators create an atmosphere in which learners acquire new skills in a supportive, caring, and nonthreatening environment. A well-designed nursing skills laboratory should closely reflect the clinical environment where learners will care for their patients. The skills laboratory is a place where learners can practice the principles and technical skills necessary for safe patient care. Learners should be given the opportunity in a nursing skills laboratory to develop their skills from beginner to proficient. The skills laboratory is an area where learners are taught through activities that support multiple learning styles. Learners are also taught the principles of evidence-based practice (EBP) as it applies to nursing skills. The learning that takes place in the skills laboratory will be transferred to the clinical setting and will be the foundation on which professional practice is built.

Virtual clinical learning has been shown to be an effective substitute for actual face-to-face clinical learning when there is lack of appropriate opportunities, such as occurred during the COVID-19 pandemic (Fogg et al., 2020). Transitioning skills laboratory learning to virtual learning requires more specific planning, including guaranteeing that students have the proper equipment needed to facilitate this process, such as skills packets. Skills packets may contain such items as Foley catheterization kits, nasogastric tubes, colostomy bag, wound care, and sterile dressing materials. Virtual simulation products such as Lippincott's© vSIM© for Nursing and Assessment Technology Institute® (ATI), LLC, Skills Modules provide the initial instruction, which is followed up by live virtual sessions. During these live sessions, the clinical instructor demonstrates procedures/skills and then provides the student an opportunity to perform these procedures/skills virtually. Verification of skills is documented through an in-person acquisition of skills competency. Evaluation methodologies are developed to ensure achievement of course and program objectives which should correspond with the student's ability to transfer learning to the clinical environment.

● LEARNING IN THE LABORATORY

Learning in the laboratory can best be described as experiential because nurse educators incorporate both patient information and critical thinking skills to lead to clinical reasoning, including the following:

- Creating new knowledge through the transformation of experience
- Incorporating new experiences into the learner's existing cognitive framework
- Helping learners develop critical thinking and clinical reasoning
- Creating a learning environment in the laboratory in which skills are not only demonstrated but new behaviors are learned
- Evaluate the effectiveness of deliberate practice on learning skills
- Reviewing previously taught skills using reflection, scenario-based learning, and return demonstration (Tutticci et al., 2018)
- Integrating experiential learning theory and nursing education
- Learn communication skills to demonstrate proficiency in caring for vulnerable populations (Felsenstein, 2019; Maruca et al., 2018)

The clinical learning environment (CLE) is one of the best places for students to practice the psychomotor skills needed in professional nursing. The CLE can also be used to practice nontechnical skills (NTS) such as social, cognitive, and decision-making skills (Fukuta & Litsuka, 2018). Nursing students are often very concerned about mastering skills to gain confidence in their roles. The learning skills laboratory assists learners to gain confidence in their roles. Examples of common psychomotor skills, social skills, and cognitive skills for nursing learners, from beginning to advanced, are outlined in Tables 5.1, 5.2, and 5.3.

Table 5.1 Common Psychomotor Skills

Beginning skills	■ Assessment
	  ● Head-to-toe established routine
	  ● Normal versus abnormal
	  ● Essential equipment needed for
	  ● Vital signs
	  ● Neurological evaluations
	■ Transmission-based precautions
	  ● Standard precautions
	  ● Contact precautions
	  ● Droplet precautions
	  ● Airborne precautions
	■ Medication administration
	  ● Improving students' skills of pharmacology and medication calculation are beneficial in relation to preventing medication errors (Latimer et al., 2017)
	  ● Use a variety of different teaching different methods for math calculation (Osahor et al., 2019)
	  ● Enhance medication administrator competency using realistic simulations and hands-on workshops (Owegi et al., 2021)
	  ● Mnemonics
	  ● Flashcards
	  ● Small group work
	  ● Logical step methodology
	■ Nursing skills (examples)
	  ● Bed bath
	  ● Mobility
	  ● Transfers
	  ● Bed making
	  ● Infection control

Advanced skills	■ Application of patient assessment with medication administration
	■ When to refuse to administer an ordered medication
	■ Appropriate steps to take when medications are not given
	■ Nursing skills (examples)
	  ● Wound care
	  ● Urinary catheter insertion
	  ● Nasogastric tube placement and care
	  ● Tracheostomy care and suction
	  ● Chest tubes
	  ● Intravenous therapy

Table 5.2 Social Skills

Social skills	▪ Verbal communication ▪ Nonverbal communication ▪ Active listening ▪ Team work ▪ Compassion ▪ Inspire trust ▪ Empathy ▪ Cultural awareness ▪ Patient education ▪ Open mindedness ▪ Flexibility ▪ Leadership ▪ Delegation

Table 5.3 Cognitive Skills

Cognitive skills	▪ Critical thinking ▪ Clinical decision making ▪ Problem-based learning ▪ Inquiry ▪ Patient perspective ▪ Clinical reasoning ▪ Creativity ▪ Transfer of knowledge ▪ Application of evidence-based practice

LABORATORY SAFETY

It is critically important to maintain a safe environment in the clinical learning laboratory. Safety of all occupants must be considered. Users of the clinical laboratory must be aware of all safety guidelines. Physical safety includes but is not limited to:

▪ Absence of latex products
▪ Use of mock medications—no real medication should be used—with clear indication on the label that the medication is not for human consumption
▪ Policies and procedures in place should staff, faculty, or learner experience an illness, accident, or injury
▪ Properly functioning equipment with guidelines for maintenance of equipment— remove any broken, damaged, or malfunctioning equipment from the clinical laboratory

■ Clean environment—adhere to infection control principles
■ Appropriate personal protective equipment (PPE) if needed
■ Appropriate sharps disposal—do not overfill sharps containers; remove and dispose when maximum capacity reached
■ Adherence to occupancy limits—overcrowding can create a hazard in the event of a fire and low-residency regulations should there be a need due to a widespread infectious outbreak
■ Fire safety plan—clear egress without obstacles

EVIDENCE-BASED TEACHING PRACTICE

Henderson et al. (2018) used Check-in and Check-out (CICO) to help students prepare for clinical practice. This three-part process uses briefing, practicing clinical skills, and debriefing to engage students in active learning. The CICO process creates a collaborative connection between student and teacher in the clinical learning laboratory and encourages student expression and feedback.

SKILLS LABORATORY LEARNING ACTIVITIES

The basic principles of skills learning are as follows:

■ Learning the steps of skills
■ Providing a full explanatory demonstration by faculty
■ Using an evidence-based skills video to view prior to demonstration
■ Progressing from skill acquisition to skill retention (Nicholls et al., 2016)
■ Understanding the scientific basis for the skill
■ Using current evidence-based skills
■ Ensuring a safe environment during the implementation of the skill
■ Demonstrating safety when performing the skill including:
  ● Safety for simulated patient, learner, and faculty
  ● Equipment safety
  ● No distractions
    ● No talking
    ● Simulating visitors/providers should not move about room
    ● Determine appropriate use of mobile devices (Alsayed et al., 2020)
■ Using multimedia to teach nursing skills (i.e., video podcasting, which has been found to increase the learner's confidence in performing clinical skills (Stone et al., 2020)
■ Using computer programs

- Recording skills on video when possible and ensuring student privacy and confidentiality
- Learning management systems to embed video, animation, and so on
- Using virtual reality simulations including: Adult Virtual I.V. ® (Intravenous) trainer; Lippincott's© vSIM© for Nursing; Assessment Technology Institute® (ATI), LLC, Real Life Cases; National League for Nursing's Advancing Care Excellence for Seniors (ACE.S), etc.
- Utilizing deliberate practice until proficient

DELIBERATE PRACTICE

Deliberate practice refers to the repeated practice of a structural activity with the objective of advancing performance. The expert performance approach is the basis of deliberate practice in which mastery is achieved through consistent repetitive practice of a skill (Owen et al., 2017).

- Rapid cycle deliberate practice has learners repeat required skills until proficient, reducing the amount of time it takes to learn a skill (Lemke et al., 2019; Ozkara et al., 2021). Activities are developed to conquer explicit weaknesses, with faculty evaluating skills throughout the experience to improve performance (Owen et al., 2017). Faculty facilitate repetitive practice with peer mentoring to assist and expedite skill competence and retention (Ross, 2019).

▶ NURSING STUDENT PORTFOLIOS SHOULD INCLUDE CLINICAL SKILL ACHIEVEMENT

Portfolios can be hard copy or electronic and include:

- Learner's knowledge, skills, and accomplishments with teaching assessment, progression, and evaluation along with career objectives and professional goals (Chang et al., 2017)
- Documentation of competency
- Verification by faculty
- Used in conjunction with résumé for job search

◎ **Critical Thinking Question**

What are the essential components of the learner's portfolio that the nurse educator should encourage collection of in order to enhance their chances of employment post-graduation?

▶ PRACTICE COMPUTER DOCUMENTATION

- Informatics competencies can be effectively practiced in the clinical skills lab (Monsen et al., 2019)
- Computer documentation practice in the learning laboratory gives students the opportunity to Practice assessment and procedural documentation improving computer literacy (Mollart et al., 2020)
- Computerized charts used in the clinical skills laboratory can help learners' use clinical reasoning to understand the context whereby a skill is necessary for a patient with a specific healthcare condition
- Computerized medication administration record (MAR) includes development in:
  - Scanning bar codes
  - Scanning quick response (QR) codes—this technology is newer than bar code scans and holds more information than a bar code (Figure 5.1)
  - QR codes can be strategically placed in the skills learning lab with instructor-led information at each skills station (Shustack, 2018)

TEACHING GEM Learners may be more successful in learning a skill if they understand the physiological concept behind the task and if the skill is embedded in a case study.

Figure 5.1 An optically readable quick response (QR) two-dimensional bar code

▶ PRACTICE THE SKILL OF DELEGATION

- Critical thinking related to delegation can be practiced in the skills laboratory, including responsibility and accountability of delegation
- Understanding the rules for delegating skills or tasks to unlicensed assistive personnel (UAP)
- Stating the requirements governing delegation to UAP or licensed practical nurses (LPNs)

TEACHING GEM Virtual reality-based skills training is emerging as an effective teaching method used to train learners in psychomotor skills (Bayram & Caliskan, 2019).

● EQUIPMENT NEEDED TO ENSURE LEARNING OUTCOMES

Both learners and nurse educators need to know the safe operation of all laboratory equipment. The purchase and maintenance of equipment must be an ongoing, thoughtful process for program directors and nurse educators. Equipment is often referred to using the following terms:

- Low fidelity—technical skills performance—anatomical models
- Mid-fidelity—limited computer operations—heart and lung sounds
- High fidelity—complex computer systems with ability to change physiology (Daley et al., 2018)

Some basic tenets of equipment use and maintenance are listed in the following:

- Safety of all equipment must be established prior to use
- Equipment similar to what the learner will experience in a clinical environment should be used
- Faculty may need additional education and training to use new equipment
- Invite a guest lecturer or representative of the technology company to demonstrate the equipment to learners
- Allow learners time to practice with equipment before testing their knowledge
- Make sure all equipment is functioning as desired prior to using for skills. Someone should be identified as a technological resource to troubleshoot technical malfunctions if needed

▶ EQUIPMENT LEARNERS NEED

Learners are instructed to purchase equipment to be used in both the skills laboratory and their clinical practice. Some programs have the learners purchase a tote bag of equipment that will be needed, whereas other programs ask the learners to purchase separate items such as:

- Watch with a second hand (water-resistant is preferred)
- Mobile device used to reference skills, medications, lab values, patient education material, evidence-based practice (EBP) guidelines, and so forth, per institution policy
- Stethoscope (must include bell-listening device)
- Penlight
- Name tag
- Ink pen (black only)

● LABORATORY ATTIRE, APPEARANCE, AND BEHAVIOR

Because the skills laboratory is a simulation of a clinical setting, most nurse educators believe that laboratory attire should be professional (Tomlinson & Jackson, 2021) and include the following:

- Laboratory coat
- Student uniform or street clothes reflecting professional attire
- Shoes need to be flat, comfortable, and enclosed

▶ PERSONAL APPEARANCE

Personal appearance should also simulate the expectations of the clinical environment, including:

- No artificial nails
- No nail polish
- Hair secured to nape of neck or put up
- No excessive perfume
- No dangling jewelry (safety hazard)

▶ INTEGRITY

Nursing learners are asked to adhere to the code of conduct that is determined by the institution and is recorded for their reference in the organization's student handbook or program guide. The essential attributes of integrity for a skills laboratory include:

- Honesty
- Ethical behavior
- Professionalism (Devine & Chin, 2018)

▶ LEARNERS WITH DISABILITIES

Learners with disabilities in the Skills Learning Lab:

- All learners should be held to the same academic standards regardless of disability
- Accommodations are in place to make sure that learners with disabilities have the same opportunity to achieve these standards
- According to the Americans with Disabilities Act (ADA), an institution may have to modify policies and practices that may discriminate against learners with disabilities
- The ADA does not require that the academic standards be altered
- Determining if a learner can practice safely is standard criteria for progression
- An institution must define safe practice (Meeks et al., 2020)
- Learners identified as having a disability and requiring accommodations in the learning lab may require a specific plan to address their identified learning need (L'Ecuyer, 2019)

⬤ EVALUATION AND REMEDIATION

Evaluating the skills acquired by the learner is a time-consuming and important task for the nurse educator, which commonly includes the following components:

- Skills checklists
  - Clarify and justify those skills required to be competent
  - Prepare a review of each skill when completed and discuss with student
- Importance of modeling experts who perform skills or tasks with accuracy and consistency
  - Careful answers to questions
  - Emphasize important information
  - Asks questions that elicit reasoning
  - Recognize strengths and weaknesses
  - Guide students to useful resources
  - Being organized (Parvan et al., 2018)
- Agency-based policy and procedure manual
  - Pass or fail skill evaluation with explanation of errors
    - Able to perform with or without assistance from the faculty
    - If with assistance or with questions from faculty, determine how much facilitation should be offered by faculty
- Allow to repeat skill at a later date after remediation
  - Educator may want to have a different or additional laboratory faculty member evaluate a repeated skill
- Evaluate learner ability to practice safely in a clinical environment
  - Evaluate a chosen practice skill
  - Determine how well the skills are developed:
    - Identify and intervene when at-risk students are identified (Donnell et al., 2018)
    - Is the learner competent to complete the skill in any clinical setting?
- Evaluate using all learning domains—cognitive, psychomotor, and affective

---

EVIDENCE-BASED TEACHING PRACTICE

Learners with disabilities in the Skills Learning Lab (1) All learners should be held to the same academic standards regardless of disability (2) Accommodations are in place to make sure that learners with disabilities have the same opportunity to achieve these standards (3) According to the Americans with Disabilities Act (ADA), an institution may have to modify policies and practices that may discriminate against learners with disabilities (4) The ADA does not require that the academic standards be altered (5) Determining if a learner can practice safely is standard criteria for progression (6) An institution must define safe practice (Meeks et al., 2020) (7) Learners identified as having a disability and requiring accommodations in the learning lab may require a specific plan to address their identified learning need (L'Ecuyer, 2019).

▶ REMEDIATION

- Required by faculty for improved performance
- Open skills practice
  - Learners require open laboratory practice time
  - Improves learners' skills, knowledge, and clinical reasoning
  - Learners may wish to learn a skill practiced at their clinical site (Herrman, 2015)
- Student-centered approach includes:
  - Individualized instruction
  - Peer tutoring (Li et al., 2018)
  - Evaluation of improvement

TEACHING GEM Remediation helps to improve retention in academic programs, decrease attrition, and improve student success (Thilges & Schmer, 2020).

⬤ INTEGRATING RESEARCH IN THE SKILLS LABORATORY

The skills laboratory is a great place to support nursing research by demonstrating how research is translated into practice and by developing the thinking process needed for clinical reasoning needed after graduation. It has been documented that learners feel more equipped to perform patient-centered care and less prepared to perform quality improvement skills (Cengiz & Yoder, 2020). Therefore, it is essential to:

- Incorporate EBP into nursing research courses (Cardoso et al., 2021)
- Increase EBP for skill development
- Understand the need for EBP skills and incorporate objective structural clinical examinations (OSCEs) skills in the lab
  - Develop reliable methods of evaluating critical clinical skills and competency
  - Foster development of communication for the healthcare setting, which requires an understanding of cultural values and norms (Henderson & Barker, 2018)

EVIDENCE-BASED TEACHING PRACTICE

Kohtz et al. (2017) replicated a study that looked at the physical assessment skills taught to undergraduate nursing students in comparison to the physical assessment skills actually used in practice. The results of this research showed that nurse educators need to differentiate between what the learner needs to know and provide the opportunity for the learner to achieve the competency of those skills most needed to provide optimal patient outcomes.

⬤ NURSING SKILLS LABORATORY MANAGEMENT

Management of a skills laboratory includes consideration of:

- Supplies and equipment meeting the curricular needs
- Adhering to safe lab practice guidelines maintained

- Ensuring adequate space is given for student practice and testing
- Providing faculty and student orientation to laboratory equipment and laboratory policy
- Defining faculty role in the skills laboratory
- Consistently demonstrate skills taught
- Ensuring the laboratory design is learner-centered
- Creating opportunities for remediation and skills practice
- Maintaining revenue for disposable supplies, equipment maintenance, and upgrades
- Organizing laboratory staff management
- Supporting skills based on EBP
- Collaborating with clinical facilities to assist with the computer learning objectives
- Educating faculty to ensure competency with existing equipment and with any new equipment obtained

---

TEACHING GEM Permitting students to use mobile technology is a way to access evidence-based nursing resources (George et al., 2017).

CASE STUDIES

CASE STUDY 5.1

A learner in the skills laboratory is having trouble donning sterile gloves because of excessively sweaty hands. As a nurse educator, how would you handle this situation? Is it a functional issue? Larger gloves, different types of gloves, and a small amount of powder on hands? Is it a psychological issue? Anxiety? Send to student services, provide relaxation techniques? Is it a physiological issue? allergy? Is a health workup indicated?

CASE STUDY 5.2

A learner has to care for a transgender patient for the first time (Montes-Galdeano et al., 2021). The learner has been raised in a very strict religious home and is having difficulties understanding how to approach the patient. How would you instruct the learner to meet and care for this patient?

CASE STUDY 5.3

During a health assessment skills lab, the learner consistently palpates the abdomen prior to auscultation. The learner states, "I just cannot remember the correct order; does it really matter?"
How would you address this question and help the student perform this skill correctly?

CASE STUDY 5.4

A learner in the skills lab becomes extremely anxious and disrupts the learning environment when you discuss the need for personal protective equipment in relation to potential health risks when caring for patients. How do you proceed with addressing this student's anxiety when maintaining the continuity of the skills lab for the other learners?

1. Which of the following demonstrates the practice of social skills in a clinical learning laboratory?

   A. The learner applies what they learned about handwashing from a research article when doing a wound dressing change procedure

   B. During a case-based activity, the learner holds a patient's antihypertensive medication when they determine the blood pressure on a mid-fidelity manikin is 82/54

   C. Learners are given wheelchairs and crutches and told to navigate the lab, bathroom, and lunchroom using this equipment

   D. A standardized patient actor of Asian descent comes to the lab to speak to the learners about how their culture impacts healthcare decisions

2. Which of the following strategies would be the best for senior-level nursing learners to gain confidence in starting an intravenous (IV) access on a patient?

   A. Ensure a working arm is available with the properly simulated medication vial and the correct needle and syringe

   B. Use a mid-fidelity manikin with a simulated IV taped to the forearm

   C. Have the learner verbalize the proper sequence of IV push medication administration

   D. Have an injection pad available and a simulated vial of the prescribed medication

3. Which of the following activities would be the best to measure senior nursing students' high-level clinical decision-making?

   A. Learners are able to choose the correct supplies from a variety of needles and syringes when practicing intramuscular (IM) injections

   B. Learners gather all necessary supplies and equipment prior to performing tracheostomy care and suctioning

   C. Learners are given a medical record and history from a simulated patient and need to administer medication

   D. Learners are required to teach a nursing skill to their peers in the clinical skill laboratory

4. A learner who is about to perform tracheostomy suctioning in the clinical skills laboratory on a task trainer alerts the clinical instructor that the cord on the portable suction machine is frayed and a wire is exposed. What is the priority intervention in this situation?

   A. Report the defect to the lab director or lab coordinator

   B. Complete a repair order form and tape it to the suction machine

   C. Unplug the suction machine

   D. Find another suction machine for the learner to use for the procedure

1. D) A standardized patient actor of Asian descent comes to the lab to speak to the learners about how their culture impacts healthcare decisions

Cultural awareness and cultural competence are essential social skills that can be practiced in the clinical laboratory environment. Applying what was learned from a research article is an example of evidence-based practice. Holding a patient's medication based on assessment data is an example of clinical decision-making. Experimenting with medical equipment used by a patient is an example of understanding the patient perspective.

2. A) Ensure a working arm is available with the properly simulated medication vial and the correct needle and syringe

Designing an activity that will closely resemble a real clinical setting is the best strategy for learner demonstration and practice. A working IV arm with medications that closely resemble the actual medication the learner will administer with the correct needle and syringe will help the learner build confidence. A simulated IV setup will not function like a real IV infusion. Verbalizing the proper sequence does not engage psychomotor skill practice. An injection pad is for subcutaneous and intramuscular injection practice.

3. C) Learners are given a medical record and history from a simulated patient and need to administer medication

Providing the learner with a medical record and history will provide the necessary information to make decisions about required medications, exercising the learners' clinical decision-making skills. When a learner is task with choosing the correct need and syringe for an intramuscular injection, they are utilizing comprehension skills. Gathering supplies for a nursing skill is an example of linear progression learning. Peer mentoring helps the learner with skills competence and retention.

4. C) Unplug the suction machine

To ensure the safety of the learner, the instructor, and the lab space, the defective equipment should be unplugged from the power source. The clinical instructor will report the defect to the lab director or coordinator, complete a repair order form and affix it to the defective equipment, and locate another suction machine for the learner to continue to practice the skill after the defective piece of equipment is removed from the lab area.

5. Utilizing a mid-fidelity manikin in the clinical learning environment to test a learner's understanding of prioritization, a nursing instructor determines a learner needs remediation when they perform which of the following skills out of sequence?

   A. Tracheostomy suctioning: Verify order, gather supplies, assess patient, place Ambu bag at the head of the bed

   B. Intermittent urinary catheterization: Inspect the integrity of package, place patient in supine position, and drape patient

   C. Subcutaneous medication administration: Gather supplies; check patient identifier, medication, expiration date, dose, route, time, and allergies; draw up medication; and perform hand hygiene

   D. Intravenous (IV) via gravity infusion: Calculate correct IV fluid drip rate, verify type, volume, and expiration date of solution, and check solution for particles, cloudiness, or discoloration

6. A learner comments that the steps of a skill learned in the clinical learning environment are different from what they saw the nurses practice in a clinical setting. What would be the clinical educator's best response to this learner?

   A. "Describe to me what you saw in practice that was different from what you learned in the skills laboratory"

   B. "Can you tell me the name of the nurse? I will speak to their supervisor"

   C. "There are many different ways to do the same skill"

   D. "Please go back and review the proper steps of the procedure"

7. Which activity demonstrates the principles of evidence-based practice applied to nursing skills?

   A. A learner completes a survey for a doctoral student's PhD dissertation at the end of a skills laboratory

   B. A learner chooses a smaller gauge intravenous catheter for packed red blood cell transfusion, which increases patient comfort

   C. A learner is sent to the nursing program chair for failing their clinical skills test

   D. Learners give feedback about their clinical lab faculty at the end of a course

8. During a skills demonstration by the clinical faculty, a learner in the skills laboratory is seen holding their personal mobile device in a manner suggesting they may be filming the demonstration. Video recording in the skills laboratory is prohibited by the school's policy without explicit permission from the clinical laboratory faculty and is clearly stated in the student handbook. What is the best immediate action in this situation?

   A. Stop the skills demonstration and send the learner home

   B. Remind the learners that filming is not permitted in the clinical learning laboratory and continue the demonstration

   C. Ignore the behavior and take note of which learner was using a mobile device

   D. Remind the learners that use of a mobile device is not permitted in the skills laboratory without permission and ask the learner to put their device away

(See answers next page.)

5. C) Subcutaneous medication administration: Gather supplies; check patient identifier, medication, expiration date, dose, route, time, and allergies; draw up medication; and perform hand hygiene

Hand hygiene should be performed prior to drawing up medication in a syringe in the process of administering subcutaneous medications. Steps outlined in tracheostomy suctioning, intermittent urinary catheterization, and intravenous gravity infusion are all in the proper sequence.

6. A) "Describe to me what you saw in practice that was different from what you learned in the skills laboratory"

Asking the learner to describe what they saw in practice will help the clinical instructor better understand the issue and how to proceed next. If the skill performed in the clinical setting by the nurse puts the patient's safety at risk, it may warrant a conversation with the nurse or the nurse's supervisor, but only after the clinical instructor understands the discrepancy in practice. Although there may be variations in how to perform a clinical skill, this response does not determine the root of the issue. Telling the learner to review the procedure does not elicit any actionable information regarding the issue.

7. B) A learner chooses a smaller gauge intravenous catheter for packed red blood cell transfusion, which increases patient comfort

Choosing a smaller-gauge catheter for a blood transfusion to increase patient comfort is an example of evidence-based practice. Completing a survey for a PhD candidate is an example of research. Sending a learner to a program chair due to a failure is an example of a school's policy for clinical lab failures. Learners giving feedback about faculty is an example of an evaluation strategy.

8. D) Remind the learners that use of a mobile device is not permitted in the skills laboratory without permission and ask the learner to put their device away

Stopping the learner from using their mobile device and asking them to put it away is the necessary initial action. The learner may receive disciplinary action for their actions, but stopping the behavior is the first step. Reminding the learners that filming is not permitted is important, but this assumes the learner is using their device to film. Reminding all learners does not directly address the learner using the mobile device. Ignoring the behavior will give the learners the message that this behavior is permissible.

9. A learner is sent to the clinical learning laboratory for remediation due to repeated lapses in sterile technique during wound dressing changes. Which of the following activities will help this learner achieve competence in proper sterile technique?

    A. Record the learner performing a sterile dressing change and have the learner watch the video
    B. Have the learner watch an evidence-based video of how to properly perform a sterile dressing change
    C. Employ a rapid cycle deliberate practice strategy with repeated feedback until the learner becomes proficient
    D. Have the learner review a skills checklist of the necessary steps of sterile wound dressing change

10. Learners complain to the clinical laboratory manager that there are differences in how skills are taught by different laboratory faculty. What would be the best initial approach to these learners?

    A. Describe the faculty orientation program to the learners
    B. Tell the learners that their faculty are skilled nurses and they should follow what is being taught
    C. Ask the learner to describe what the discrepancy is by giving examples
    D. Promise the learners that their complaints will be kept confidential

(See answers next page.)

9. C) Employ a rapid cycle deliberate practice strategy with repeated feedback until the learner becomes proficient

Rapid cycle deliberate practice is the best strategy when the skill is a structured activity, and the objective is to master a specific skill. Recording the learner while they perform the skill and having the learner watch the video do not offer the learner any feedback about what they may be doing incorrectly. Watching a video about how to perform the skill does not address what the learner is doing incorrectly or how the learner will master the skill. The learner may know all of the steps on the checklist; however, they were sent for contaminating the sterile field, not because they did not know the steps of the procedure.

10. C) Ask the learner to describe what the discrepancy is by giving examples

More information is needed by the laboratory manager before they decide on a strategy to address the issue. Although all lab faculty should be skilled, there may be times when they are giving misinformation and need to be corrected. Although you may keep the learners' identities confidential, this response does not address the issue of a potential lack of consistency in skills demonstration by the lab faculty.

REFERENCES

Alsayed, S., Bano, N. & Alnajjar, H. (2020). Evaluating practice of smartphone use among university students in undergraduate nursing education. *Health Professions Education 6*(2), 238–246. 10.1016/j.hpe.2019.06.004

Bayram, S. B., & Caliskan, N. (2019). Effect of a game-based virtual reality phone application on tracheostomy care education for nursing students: A randomized controlled trial. *Nurse Education Today, 79*, 25–31. 10.1016/j.nedt.2019.05.010

Blackburn, L., Acree, K., DiGiannantoni, E., Renner, E., Sinnott, L. T. (2020). Microbial growth on the nails of direct patient care nurses wearing nail polish. *Oncology Nursing Forum, 47*(2), 155–164. 10.1188/20.ONF.155-164

Cardoso, D., Rodrigues, M., Pereira, R., Parola, V., Coelho, A., Ferraz, L., Cardoso, M. L., Ramis, M. A., & Apostolo, J. (2021). Nursing educators' and undergraduate nursing students' beliefs and perceptions on evidence-based practice, evidence implementation, organizational readiness and culture: An exploratory cross-sectional study. *Nurse Education in Practice, 54*, 103122. h10.1016/j.nepr.2021.103122

Cengiz, A., & Yoder, L. (2020). Assessing nursing students' perceptions of the QSEN competencies: A systematic review of the literature with implications for academic programs. *Worldviews on Evidence-Based Nursing: Linking Evidence to Action, 17*(4), 275–282. 10.111/wvn.12458

Chang, C. P., Lee, T. T., & Mills, M. (2017). Clinical nurse preceptors' perception of e-portfolio use for undergraduate students. *Journal of Professional Nursing, 33*(4), 276–281. 10.1016/j.profnurs.2016.11.001

Daley, B. J., Berman, S. B., Morgan, S., Kennedy, L., & Sheriff, M. (2017). Concept maps: A tool to prepare for high fidelity simulation in nursing. *The Journal of Scholarship of Teaching and Learning, 17*(4), 17–30. 10.14434/josotl.v17i4.21668

Devine, C. & Chin, E. (2018). Integrity in nursing students: A concept analysis. *Nurse Education Today, 60*, 133–138. 10.1016/j.nedt.2017.10.005

Donnell, W. M., Walker, G. C., & Miller, G. (2018). Statewide at-risk tracking and intervention for nurses: Identifying and intervening with nursing students at risk of attrition in Texas. *Nursing Education Perspectives, 39*(3), 145–150. 10.1097/01.NEP.0000000000000281

Felsenstein, D. R. (2019). Providing culturally sensitive nursing care for vulnerable immigrant populations. *Creative Nursing, 25*(2), 133.

Fukuta, D., & Litsuka, M. (2018). Nontechnical skills training and patient safety in undergraduate nursing education: A systematic review. *Teaching and Learning in Nursing, 13*(4), 233–239. 10.1016/j.teln.2018.06.004

Fogg, N., Wilson, C., Trinka, M., Campbell, T., Thomson, A., Merritt, L., Tietze, M. & Prior, M. (2020). Transitioning from direct care to virtual clinical experiences during the COVID-19 pandemic. *Journal of Professional Nursing*, Published Online Date: October 2, 2020. 10.1016/j.profnurs.2020.09.012

George, T. P., DeCristofar, C., Murphy, P. F., & Sims, A. (2017). Student perceptions and acceptance of mobile technology in an undergraduate nursing program. *Healthcare, 5*(3), 35. 10.3390/healthcare5030035

Handeland, J., Prinz, A., Ekra, M., & Fossum, M. (2021). The role of manikins in nursing students' learning: A systematic review and metasynthesis. *Nurse Education Today, 98*, 1–11. 10.1097/01.NEP.0000000000000515

Henderson, A., Harrison, P., Rowe, J., Edwards, S., Barnes, M., & Henderson, S. (2018). Students take the lead for learning in practice: A process for building self-efficacy into undergraduate nursing education. *Nurse Education in Practice, 31*, 14–19. 10.1016/j.nepr.2018.04.003

Henderson, S., & Barker, M. (2018). Developing nurses' intercultural/intraprofessional communication skills using the EXCELLence in cultural experiential learning and leadership social interaction maps. *Journal of Clinical Nursing, 27*(17-18), 3276–3286. 10.1111/jcon.14089

Herrman, J. (2016). Creative lab skills. In J. Herrman (Ed.), *Creative teaching strategies for the nurse educator* (2nd ed., pp. 175–176). F. A. Davis.

Kenery, S. & Briyana, L. (2020). Differences in psychomotor skills teaching and evaluation practices in undergraduate nursing programs. *Nursing Education Perspectives, 41*(2), 83–87. 10.1097/01.NEP.0000000000000515

Kohtz, C., Brown, S., Williams, R. & O'Connor, P. (2017). Physical assessment techniques in nursing education: A replicated study. *Journal of Nursing Education, 56*(5), 287–291. 10.3928/01484834-20170421-06

Latimer, S., Hewitt, J., Stanbrough, R. & McAndrew, R. (2017). Reducing medication errors: Teaching strategies that increase nursing students' awareness of medication errors and their prevention. *Nurse Education Today, 52*, 7–9. 10.1016/j.nedt.2017.02.004

Leach, M. J., Hofmeyer, A., & Bobridge, A. (2016). The impact of research education on student nurse attitude, skill and uptake of evidence-based practice: A descriptive longitudinal survey. *Journal of Clinical Nursing, 25*(1/2), 194–203. 10.1111/jocn.13103

LeClair-Smith, C., Branum, B., Bryant, L., Cornell, B., Martinez, H., Nash, E., & Phillips, L. (2016). Peer-to-peer feedback: A novel approach to nursing quality, collaboration, and peer review. *JONA: The Journal of Nursing Administration, 46*(6). 321–328. 10.1097/NNA.0000000000000352

Li, T., Petrini, M. A., & Stone, T. E. (2018). Baccalaureate nursing students' perspectives of peer tutoring in simulation laboratory, a Q methodology study. *Nurse Education Today, 61*, 235–241. 10.1016/j.nedt.2017.12.001

Maruca, A. T., Diaz, D. A., Stockmann, C., & Gonzalez, L. (2018). Using simulation with nursing students to promote affirmative practice toward the lesbian, gay, bisexual, and transgender population: A multisite study. *Nursing Education Perspectives, 39*(4), 225–229. 10.1097/01.NEP.0000000000000302

Monsen, K. A., Bush, R. A., Jones, J., Manos, E. L., Skiba, D. J., & Johnson, S. B. (2019). Alignment of American Association of Colleges of Nursing graduate-level nursing informatics competencies with American Medical Informatics Association health informatics core competencies. *Computers, Informatics, Nursing, 37*(8), 396–404. 10.1097/CIN.0000000000000537

National League for Nursing. (2021). Certified Nurse Educator (CNE) 2021 candidate handbook. http://www.nln.org/docs/default-source/default-document-library/cne-handbook-2021_revised_07-01-2021.pdf?sfvrsn=2

National League for Nursing. (2021). Certified Nurse Educator Novice (CNEn) 2021 candidate handbook. http://www.nln.org/Certification-for-Nurse-Educators/cne-n/cne-n-handbook

Nicholls, D., Sweet, L., Muller, A. & Hyett, J. (2016). Teaching psychomotor skills in the twenty-first century: Revisiting and reviewing instructional approaches through the lens of contemporary literature. *Journal of Medical Teacher*, *38*(10), 1056–1063. 10.3109/0142159X.2016.1150984

Parvan, K., Hosseini, F., & Bagherian, S. (2018). The relationship between nursing instructors' clinical teaching behaviors and nursing students' learning in Tabriz University of Medical Sciences in 2016. *Education for Health*, *31*(1), 32–38. 10/4103/1357-6283.239044

Power, T., Virdun, C., White, H., Hayes, C., Parker, N., Kelly, M., Disler, R. & Cottle, A. (2016). Plastic with personality: Increasing student engagement with manikins. *Nurse Education Today*, *38*, 126–131. 10.1016/j.nedt.2015.12.001

Ross, J. (2019). Repetitive practice with peer mentoring to foster skill competence and retention in baccalaureate nursing students. *Nursing Education Perspectives*, *40*(1), 48–49. 10.1097/01.NEP.0000000000000358

Shelton, C. (2016). Students who developed logical reasoning skills reported improved confidence in drug dose calculation: Feedback from remedial maths classes. *Nurse Education Today*, *41*, 6–11. 10.1016/j.nedt.2016.03.007

Shustack, L. (2018). Virtually engaging millennial nursing students through QR codes. *The Journal of Nursing Education*, *57*(11), 699–700. 10.3928/01484834-20181022-15

Stone, R., Cooke, M. & Mitchell, M. (2020). Exploring the meaning of undergraduate nursing students' experiences and confidence in clinical skills using video. *Nurse Education Today*, *86*. 10.1016/j.nedt.2019.104322

Thilges, N., & Schmer, C. (2020). A concept analysis of remediation. *Teaching and Learning in Nursing*, *15*(1), 98–103. 10.1016/j.teln.2019-09.004

Tutticci, N., Lewis, P. A., & Coyer, F. (2016). Measuring third year undergraduate nursing students' reflective thinking skills and critical reflection self-efficacy following high fidelity simulation: A pilot study. *Nurse Education in Practice*, *18*, 52–59. 10.1016/j.nepr.2016.03.001

West, M., Wantz, D., Campbell, P., Rosler, G., Troutman, D. & Muthler, C. (2016). Contributing to a quality patient experience: Applying evidence based practice to support changes in nursing dress code policies. *The Online Journal of Issues in Nursing*, *21*(1), 4. 10.3912/OJIN.Vol21No01Man04.

Facilitating Learning in the Clinical Setting

Marylou K. McHugh and Tracy P. George

Live as if you were to die tomorrow. Learn as if you were to live forever.
—Mahatma Gandhi

> ## ▶ LEARNING OUTCOMES
>
> This chapter addresses the Certified Nurse Educator Exam and the Certified Nurse Educator Exam Content Area 1: Facilitate Learning
> - Discuss the goals of clinical education
> - Explain the different types of clinical learning activities
> - Describe the purpose of pre- and post-clinical conference
> - Analyze evaluation methods appropriate to measuring clinical outcomes of learners

Clinical education is a "core component of nursing education" (Dahlke, O'Connor, Hannesson, & Cheetham, 2016, p. 145). Clinical education is more than just being a proficient practitioner; it is synthesizing nursing and educational knowledge to guide learners. The clinical learning environment (CLE) includes not only the physical setting but also the psychosocial aspects and interactions with others, the organizational culture, and the intended teaching and learning (Flott & Linden 2016).

The CLE allows students to learn skills as they socialize into their professional roles as nurses (Shivers, Hasson & Slatter, 2017). However, nursing students in one study reported that the CLE was stressful due to:

- Heavy patient loads
- Limited resources
- Health and safety risks
- Few learning opportunities
- Poor communication

The characteristics just listed may not support socialization into the professional nursing role (de Swardt, 2019). Trusting relationships, teamwork, effective communication, proper planning, and leadership may lead to improved socialization into the nursing role (de Swardt, 2019). Nursing students should feel accepted, and their contributions are valued in the CLE (Flott & Linden, 2016).

Appropriate CLEs need to be planned throughout the curriculum and should grow in skill and complexity. The CLE must be congruent with the desired course, curriculum, and course and program outcomes (Billings & Halstead, 2020). The CLE provides practical implementation of the taught didactic content.

When selecting the CLE, the clinical nurse educator should consider:

- The ability of the site to meet the course outcomes
- The level of the learner
- Whether the clinical nurse educator is permitted to schedule learning activities at the site
- The availability of appropriate role models at the site
- The location and type of facility
- Orientation and agency requirements
- Presence of a positive relationship among staff, learners, and clinical nurse educators
- The ability of learners to participate in interprofessional clinical activities (Oermann, Shellenbarger, & Gaberson, 2018)

The learning outcomes of clinical nursing education are to assist learners to:

1. Apply theoretical learning to patient care situations using critical thinking skills to recognize and resolve patient care problems. Use the nursing process to design therapeutic nursing interventions and evaluate their effectiveness.
2. Develop communication skills when working with patients, their families, and other healthcare providers.
3. Demonstrate skill in the safe use of therapeutic nursing interventions when providing care to patients.
4. Evaluate and utilize evidence-based practices and research findings in designing patient care.
5. Evince caring behaviors in nursing actions.
6. Recognize and respect the varied beliefs, values, and customs of individual patients inherent in an increasingly diverse population.
7. Consider the ethical implication of clinical decision-making and nursing actions.
8. Gain a perspective of the contextual environment of healthcare delivery.
9. Develop a beginning mastery of technology as it is utilized in patient care settings.
10. Experience the various roles of the nurse within the healthcare delivery system.
11. Develop the skills necessary to continuously update knowledge in the practice nursing (O'Connor, 2015).

SELECTING APPROPRIATE CLEs THROUGHOUT THE CURRICULUM

CLEs usually include acute care hospitals, outpatient clinics, other community-based sites, and simulation laboratories (Flott & Linden, 2016). Nursing practice is shifting from acute care to community-based settings, so rotations in community health settings, such as ambulatory care, hospice, summer camps, occupational locations, long-term care, and homeless shelters, are being utilized more frequently (Billings & Halstead, 2020).

Normally, clinical groups in acute settings consist of 8 to 10 learners (Scholtz, 2007). The number of learners that can be supervised in an acute or non-acute setting is usually dictated by the state board of nursing in which the educational program resides. Some clinical agencies may also dictate the number of students they can accommodate in certain clinical settings.

> **TEACHING GEM**   During unusual times, such as a pandemic, numbers of students in CLE may decrease due to the stress placed on the healthcare system. Decreased numbers may assist not only the healthcare organization but also student stress.

According to McNelis et al. (2014), nurse educators may need to optimize the CLE so that students obtain experiences that foster critical thinking skills, clinical reasoning, patient safety, and quality care. In a multi-methods study of 30 final-semester nursing students and six faculty members from three different sites on the CLE, four themes emerged:

1. Missing opportunities for learning in a clinical setting
2. Getting the work done as the measure of learning
3. Failing to enact situation-specific pedagogies to foster clinical learning
4. Failing to engage as part of the team (McNelis et al., 2014)

One approach is to provide students the opportunity to work with interprofessional team members. Turner (2015) developed an interprofessional clinical experience in a medical–surgical course, in which each of the nursing students collaborated with respiratory therapists, physical therapists, and emergency medical technicians, with positive feedback from students.

In certain areas of the United States, there is a shortage of clinical sites resulting from competition from multiple nursing programs, a lack of consistent student experiences in the clinical setting, and difficulty recruiting nursing faculty, which has led to an increased use of simulation in some programs (Andrew & Baxter, 2019). Andresen and Levin (2014) developed alternative clinical learning activities, including simulation, service-learning experiences, and collaborative learning activities, which were developed to meet the course objectives. In addition to increasing the enrolment capacity of students, there was an improved quality and variety of clinical experiences while maintaining high student satisfaction.

Although the simulation-based training of basic nursing care takes place in modern school simulation labs, it will always be secondary to real-life practice. Therefore, there is a need for further research that will develop and implement models of preceptorship with clear guidelines and different learning activities that can improve theoretical and practical knowledge in relation to the basic nursing care education students receive during the process of becoming professional nurses. (Lillelroken, 2019).

Virtual CLEs are also being used to provide online clinical experiences in various settings such as community sites and specialty inpatient units (Andersen et al., 2018; Duff, Miller, & Bruce, 2016). Virtual CLEs were used extensively in nursing education during the conoravirus (COVID-19) pandemic. Virtual clinical experiences may encourage critical thinking, clinical reasoning, communication, and interprofessional teamwork (Peddle, Bearman, & Nestle, 2016).

Telehealth is a growing modality of care in the United States (National Council of State Boards of Nursing, 2017). Tele health can be utilized as clinical experiences, which allows students to gain experiences (Wynn, 2019). The American Telemedicine Association (2019) recommends that telehealth be included in all levels of nursing education, including baccalaureate-level programs. In 2018, the National Organization of Nurse Practitioner Faculties (NONPF) published a white paper encouraging the inclusion of telehealth into nurse practitioner programs (Rutledge et al., 2018).

EVIDENCE-BASED TEACHING PRACTICE

In a study of 27 sophomore nursing students, who completed a psychiatric nursing telehealth experience, students rated as "agree" or "strongly agree" to the following statements in the post-survey: "This activity improved my understanding of health informatics" (96%); "This activity improved my clinical decision-making skills" (89%); and "This activity improved my communication skills" (93%) (Wynn, 2019).

To ensure that the goals are met, Infante (1975) suggested that the essential elements of any CLE should include:

- Opportunity for patient contact
- Objectives for activities
- Competent guidance
- Individuation of activities
- Practice for skill learning, both motor and cognitive
- Encouragement of critical thinking and clinical reasoning
- Opportunity for problem-solving
- Opportunity for observation
- Opportunity for experimentation
- Development of professional judgment or decision-making
- Encouragement of creative abilities
- Provision for the transfer of knowledge
- Participation in integrative activities
- Utilization of the team concept

CHOOSING AND EVALUATING THE CLE

Faculty choose and evaluate the clinical area carefully in order to meet the goals of the curriculum. Chan (2002) identified six attributes that the clinical area should offer students:

- Individualization—students can make decisions and are treated differently according to their ability or interest.
- Innovation—the faculty is able to plan new and interesting learning techniques and activities.
- Satisfaction—students enjoy the clinical placement and leave with a sense of satisfaction.
- Involvement—students can participate actively and attentively in the learning activities.
- Personalization—students have opportunities to interact with clinicians who are concerned with the students' welfare.
- Task orientation—assignments are clear and meet the learning objectives for the day.

ATTRIBUTES OF CLINICAL EDUCATORS

Oermann and colleagues (2018) state that an effective clinical educator needs to:

- Be familiar with the practice area
- Exhibit clinical competence
- Effectively teach students in the clinical area
- Relate well to students
- Demonstrate enthusiasm
- Act as a role model
- Provide feedback on student performance
- Be available to students in the clinical area when needed

Hanson and Stenvig (2008) developed a list of attributes needed for nurse educators to be successful clinical instructors. These include the following:

- Educator knowledge attributes
  - Knowledge of theory and clinical practice
  - Knowledge of the facility
  - Knowledge of the learner

- Educator interpersonal presentation attributes
  - Positive educator attitude
  - Encouraging demeanor
  - Organizational skill
  - Serve as a primary resource
  - Available and approachable

- Learning activities attributes
  - Managing paperwork
  - Keeping learners challenged
  - Post conference planning
  - Firm knowledge of the technology or computer charting system used by the facility

Kan and Stabler-Haas (2014) state that learners will expect that clinical nurse educators have attributes that can be expressed with the acronym CAP:

- C = Consistent
- A = Approachable
- P = Proficient

TEACHING GEM Professional relationships with staff are very important for the learning experience. Clinical nurse educators need to focus on education and stay clear of unit conflicts. Professional role modeling is essential for the role of clinical nurse educator. Remembering at all times that you are a "guest" is helpful (Kan & Stabler-Haas, 2014).

EVIDENCE-BASED TEACHING PRACTICE

In a study of undergraduate students (N = 165) using Carl Rogers' Person Centered Model, realness was the attribute that was most likely to facilitate positive interpersonal relationships with students. Nurse educators who are genuine may be better able to motivate students, develop positive relationships with students, and encourage positive attitudes about the course (Bryan, Lindo, Anderson-Johnson, & Weaver, 2015).

PART-TIME CLINICAL EDUCATORS

Nursing programs frequently utilize part-time clinical faculty members. Although clinical nurse educators may not be as visible as classroom nurse educators, their role is vital in the education of nursing students. Transitioning from a staff nurse position to the role of the clinical nurse educator can be challenging. In a study of 10 clinical nurse educators, Clark (2013) identified five themes relevant for nurses' socialization to the role of clinical nurse educator:

- Beginning the role
- Employing strategies to survive in the role
- Coming to a turning point in the role
- Sustaining success in the role
- Finding fulfillment in the role

Many of the part-time clinical educators are new to their role. In a study of 15 clinical educators and 17 preceptors, investigators identified the need for additional support and mentoring in the area of teaching (Dahlke et al., 2016). Rice (2016) found that a one-day clinical adjunct orientation increased the knowledge of attendees and may better prepare new nurse educators for their roles. However, it may be difficult to provide face-to-face orientation sessions because of the work schedules of the full-time and part-time nurse educators. In a study of 17 part-time nurse educators, the learning management system (LMS) was used to provide an online orientation to the role of the clinical educator (Fura & Symanski, 2014).

TEACHING GEM During times of a pandemic and due to conflicting work schedules of clinical educators, virtual orientation programs have developed.

The retention of part-time clinical faculty is necessary for consistency and the achievement of student learning outcomes. In a national web-based survey (N = 533), part-time nursing faculty reported that enjoyment of teaching, pay and benefits, support, and being a valued member of the program were reasons they continued in their role (Carlson, 2015). Conflicts with a job and family responsibilities, low pay, and a heavy workload were cited as reasons not to continue working as a clinical nurse educator.

PRECEPTING

Precepting is a term used to describe the pairing of learners with experienced nurses to collaborate on the delivery of care. Many educational units use this model in their senior nursing courses, advanced nursing curricula, and dedicated educational units (DEUs). When precepting a nursing student, frequent and specific feedback is necessary, and the preceptor needs to report any issues to the faculty member (Ingwerson, 2014).

TEACHING GEM For high-acuity patients, learners can be assigned to teams to increase safe supervision.

Assets of precepted experiences include:

- Flexible hours (learners may be able to work evenings, nights, and weekends if they follow their preceptor's schedule)
- Role modeling (preceptors show learners not only how to provide nursing care but how nurses think and act)
- Clinical advancement (precepting contributes to the expectations of advancing on a clinical ladder track; Woolsey & Bracy, 2012)
- Preceptors may be better able to determine appropriate assignments for students because of the close one-to-one working relationship that is established (Haitana & Bland, 2011)
- Socialization into the role of nursing is facilitated by a preceptor's mentorship and a close working relationship

Disadvantages of using a preceptorship model include:

- Lack of time for staff nurses to teach (Carlson, Pilhammar, & Wann-Hansson, 2010)
- Understanding that developing a personal friendship may not serve the preceptor well when evaluations need to be completed (Kan & Stabler-Haas, 2014)
- Preceptors need to be chosen carefully and should want to be involved in nursing education
- Preceptors need to be educated about precepting activities as well as about evaluation principles because often they are asked to evaluate the learner

---

EVIDENCE-BASED TEACHING PRACTICE

Kol (2018) found that preceptors need preparation courses to include clinical teaching skills in order to increase their effectiveness and minimize their frustration. There also needs to be greater collaboration between faculties and clinical settings to develop skills related to basic nursing care.

DEDICATED EDUCATIONAL UNITS

DEUs are nursing units in which the staff nurses actually become the clinical instructors for the learners. They are similar to precepting learners but foster an entire unit in which all or most of the nurses are preceptors. The staff nurses work closely with clinical nurse educators and have been educated in instructing learners. Some outcomes of DEUs include student and faculty satisfaction, sharpening of clinical skills, increased teamwork, and improved critical thinking skills and clinical

Competence DEUs are actively studied, and the preliminary results are favorable for the learners and for patient care safety (Harris, Keller, & Hinton, 2018).

DEUs are increasing in popularity for several reasons. They:

- Increase patient safety
- Assist with the nurse educator shortage
- Promote learner attainment of competencies in a one-on-one situation
- Assist staff nurses to fulfil the teaching portion of their professional roles (Mulready-Shick, Kafel, Banister, & Mylott, 2009)

EVIDENCE-BASED TEACHING PRACTICE

In a study of 41 nursing students and 22 nurses on a DEUs at a large academic medical center, pre- and post-surveys were used to obtain nursing student and nursing staff perceptions of their experiences on the DEUs. Nurses felt that the DEU was a satisfying and rewarding work environment (Fusner & Melnyk, 2019).

LEARNING ACTIVITIES FOR THE CLINICAL SETTING

One of the goals of the clinical instructor is to assist learners as they reflect on their practice (Baker, 1996). A reflective learning practice includes:

- A sense of inner discomfort triggered by a live experience
- Identification or clarification of the concern makes the nature of the problem or issue more evident
- Openness to new information from internal and external sources, along with the ability to observe and take information from a variety of perspectives; there is a willingness to forego a quick resolution concerning a problem
- Resolution occurs through insight, whereby the learner feels they have changed or learned something that is personally significant
- A change is experienced in self as a result of internalization of a new perspective
- A decision is made whether to act on the outcome of the reflective process by determining whether the insight can be operationalized (p. 20).

There is a whole set of strategies available for the clinical nurse educator, that is different from those available to the classroom nurse educator. Table 6.1 presents selected clinical teaching and supervision activities, along with some clinical tips for implementing these activities.

EVIDENCE-BASED TEACHING PRACTICE

In a qualitative study with 16 undergraduate nursing students and 15 clinical instructors, reflection, preparation, motivation, trust, sense of belonging in a community, and contextual factors were identified as essential to supporting nursing students' learning (Nyqvist, Brolin, Nilsson & Lindström, 2020).

Table 6.1 Clinical Teaching

Learning Activities	Tips for Implementing Activities
Demonstration	The instructor demonstrates physical skills as well as reasoning skills and can encourage the learner to be attentive to his or her own mental work
War stories/personal experiences	War stories describe particularly memorable events in a nurse's past practice, which now serve as a paradigm for the learners' current practice
Questioning	This is a constant in clinical practice. A form of Socratic questioning will stimulate the students to think the problem through and will elicit formative evaluation
Listening	Clinical nurse educators must pay careful attention to what the learners are saying in the clinical area. Paraphrase the learners' comments to ensure clear communication
Supervision of Learner Performance of Technical Skills	
Process of skill mastery	Learners are at very low levels of skill mastery and will need to go through the sequential steps for all procedures. For information on this process, see Benner (1982)
How to let go	Clinical nurse educators need to allow the learners to work through their technical skills. Although taking over is a natural skill, do this only if it is absolutely necessary, then allow the learner to assume an assistant role. Process the experience with the learner. Allow learners to ask the patients what works best for them
When to jump in	The clinical instructor should be prepared to intervene when the learner's actions, inaction, or ineptitude jeopardize patient safety. Be calm and assertive. Remember to help the learner work through the situation in a way that does not destroy self-esteem
Ensuring that patient needs are met	Help learners set priorities so that all care is delivered in a timely manner. Keep the context of the whole situation in mind. The timing of all procedures, as well as the schedule, should be addressed. If the learner is caring for more than one patient, help the learner to set priorities. Make sure that the learner allows enough time for all activities

(continued)

Table 6.1 Clinical Teaching (*continued*)

Learning Activities	Tips for Implementing Activities
Promoting the Integration of Theory and Practice	
Case studies	If patients are not available to meet the clinical objectives, preparing case studies that include some of the prescribed outcome will assist the learner
Seminars	Seminars based on patient problems that learners have encountered can be used to foster integration. Several learners who care for the same patient on different days can work as a group with patients
Nursing rounds	Nursing rounds involve a group. They provide an opportunity for all learners to reflect on clinical events. Although background information and conclusions are discussed away from the bedside, the patient can add to the discussion by articulating his or her experience and expectations
Written assignments	Major nursing care plans, care maps, synthesis papers, and journaling may be part of the clinical experience. Clinical and classroom nurse educators must collaborate so that learners are clear about the assignment
Developing Critical Thinking Skills and Reflective Practice	
Strategies for promoting critical thinking and reflective practice	Clinical instructors must use higher-order cognitive questioning that includes "why" instead of "what." Debrief all of the experiences in post-clinical conferences. Process recordings and self-evaluations to assist the learners to think at higher cognitive levels

Learning activities used by effective clinical nurse educators include:

- Questioning
- Role-playing
- Interactive discussions (Kan & Stabler-Haas, 2014)

EVIDENCE-BASED TEACHING PRACTICE

Nafei, Markani, Motearafi, Moghadam, and Sakaei (2015) studied critical thinking skills in undergraduate students ($N = 24$). They found that the use of reflective journals significantly increased students' critical thinking skills when compared to a control group that did not use journaling.

TEACHING GEM "Ah ha" moments are especially important to focus on in the clinical domain. These moments occur when the learner successfully integrates the application of concepts. Many times, "ah ha" moments are a result of faculty's questioning, which produces critical thinking in the learner (Kan & Stabler-Haas, 2014).

EVIDENCE-BASED TEACHING PRACTICE

In a systematic review of 19 articles, McCutcheon, Lohan, Traynor, and Martin (2015) found that online learning was as effective as traditional teaching methods in teaching clinical skills in undergraduate students. However, there is a lack of evidence on the use of blended learning in the development of clinical skills in undergraduate nursing students.

MAKING LEARNER ASSIGNMENTS

All learners as well as clinical nurse educators should have an orientation to the unit on which students will be learning. Many times, meeting the nurse manager or director and understanding his or her expectations is a great way to start a clinical rotation. Some aspects that may be included in orientation are:

- Icebreakers and tours
- Defining and reviewing goals
- Understanding course requirements
- Evaluating math skills for medication calculations
- Reviewing the learners' responsibilities (Kan & Stabler-Haas, 2014)

◎ **Critical Thinking Question**

Many nurse educators use scavenger hunts to familiarize the learners with the unit. What activity can be used to familiarize learners with interdisciplinary communication?

Patient assignments should assist the learner to tie the course's didactic content to practical applications. Factors to consider are:

- The skill level of the learner
- The acuity of the patient
- The number of learners in the clinical group
- The availability of patients whose conditions directly meet the objectives of the day

Types of assignments can also differ to meet the clinical objectives and include:

- **Dual assignments**: These should be used when the complexity of care is more than one learner can handle. The clinical nurse educator is responsible for making sure each student is clear about each learner's role in this situation.
- **Observational assignments**: These should be used to augment the learner's appreciation of the various procedures that patients experience but when there is no reason for the learner to practice these procedures. Faculty can send learners to observe the operating room, radiology or laboratory departments, clinics, and so on.

When making clinical assignments, the following considerations may be useful (O'Connor, 2015):

1. Assess available clinical material

   - What experiences are available in the clinical setting?
   - What potential learning opportunities are presented in relation to specialty-specific theoretical content, skill development, and overriding curricular content (e.g., interpersonal communication, patient teaching, advocacy, and life span development)?

- What anticipated patient events (e.g., absence from the unit for prolonged testing, imminent discharge) might interrupt or interfere with student learning?
- Have staff voiced concerns or cautions regarding specific patient care assignments?

2. What are the curricular goals and related clinical outcomes for this experience?

- What is the primary focus of learning for this clinical experience?
- Can that focus be described as a larger concept of which the specific patient case at hand is an example?
- What other learning can be extracted from the situation? Scan curricular goals and clinical objectives to identify two or three other objectives that might be addressed in the experience.
- Does the student have sufficient background knowledge, either from previous courses or experiences or from the concurrent theoretical class, to deal with the situation? If not, can sufficient theory be provided to permit the student to function safely and effectively in an otherwise excellent learning situation?

3. What is the overall environment for learning?

- Can connections be made between the proposed assignment and the previous experiences of the learner that will help to integrate the experiences?
- What lessons might be drawn from the specific clinical setting that can be carried over into another setting (e.g., what information from the patient setting would be helpful to the nurse providing care for the patient in a community setting or to the nurse providing care for a nursing home resident admitted to the hospital for an episodic illness)?
- What staffing issues need to be considered in making the assignment (e.g., short staffing because of illness or planned meetings) that may impact the learning experienced?

4. What do you, as the instructor, feel comfortable managing?

- Where do you anticipate needing to spend the most time with specific students and/or specific patient care assignments?
- Does the overall assignment short-change any students or create safety issues?
- What patient events can or might happen in the course of the clinical day? If one or more of these events were to occur, would this be manageable given the assignments planned for all students in the group?

5. What are the characteristics of the learner group and individual learners?

- What previous experiences have the students had that can be drawn on when managing the proposed clinical assignment?
- What is the performance level of individual students? Is each student capable of managing the proposed assignment?
- Has each student had opportunities to progress toward achieving clinical outcomes?

- What level of independent functioning has each student achieved? Will one or several students require more attention than others?
- What learning needs have individual students expressed? Are these addressed in the assignment?
- Have students voiced any specific needs or desires in relation to clinical assignments? Can these be accommodated?
- What is the level of student confidence? Anxiety?
- Can each student function safely? If not, what precautions must be taken as the student proceeds through the clinical day?
- Are there any special needs of patients that can be matched to a student's special abilities?

6. What backup plans are available?

- Can students be paired in providing care without diluting the experience?
- Can students be assigned multiple patients to provide opportunities to practice planning and priority setting when challenging clinical situations are not available?
- Are there any off-unit experiences available that address clinical objectives?
- Can students focus on a single skill set with multiple patients?
- Can case studies and "what if" scenarios be developed to use "down time" effectively (O'Connor, 2015)?

Alternative assignments need to be considered if the clinical site does not support the learners' needs because of lack of patients or an unplanned accreditation visit that curtails student activity in some places. Alternative assignments should meet the course outcomes. Alternative assignments can also be used for makeup days for learners who are absent from clinical assignments. Some alternative assignments may be:

- Observational experiences if they are congruent with the course outcomes
- Case studies about patients who manifest conditions that are consistent with course content (O'Connor, 2015)

LEGAL CONSIDERATIONS OF CLINICAL EDUCATION

Understanding the legal ramifications of clinical instruction is important. Many novice nurse educators say that the learner "is working under my license." This is not accurate; the only person who can be working under a license is the person to whom the license is issued. Some guidelines to remember for legal considerations are as follows:

- The staff nurse is ultimately responsible for the patient.
- The nurse educator needs to supervise new procedures.
- Staff nurses, if they choose, can supervise learners.
- Clinical nurse educators should be familiar with the student handbook of the educational unit on which they are working because it outlines what is "unsafe practice."

- Clinical nurse educators should be familiar with the nursing educational program's evaluation forms and program goals.
- Clinical nurse educators should know their learners and the learners' capabilities in order to properly supervise them.

HEALTH INSURANCE PORTABILITY AND ACCOUNTABILITY ACT (HIPAA)

Confidentiality is another issue when teaching in the clinical domain. Learners need to maintain competence in understanding the Health Insurance Portability and Accountability Act (HIPAA), and no patient care issues can be discussed outside the clinical unit's realm (Kan & Stabler-Haas, 2014). Additional precautions must be taken when using mobile electronic devices (MEDs) as reference portals. Devices that are internet accessible can be a threat to patient confidentiality if used wrongly (Wittmann-Price, Kennedy, & Godwin, 2012).

Nursing students should not share information from the clinical setting on social media. There is a risk of breach of confidentiality when nursing students make posts on social media about a patient (Westrick, 2016). As a result of professional boundaries, students should not become "friends" on social media with patients (Ashton, 2016). It is important to remind nursing students that they should be careful about what they post on social media. Posts can be scrutinized by potential employers or by the nursing program.

PRE- AND POST-CLINICAL CONFERENCES

The clinical day requires thought and preparation for the learners to successfully apply to patient care the knowledge that they have learned in the classroom. The clinical nurse educator needs to reserve space that is accessible and private to facilitate pre- and post-clinical conferences. The preclinical conference is a time to review the clinical outcomes, the kinds of patients the learners will care for, the degree of the preparation the learners have done, and any procedures that may be part of the day. Whether this is done in a formal setting with all learners present or done informally and individually with each learner depends on the level of the learner and the instructor's preference. The goal is to be sure that all learners are adequately prepared. The post-clinical conference is a time for learners to process the day's experiences to debrief and reflect. According to O'Connor (2015), there are several purposes to post-clinical conferences:

- Providing a time for students and instructor to pause and reflect on the day's events, their meaning, and the relation between what has been observed and experienced and what was taught in the classroom or discussed in assigned readings
- Contributing to the achievement of the course and to clinical outcomes by making explicit the connections between clinical activities and the goals for learning
- Examining commonalities and differences in patient responses to illness and its treatment within the clinical specialty

- Permitting students to vicariously share in their peers' experiences, broadening their exposure to the clinical situations they might encounter in practice
- Promoting affective learning through debriefing that allows students to express feelings and attitudes about the experiences they encountered during the day's activities
- Providing students with the experience of the effective use of the group process (O'Connor, 2015).

REFLECTIVE TECHNIQUES AS PART OF THE CLINICAL POST-CONFERENCE

The NLN, in collaboration with the International Nursing Association for Clinical Simulation and Learning (INACSL), believes that "integrating debriefing across the curriculum not just in simulation has the potential to transform nursing education" (2015, p. 2). Critical reflection via debriefing can be a powerful method to guide a post-conference discussion. It helps the student to:

- Examine information to see the whole of reality
- Promote "knowing how" and "knowing why" rather than "knowing what"
- Reframe the context of the situation
- Attach meaning to information

A good debriefing is a theory driven with formal training and ongoing assessment competencies for faculty (NLN, 2015). Two of the most commonly used methods are:
Debriefing with Good Judgement (Rudolph, Simon, Dufresne, & Raemer, 2006) focuses on:

- Creating a context for adult learners (including the instructor) to learn important lessons that will help them move toward key objectives, determined either unilaterally by the instructor or collaboratively with the trainee and
- Widens to include not only the trainees' actions but also the meaning-making systems of the trainees, such as their frames, assumptions, and knowledge

Debriefing for Meaningful Learning (Dreifuerst, 2012) has six components:

- Engage (the participants)
- Explore (options reflecting-in-action)
- Explain (decisions, actions, and alternatives using deduction, induction, and analysis)
- Elaborate (thinking like a nurse and expanding analysis and inferential thinking)
- Evaluate (the experience reflecting-on-action
- Extend (inferential and analytic thinking, reflecting-beyond-action)

Students must feel safe. Faculty must correct errors in judgment while helping students feel valued. What is said in post-conference must stay in post-conference.

> **TEACHING GEM** Unfolding case studies, books are excellent mechanisms to promote critical thinking and can be used as an alternative assignment when a learner misses clinical instruction (Wittmann-Price & Cornelius, 2011, 2013; Wittmann-Price & Thompson, 2010).

THE AFFECTIVE DOMAIN IN CLINICAL PRACTICE

The American Association of Colleges of Nursing (AACN; 2008) identified five core values that epitomize the caring, professional nurse.

1. **Altruism** is a concern for the welfare and well-being of others. In professional practice, altruism is reflected by the nurse's concern and advocacy for the welfare of patients, other nurses, and other healthcare providers.
2. **Autonomy** is the right of self-determination. Professional practice reflects autonomy when the nurse respects patients' rights to make decisions about their healthcare.
3. **Human dignity** is respect for the inherent worth and uniqueness of individuals and populations. In professional practice, concern for human dignity is reflected when the nurse values and respects all patients and colleagues.
4. **Integrity** is acting in accordance with an appropriate code of ethics and accepted standards of practice. Integrity is reflected in professional practice when the nurse is honest and provides care based on an ethical framework that is accepted within the profession.
5. **Social justice** is acting in accordance with fair treatment regardless of economic status, ethnicity, age, citizenship, disability, or sexual orientation.

These core values come into play in the clinical area; the clinical nurse educator must be alert to demonstrating how these values inform patient care. Opportunities to apply ethical principles are present in every clinical experience, but often learners need to be prompted to examine their performance and attitudes in light of these values.

STRATEGIES FOR EVALUATING LEARNING IN THE CLINICAL AREA

Although evaluation of learner performance in the clinical area is vital, the clinical nurse educator needs to remember that teaching is primary. Learners need clear definitions of safe and unsafe behaviors, and faculty need to give very specific rationales for their decision to give an unsatisfactory grade. On the other hand the teacher should remember that often the first time a learner performs a procedure and may need some coaching. There is a fine line between teaching and evaluating in the clinical area. Table 6.2 presents a variety of evaluation methods that are useful when evaluating learners' clinical performance, which include:

- Observation of learners as they perform in the clinical area
- Learners' written work that is used to reveal intellectual processes that guide learners' clinical performance
- Oral presentations
- Simulations

- Learner self-evaluation
- Testimonials/feedback from staff

Frequent feedback (daily if possible) is essential for learners to have the opportunity to improve on areas found to be deficient. Without positive and frequent feedback, the goal of the clinical experience can be lost. Remember, most clinical evaluations are done using a pass/fail mechanism; therefore, the formative evaluations done during the course inform the summative evaluation of pass/fail at the end of the course.

Table 6.2 Evaluation Methods

Observations of Learners as They Perform in Clinical Settings	
Anecdotal notes	Data obtained through observation and recorded for later evaluation
Incident reports	Instances of unsafe behavior or unprofessional behavior; if no other instances of unsafe behavior occur, the event should be ignored unless it is a sentinel event in the learner's final evaluation
Rating scales	Provide a summary of accumulated observations of the learner's clinical performance; these scales are usually based on the course objectives
External raters	A rating done by a person who has not seen the learner perform previously
Videotapes	Videotapes can be recorded in a simulated setting; they are also of value in distance learning settings
Skills checklist	Skills checklists are usually used in the college laboratory and detail the steps for a particular skill; they can be used for teaching as well as learning
Examples of Written Work That Reveal the Intellectual Processes That Guide Learners' Clinical Performances	
Observation guides	These guides can be developed to assist the learners in observing an independent assignment or off-unit experience
Process recordings	Process recordings are used to capture interpersonal interactions between the learner and another person; they focus on communication skills
Nursing care plans and care maps	The major nursing care plan and care map details the application of the nursing process for all nursing diagnoses that the learner has identified for a selected patient
Oral presentations—include communication with staff and instructors, active participation in pre- and post-clinical conference, and formal presentations	
Simulations—may also be used for evaluation and teaching; these standardize the stimuli to which learners respond and may be in the form of a case study, the use of manikins or models, or standardized patients	
Self-evaluation—often learners provide valuable insights for their instructors when they conduct a self-evaluation	
Testimonial—verbal comments from staff, patients and, in some cases, other learners may play a part in the evaluation process; however, the instructor should validate the observation for himself or herself	

Clinical nurse educators often use a clinical evaluation form that ranks learner behavior in all three domains—cognitive, affective, and psychomotor or knowledge, skills, and attitudes. One of the more well-known ranking scales was devised by Bondy (1983), which rates learner performance as:

- Independent—indicating the learner is proficient and does not waste unnecessary time when completing patient care
- Supervised—the learner expends some extra energy and takes some extra time to complete care, but is safe
- Assisted—the learner needs frequent cues and expends unnecessary energy but is safe most of the time
- Marginal—at this level, the learner is inefficient and not safe alone
- Dependent—the learner is unsafe and needs continuous verbal cues

Walsh, Jairath, Paterson, and Grandjean (2010) developed a clinical evaluation tool based on the Quality and Safety Education for Nurses (QSEN) that includes rating of the following:

- Provides patient-centered care (caring, spirituality, human dignity, and ethics)
- Exhibits teamwork and collaboration (communication and roles)
- Incorporates evidence-based practice (critical thinking)
- Promotes quality improvement (leadership, assessment)
- Promotes safety (skill)
- Uses informatics (decision-making)

THE CLINICAL EVALUATION PROCESS

Clinical evaluation is a process by which judgments are made about learners' competencies in practice. This practice may involve care of patients, families, and communities; other types of learning activities in the clinical setting; simulation activities; performance of varied skills in the learning laboratories; or activities using multimedia. (Oermann, Shellenbarger, & Gaberson, 2018)

In the clinical setting, learners are evaluated by the observation of the educator, rating scales, rubrics, skills checklists, journals, logs, and various other types of sources. The major thing to remember is that clinical evaluations should always be based on the objectives/outcomes for the course, and the criteria need to be clearly defined.

There are a few principles to keep in mind regarding the clinical evaluation process

- Objectives/outcomes and expectations should be shared with the learner at the beginning of the course and referred to throughout the clinical experience.
- The objectives and criteria can be used in multiple settings, such as the clinical skills laboratory, simulation learning, and clinical experiences in the practice setting.
- In some nursing programs, the clinical evaluations are conducted at mid-semester or mid-rotation (formative evaluation) and at the end of the experience (summative

evaluation). In other programs, daily or weekly evaluations are done after the clinical experience to show progress toward meeting objectives (formative evaluation) and are used to determine whether or not objectives have been achieved at the end of the experience (summative evaluation).

- The clinical grade may be assigned as pass/fail, satisfactory/unsatisfactory, or as a numerical grade in the course. In the course syllabus, nurse educators must document how the grade is calculated. Usually, the learner must achieve a passing or satisfactory grade in the clinical course to pass the nursing course; failure to achieve a satisfactory grade in clinical results in failure of the course in many nursing programs regardless of the grade achieved in the theoretical component of the course.
- The nurse educator should keep anecdotal notes throughout the clinical experience for each learner based on his or her performance for each experience within the confines of the objectives or outcomes. Anecdotal notes are not shared with the learner as they are strictly for the nurse educator's reference.
- If a learner is not doing well in any aspect of the clinical, course conferences should be held with the learner on a regular basis and a formal note, plan, or contract may need to be written that clearly outlines the expectations and what the learner needs to do to meet the objectives. The learner should sign the notes after such meetings.

Feedback is an important aspect of the clinical evaluation. Learners should receive feedback throughout the clinical experience regarding their performance in the clinical setting, areas of strengths, and areas that need improvement. As stated earlier, the learner is judged in the clinical setting by the nurse educator based on objectives, outcomes, competency achievement, and knowledge. Oermann et al. (2018) suggest the following principles regarding feedback in the clinical evaluation process:

- The feedback provided by the nurse educator should indicate specific areas of knowledge, competency, skill performance, critical thinking, and judgment that need further development or improvement.
- If the learner needs to improve performance in areas of psychomotor skills or use of technologies, the educator should explain where errors were made, demonstrate to the learner the correct procedure, then allow the learner the opportunity to practice the skill in the presence of the educator.
- Feedback should be given to the learner at the time of learning or as close to it as possible.
- The amount of feedback needed is dependent on the individual learner and the level of progression within the nursing program.
- Positive reinforcement is essential to promote learning in the clinical setting.

EVIDENCE-BASED TEACHING PRACTICE

Clinical nurse educators have an important role in clinical education. Higher self-efficacy levels of students ($N = 236$) were associated with faculty members who gave suggestions for improvement, provided feedback on strengths and weaknesses, observed students frequently, offered clear expectations, gave positive feedback, and offered constructive criticism (Rowbotham & Owen, 2015).

STRATEGIES FOR DEALING WITH UNSAFE OR UNSATISFACTORY LEARNER BEHAVIOR

Unfortunately, clinical nurse educators must deal with unsatisfactory and, at times, unsafe learner behavior. Unsatisfactory behavior by a learner can be exhibited in any of the three learning domains:

1. Cognitive—the learner is just not making the connection in applying theory to practice, demonstrated by thought processes that do not prioritize, delegate, or recognize significant patient care needs
2. Affective—the learner's behavior is unprofessional in appearance (per the student handbook) or there is a habit of tardiness or there are communication (verbally and nonverbally) issues
3. Psychomotor—the learner's behavior is not up to par when performing skills such as gloving, sterilizing, dressing changes, or other procedures

Unsafe behavior may include a sentinel event; this is an occurrence that poses a real risk to the physical or psychological safety of patients. Sometimes it is difficult to determine the difference between unsatisfactory or unsafe behavior. When behavior is unsafe, the clinical nurse educator has an obligation to step in and protect both the patient and the learner.

Documentation and remediation of unsatisfactory behavior are necessary. Many times, the learner can be sent back to the skills laboratory for remediation. Correction of the unsatisfactory behavior is usually expected within a specific time period. A mechanism for documenting the need for remediation is a "learning contract" that specifies the following:

- What behaviors need remediation?
- How the remediation will be completed?
- What the time frame is for remediation completion?
- What consequences can be expected if remediation is not completed or the behavior is repeated?

Another common unsatisfactory and potentially unsafe learner behavior is not being prepared for the clinical day. Although many educational units do not participate in "pick up" or recording information about the patient the day before clinical because of security and unit congestion issues, the learner is expected to know the basic information needed to participate in care. Many times, the nursing staff on the unit will also comment on an unprepared learner. The staff on a clinical unit who are familiar with learners are keen observers and can be an evaluative asset (Kan & Stabler-Haas, 2014).

FOSTERING DIVERSITY IN THE CLE

Minority nursing students may have higher attrition rates. One factor in attrition is not having a sense of "belonging," so it is important for clinical nurse educators to foster that sense of "belonging." Minority students may experience discrimination and bias by patients, nursing staff, other students, and clinical nurse educators. Discriminatory words by patients, nurses, other students, and faculty are hurtful to students, as are gestures, expressions, and certain tones of voice. Experiences in the clinical setting are important to professional integration and socialization of students (Graham, Phillips, Newman, & Atz, 2016). Instructors need to intervene when students are exposed to discriminatory actions by patients and/or nurses (Sedgwick, Oosterbroek, & Ponomar, 2014). Nurse educators need to create environments in which diversity is welcomed and fostered (National League for Nursing, 2018).

EVIDENCE-BASED TEACHING PRACTICE

In a review of 30 studies, Metzger, Dowling, Guinn, and Wilson (2020) found that minority nursing students experience discrimination from peers, faculty, and clinicians in the classroom, the clinical setting and/or the university as a whole, which can result in a lack of belongingness. All of the components of nursing students' learning act as facilitators or barriers to a sense of belongingness.

CASE STUDY

CASE STUDY 6.1

A learner at the midpoint of the first senior semester is on an acute care CLE and is assigned three patients. The learner cannot prioritize care and spends an excessive amount of time and energy in organizing the day's tasks. The learner is provided with a formative evaluation and does not improve enough to be passed to the final semester. The learner seeks a grade appeal because the clinical nurse educator was unfair and assigned the learner patients who were more acutely ill than those assigned to other learners. The college's grade appeal committee upholds the clinical nurse faculty member's decision, and the learner will have to repeat the course the following.

What suggestions do you have that would increase the learner's chance of success and promote a fair evaluation process?

1. A new clinical faculty member has extensive clinical experience but has never worked as a nurse educator. In order to prepare the new clinical faculty member, the best action for the course coordinator would be to:

   A. Invite the new clinical faculty member to attend the clinical orientation for new clinical faculty

   B. Invite the new clinical faculty member to attend a lecture for the course

   C. Encourage the new clinical faculty member to take a course on nursing education

   D. Take the new clinical faculty member to the acute care facility to introduce them to the unit

2. What is the best activity for the nurse educator to use in order to promote critical thinking in post-conference?

   A. Complete a case study

   B. Have students look for evidence-based guidelines on sepsis and discuss them with the group

   C. Demonstrate proper use of personal protective equipment (PPE)

   D. Ask students to reflect on their experiences and what they learned

3. The patient has a medication ordered that is not familiar to the nursing student. What should the clinical nurse educator do in this situation?

   A. Have the student ask a staff nurse on the unit about the medication

   B. Advise the student to look up the medication in an electronic database

   C. Encourage the patient's primary nurse to administer the medication and have the student observe

   D. Instruct the student to administer the medication without further information

4. There is a shortage of clinical placements for the undergraduate psychiatric nursing course. The new mental health clinical instructor needs further understanding of the course learning outcomes when the students are assigned to:

   A. Medical surgical floor

   B. Virtual simulation experience

   C. Simulation experience

   D. Telehealth experience

1. A) Invite the new clinical faculty member to attend the clinical orientation for new clinical faculty

The clinical faculty orientation is the best answer because it will familiarize the new clinical faculty member with the expectations and role. Attending a lecture or introducing the faculty member to the unit may not be as useful. There may not be time to take coursework on nursing education prior to the start of the semester, although that may be useful.

2. D) Ask students to reflect on their experiences and what they learned

Asking students to reflect on their clinical experiences is the best answer because it encourages students to think about what went well or poorly so that they can improve in future clinical experiences. Having students complete a case study may not promote critical thinking. Researching evidence-based guidelines will promote knowledge about sepsis but not critical thinking. Demonstrating the proper use of PPE does not promote critical thinking.

3. B) Advise the student to look up the medication in an electronic database

The student should look up all unfamiliar medications prior to administering them in order to promote patient safety. Asking a staff nurse about the medication does not promote patient safety or information-seeking by the student. Having the student watch the administration of the medication does not promote active learning. Telling the student to administer the medication without looking it up is unsafe.

4. A) Medical surgical floor

Students will be able to obtain alternative clinical experiences in the psychiatric nursing specialty through simulation, virtual simulation, or telehealth. Providing students with additional medical-surgical clinical hours will not be the student learning objectives of the psychiatric nursing course.

5. The clinical nurse educator has a nursing student in the clinical group who wears a hijab due to her religion. What should the nurse educator tell her in clinical?

   A. You must remove your hijab while in clinical. It is not part of your nursing uniform

   B. You may wear your hijab, but only if you explain it to each patient

   C. I know that the hijab is an important part of your religion, so you may continue to wear it

   D. Wearing your hijab could be an infection-control issue. Please remove it during clinical

6. At a clinical post-conference, the students are complaining about the course coordinator to the clinical nurse educator. What is the best course of action by the clinical nurse educator?

   A. Advise the students to make an appointment with the course coordinator to discuss their concerns

   B. Tell them that they heard that the course coordinator is disorganized

   C. Encourage the students to go to the university provost with their concerns

   D. Share with the students other stories heard about this instructor

7. Which of the following would indicate understanding by the nurse educator of the role of dedicated education units (DEUs)?

   A. DEUs allow academic nurse educators a place to practice as professional nurses

   B. On DEUs, staff nurses are the clinical instructors for the nursing students

   C. On DEUs, the nurse educators are the clinical instructors for the nursing students

   D. DEUs are associated with teaching the research process

8. The new clinical educator needs guidance making clinical assignments because they state they always consider:

   A. The student's skill level

   B. Patient acuity

   C. The number of patients on the unit who meet the clinical objectives

   D. The physical location of the patients on the floor

(See answers next page.)

5. C) I know that the hijab is an important part of your religion, so you may continue to wear it

Allowing the wearing of the hijab is culturally sensitive and promotes a sense of belonging and acceptance by students. Telling students that they must remove the hijab or requiring them to explain it to each patient is not culturally sensitive.

6. A) Advise the students to make an appointment with the course coordinator to discuss their concerns

Students should first be encouraged to discuss their concerns with the course coordinator prior to going to the university provost. The clinical nurse educator should not share stories or concerns about the course coordinator students in order to remain professional.

7. B) On DEUs, staff nurses are the clinical instructors for the nursing students

On DEUs, the staff nurses are the instructors and receiving training in this role. DEUs are not designed as a practice site for nurse educators. DEUs are not primarily for research education.

8. D) The physical location of the patients on the floor

The physical location should not be the primary concern when making clinical assignments. Patient acuity, student skills level, and the number of patients meeting the clinical objectives should be considered.

9. The nurse educator is concerned about a nursing student's organizational and assessment skills in the medical surgical clinical learning environment. What is the best response by the nurse educator?

A. Document the concerns on the summative evaluation

B. Complete a formative evaluation so that remediation can occur

C. Monitor the student's progress for a few more weeks to verify observations

D. Discuss the need for better organizational skills with the whole clinical group during post-conference

10. The clinical nurse educator sees a post on social media in which a nursing student describes the day on the unit and the diagnosis of a patient. What is the best response to the student about this issue?

A. Nursing students should not share any information from clinical on social media due to HIPAA concerns

B. It is acceptable to share information about clinical on social media as long as no names are provided

C. It is acceptable to post pictures on social media as long as the patient agrees

D. Nursing students can become friends with patients on social media

(See answers next page.)

9. B) Complete a formative evaluation so that remediation can occur

Completing a formative evaluation and creating a remediation plan will increase the student's chance of being successful in the course. Waiting until the final (summative) evaluation will not allow for improvement during the clinical experience. Monitoring the student further will not work toward improvement since the issue has already been identified. It may not be apparent to the nursing student that they are having issues with organization if it is brought up to the whole group and not discussed individually.

10. A) Nursing students should not share any information from clinical on social media due to HIPAA concerns

No information from clinical should be shared on social media due to HIPAA concerns. Even if names are not provided, it can be a violation of HIPAA. Pictures and friending patients are not acceptable practices.

REFERENCES

American Association of Colleges of Nursing. (2008). The essentials of baccalaureate education for professional nursing practice. Author. http://www.aacn.nche.edu/education-resources/BaccEssentials08.pdf

American Telemedicine Association. (2019). Telehealth nursing: A position statement. https://www.americantelemed.org/wp-content/themes/ata-custom/download.php?id=3444

Andersen, P., Baron, S., Bassett, J., Govind, N., Hayes, C., Lapkin, S., & Power, T. (2018). Snapshots of simulation: Innovative strategies used by international educators to enhance simulation learning experiences for health care students. *Clinical Simulation in Nursing, 16,* 8–14. 10.1016/j.ecns.2017.10.001

Andresen, K., & Levin, P. (2014). Enhancing quantity and quality of clinical experiences in a baccalaureate nursing program. *International Journal of Nursing Education Scholarship, 11*(1), 137–144. 10.1515/ijnes-2013-0053

Andrew, L. A. & Baxter, P. M. (2019). Incorporating innovative simulation activities into campus lab to enhance skill competence and critical thinking of second-semester associate degree nursing students. *Nursing Education Perspectives, 40*(1), 58–59. 10.1097/01.NEP.0000000000000321

Ashton, K. S. (2016). Teaching nursing students about terminating professional relationships, boundaries, and social media. *Nurse Education Today, 37,* 170–172. 10.1016/j.nedt.2015.11.007

Baker, C. (1996). Clinical education: A teaching strategy for critical thinking. *Journal of Nursing Education, 35,* 19–22.

Benner, P. (1982). From novice to expert. *American Journal of Nursing, 82*(3), 402–407.

Billings, D. M., & Halstead, J. A. (2020). *Teaching in nursing: A guide for faculty* (6th ed.). Elsevier.

Bondy, K. (1983). Criterion-referenced definitions for rating scales in clinical evaluation. *Journal of Nursing Education, 122*(9), 376–382.

Bryan, V. D., Lindo, J., Anderson-Johnson, P., & Weaver, S. (2015). Using Carl Rogers' person-centered model to explain interpersonal relationships at a school of nursing. *Journal of Professional Nursing, 31*(2), 141–148. 10.1016/j.profnurs.2014.07.003

Carlson, E., Pilhammar, E., & Wann-Hansson, C. (2010). Time to precept: Supportive and limiting conditions for precepting nurses. *Journal of Advanced Nursing, 66*(2), 432–441. 10.1111/j.1365-2648.2009.05174.x

Carlson, J. S. (2015). Factors influencing retention among part-time clinical nursing faculty. *Nursing Education Perspectives, 36*(1), 42–45. 10.5480/13-1231

Chan, D. (2002). Development of the clinical learning environment inventory: Using the theoretical framework of learning environment studies to assess nursing students' perceptions of the hospital as a learning environment. *Journal of Nursing Education, 41*(2), 69–76.

Clark, C. L. (2013). A mixed-method study on the socialization process in clinical nursing faculty. *Nursing Education Perspectives, 34*(2), 106–110.

Dahlke, S., O'Connor, M., Hannesson, T., & Cheetham, K. (2016). Understanding clinical nursing education: An exploratory study. *Nurse Education in Practice, 17,* 145–152. 10.1016/j.nepr.2015.12.004

de Swardt, H. C. (2019). The clinical environment: A facilitator of professional socialisation. *Health SA Gesondheid, 24,* 1–7. 10.4102/hsag.v24i0.1188

Dreifuerst, K. (2012). Using debriefing for meaningful learning to foster development of clinical reasoning in simulation. *Journal of Nursing Education, 61*(6), 326–333.

Duff E., Miller L., Bruce J. (2016). Online virtual simulation and diagnostic reasoning: A scoping review. *Clinical Simulation in Nursing, 12*(9), 377–383. 10.1016/j. ecns.2016.04.001.

Flott, E. A., & Linden, L. (2016). The clinical learning environment in nursing education: A concept analysis. *Journal of Advanced Nursing, 72*(3), 501–513. 10.1111/jan.12861

Fura, L. A., & Symanski, M. E. (2014). An online approach to orienting clinical nursing faculty in baccalaureate nursing education. *Nursing Education Perspectives, 35*(5), 324–326. 10.5480/12-868.1

Fusner, S., & Melnyk, B. M. (2019). Dedicated education units: A unique evaluation. *Journal of Doctoral Nursing Practice, 12*(1), 102–110. 10.1891/2380-9418.12.1.102

Graham, C. L., Phillips, S. M., Newman, S. D., & Atz, T. W. (2016). Baccalaureate minority nursing students perceived barriers and facilitators to clinical education practices: An integrative review. *Nursing Education Perspectives, 37*(3), 130–137.

Haitana, J., & Bland, M. (2011). Building relationships: The key to preceptoring nursing students. *Nursing Praxis in New Zealand, 27*(1), 4–12.

Hanson, K., & Stenvig, T. E. (2008). The good clinical nursing educator and the baccalaureate nursing clinical experience: Attributes and praxis. *Journal of Nursing Education, 47*(1), 38–42.

Harris, J. Y., Keller, S., & Hinton, E. (2018). Dedicated education units as a clinical rotation for nursing students: a scoping review protocol. *JBI Database of Systematic Reviews & Implementation Reports, 16*(3), 642–647. 10.11124/JBISRIR-2017-003519

Infante, M. S. (1975). *The clinical laboratory in nursing education.* New York, NY: Wiley.

Ingwerson, J. (2014). Tailoring the approach to precepting: Student nurse vs. *new hire. Oregon State Board of Nursing Sentinel, 33*(2), 11–13.

Kan, E. Z., & Stabler-Haas, S. (2014). *Fast facts for the clinical nursing instructor* (2nd ed.). Springer Publishing Company.

Kol, E. (2018). Determining the opinions of the first-year nursing students about clinical practice and clinical educators. *Nurse Education in Practice, 31,* 35–40. 10.1016j.nerj.2018.04.009

Lillelroken. D. (2019). Teaching basic nursing care: Nurse preceptors' perceptions about changing the teaching context from the clinical setting to a school simulation lab. *International Journal of Nursing Education Scholarship, 16*(1). 10.1515/ijnes-2018-0033

McCutcheon, K., Lohan, M., Traynor, M., & Martin, D. (2015). A systematic review evaluating the impact of online or blended learning vs. face-to-face learning of clinical skills in undergraduate nurse education. *Journal of Advanced Nursing, 71*(2), 255–270. 10.1111/jan.12509

McNelis, A. M., Ironside, P. M., Ebright, P. R., Dreifuerst, K. T., Zvonar, S. E., & Conner, S. C. (2014). Learning nursing practice: A multisite, multimethod investigation of clinical education. *Journal of Nursing Regulation, 4*(4), 30–35.

Metzger, M., Dowling, T., Guinn, J., & Wilson, D. T. (2020). Inclusivity in baccalaureate nursing education: A scoping study. *Journal of Professional Nursing, 36*(1), 5–14. 10.1016/j.profnurs.2019.06.002

Mulready-Shick, J., Kafel, K. W., Banister, G., & Mylott, L. (2009). Enhancing quality and safety competency development at the unit level: An initial evaluation of student learning and clinical teaching on dedicated education units. *Journal of Nursing Education, 48*(12), 716–719. 10.3928/01484834-20091113-11

Nafei, A. R., Markani, A. K., Motearafi, H., Moghadam, Y. H., & Sakaei, S. H. (2015). The effect of reflecting journaling on nursing students' critical thinking in clinical activities. *Journal of Urmia Nursing & Midwifery Faculty, 13*(1), 19–26.

National Council of State Boards of Nursing. (2017). Highlights of the 2017 environmental scan. *Journal of Nursing Regulation, 7*(4), 4–14. doi:10.1016/S2155-8256(17)30014-5.

National League for Nursing. (2016a). Achieving diversity and meaningful inclusion in nursing education. http://www.nln.org/docs/default-source/about/vision-statement-achieving-diversity.pdf?sfvrsn=2

National League for Nursing. (2021). Certified Nurse Educator (CNE) 2021 candidate handbook. http://www.nln.org/docs/default-source/default-document-library/cne-handbook-2021_revised_07-01-2021.pdf?sfvrsn=2

National League for Nursing. (2021). Certified Nurse Educator Novice (CNEn) 2021 candidate handbook. http://www.nln.org/Certification-for-Nurse-Educators/cne-n/cne-n-handbook

Nyqvist, J., Brolin, K., Nilsson, T., & Lindström, V. (2020). The learning environment and supportive supervision promote learning and are based on the relationship between students and supervisors-A qualitative study. *Nurse Education in Practice, 42*, 102692. 10.1016/j.nepr.2019.102692

O'Connor, A. (2015). Clinical instruction and evaluation: A teaching resource (3rd ed.). Jones & Bartlett. Oermann, M. H., Shellenbarger, T., & Gaberson, K., (2018). *Clinical teaching strategies in nursing* (5th ed.). Springer Publishing Company.

Peddle, M., Bearman, M., & Nestel, D. Virtual patients and nontechnical skills in undergraduate health professional education: An integrative review. *Clinical Simulation in Nursing, 12*(9), 400–410. 10.1016/j.ecns.2016.04.004.

Rice, G. (2016). An orientation program for clinical adjunct faculty. *Association of Black Nursing Faculty (ABNF) Journal, 27*(1), 7–10. https://www.pubfacts.com/detail/26930766/An-Orientation-Program-for-Clinical-Adjunct-Faculty

Rowbotham, M., & Owen, R. M. (2015). The effect of clinical nursing instructors on student self-efficacy. *Nurse Education in Practice, 15*(6), 561–566. 10.1016/j.nepr.2015.09.008

Rudolph, J., Simon, R., Dufresne, R., & Raemer, D. (2006). There's no such thing as "nonjudgmental" debriefing: A theory and method for debriefing with good judgment. *Simulation in Health Care, 1*(1), 49–55.

Scholtz, S. M. P. (2007). Management strategies in clinical care settings. In B. Moyer & R. A. Wittmann-Price (Eds.), *Nursing education: Foundations for practice excellence* (pp. 251–261). F. A. Davis.

Rutledge, C., Pitts, C., Poston, R., & Schweickert, P. (2018). NONPF supports telehealth in nurse practitioner education. https://cdn.ymaws.com/www.nonpf.org/resource/resmgr/2018_Slate/Telehealth_Paper_2018.pdf

Sedgwick, T., Oosterbroek, T., & Ponomar, V. (2014). 'It all depends': How minority nursing students experience belonging during clinical experiences. *Nursing Education Perspectives, 35*(2), 89–93. 10.5480/11-707.1

Shivers, E., Hasson, F., & Slater, P. (2017). Pre-registration nursing student's quality of practice learning: Clinical learning environment inventory (actual) questionnaire. *Nurse Education Today, 55*, 58–64. 10.1016/j.nedt.2017.05.004

Turner, S. (2015). Interprofessional clinical assignments: A project in nursing education. *Creative Nursing, 21*(3), 156–160.

Walsh, T., Jairath, N., Paterson, M. A., & Grandjean, C. (2010). Quality and safety education for nurses clinical evaluation tool. *Journal of Nursing Education, 49*(9), 517–522.

Westrick, S. J. (2016). Nursing students' use of electronic and social media: Law, ethics, and e-professionalism. *Nursing Education Perspectives, 37*(1), 16–22. 10.5480/14-1358

Wynn, S. T. (2019). Limited mental health clinical sites: Telehealth is the answer. *Journal of Nursing Education, 58*(3), 187. 10.3928/01484834-20190221-14

Wittmann-Price, R. A., & Cornelius, F. (2011). *Maternal–child nursing test success: An unfolding case study review*. Springer Publishing Company.

Wittmann-Price, R. A., & Cornelius, F. (2013). *Nursing fundamentals: An unfolding case study review*. Springer Publishing Company.

Wittmann-Price, R. A., Kennedy, L., & Godwin, K. (2012). The use of personal phones by senior nursing students to access health care information during clinical education: Staff nurses' and students' perceptions. *Journal of Nursing Education, 51*(11), 642–646. 10.3928/01484834-20120914-04

Wittmann-Price, R. A., & Thompson, B. R. (Eds.). (2010). *NCLEX-RN® EXCEL: Test success through unfolding case study review*. Springer Publishing Company.

Woolsey, C., & Bracy, K. (2012). Building a clinical ladder for ambulatory care. *Nursing Economic$, 30*(1), 45–49.

Learning With Simulation

7

Linda Wilson and Dorie Weaver

"The simulation is fiction but your decisions are real."
—John Cornele

▶ LEARNING OUTCOMES

This chapter also addresses the Certified Nurse Educator Exam and the Certified Nurse Educator Novice exam Content Area 1: Facilitate Learning

- Discuss the role of simulation learning experiences in nursing education
- Describe the types of simulation and their use in nursing education
- Describe strategies to integrate simulation into the learning environment
- Discuss the importance of evaluation of simulated experiences
- Review the opportunities for certification in simulation

● TYPES OF SIMULATION

▶ SIMULATION USING THE HUMAN PATIENT SIMULATOR

Human patient simulator (HPS) simulation includes the use of low-fidelity, mid-fidelity, and high-fidelity manikins. The fidelity of the manikin determines the complexity and realism of the manikin's capabilities. The high-fidelity manikin can cry, sweat, seize, has pupils that react to light, has changeable heart sounds, has changeable lung sounds, can physiologically react to medication administration, and much more. There are several companies that produce and sell manikins with varying fidelity. HPS simulation provides students opportunities to apply their skills and knowledge based on realistic clinical scenarios. HPS simulation allows students to practice in a safe and controlled environment where there is no threat for patient harm (Turrentine et al., 2016).

● **TEACHING GEM** Simulation is an effective teaching strategy in enhancing collaborative communication, mutual respect, problem-solving, and shared decision making when conducted utilizing a team-based, interprofessional approach. Simulation can use individuals from various professions, such as medicine, pharmacy, case management, physical therapy, and nutrition.

> **EVIDENCE-BASED TEACHING PRACTICE**
>
> Hardenberg, Rana, and Tori (2020) studied simulation and its relationship to nursing curricula. The results indicate that simulation needs to be implemented in a scaffolding manner to achieve cognitive deep learning and psychomotor skill attainment.

▶ SIMULATION USING STANDARDIZED PATIENTS

A **standardized patient** (SP) is an actor who has been trained to portray a patient in a consistent manner in a specific scenario portraying a medical condition, a psychiatric disorder, an ethical situation, or any other health care situation (Onori, Pampaloni, & Multak, 2012). The SP simulation is an excellent method of simulation because the patients can portray real emotions, such as anxiety or depression, and can even cry on demand.

SPs can be hired to work in the simulation laboratory for specific simulation experiences. If an organization cannot afford to hire SPs, it can possibly contract with the drama department at their school, a drama club in their community, or they can even seek volunteers for patients.

▶ HYBRID SIMULATION

Hybrid simulation is the term used for a simulation that uses a combination of HPS simulation and SP simulation. For example, a simulation scenario in which a baby manikin is being used as the patient and an SP is portraying the parent is considered to be a hybrid simulation.

▶ SIMULATION USING PART-TASK TRAINERS

Part-task trainers (PTT) are used to teach a specific skill or set of specific skills, usually related to clinical procedures. PTTs "range in complexity from a piece of fruit to teach injections to a torso to teach central line placement" (Arnold & Wittmann-Price, 2015, p. 170). Simulation using a PTT "usually does not include patient feedback or debriefing" (Arnold & Wittmann-Price, 2015, p. 170). Complex PTTs increase the fidelity of the learning experience by allowing the learner to use a combination of PTT in conjunction with a computer-based simulated environment (Galloway, 2009).

◎ **Critical Thinking Question**

If there are no actors or actresses available in your educational system, what other resources could be used to incorporate SPs? Perhaps senior groups, other learners, and so forth?

 ## SIMULATION CASE DEVELOPMENT

▶ HPS SIMULATION CASES

HPS simulation cases can be obtained in a variety of ways. They can be purchased as preprogrammed scenarios from a manikin vendor. The faculty can also choose to create and program their own scenarios using the simulator software. Another easy way to run scenarios is to have a faculty member adjust the actions of the manikin while the scenario is taking place based on the actions of the simulation participants. See Exhibit 7.1 for a sample template HPS case development.

> ● **TEACHING GEM** When selecting an actor for a standardized patient simulation, to be most effective, it is important to choose someone that the learner does not know.

Exhibit 7.1 HPS Simulation Scenario Template

Authors:
Date/Time of Scenario:
Case Title:
Target Audience:
Primary Learning Objectives: key learning objectives of the scenario
Critical actions checklist: a list to ensure the educational/assessment goals are met.
Environment (if using as a simulation case)

    1. Room Setup
       a. Audio visual
       b. Other equipment

Actors

    1. Roles

    For Instructor ONLY

    Authors:

    Case Title:

CASE SUMMARY

SYNOPSIS OF CASE

SYNOPSIS OF HISTORY/SCENARIO BACKGROUND

SYNOPSIS OF PHYSICAL

For Participants

HISTORY

Onset of Symptoms:

Background Info:

Chief Complaint:

Past Medical History:

Past Surgical History:

Family Medical History:

Social History:

For Instructor ONLY

(*continued*)

PHYSICAL EXAMINATION

Patient:

Age and Sex:

General Appearance:

Vital Signs:

Blood pressure:

Pulse:

Respiratory rate:

Temperature:

Head:

Eyes:

Ears:

Mouth:

Neck:

Skin:

Chest:

Heart:

Abdomen:

Extremities:

Neurological:

Mental Status:

Learner Stimulus

Hospital
Admitting Form

Name:

Age:

Sex:

Method of transportation:

Person giving information:

(continued)

Presenting Complaint:

Background:

Triage or Initial Vital Signs:

Blood pressure:

Pulse:

Respiratory rate:

Temperature:

CASE:

Critical Actions:

Additional documentation and supporting material for scenario: (i.e., Advanced Cardiac Life Support [ACLS] algorithm, APGAR scoring, etc.)

Developed by Carol Okupniak. Reprinted with permission.

▶ STANDARDIZED PATIENT SIMULATION CASES

SP simulation cases are usually written by the faculty member who is planning and running the simulation experience. Because the SPs are actors, they need a very detailed script. The SP simulation case will include the following sections: patient name, patient role, timing for the simulation encounter, setting, overview of the scenario, instructions or door sign explaining the condition of the patient in the room, opening line, patient position and attire, challenge questions, questions that might be asked during the simulation and the specific answer required, evaluation criteria/checklist items, passing score, and type of feedback.

Prior to an SP simulation experience, the SPs will participate in training for the simulation experience (Onori et al., 2012; Wilson, 2018). The training will include the review of the SP case scenario or script, opportunity for questions and answers, demonstration of physical exam techniques if indicated, and role-play to practice the scenario.

See Exhibit 7.2 for a sample template of an SP simulation case development.

Exhibit 7.2 SP Simulation Case Template

Title of the Case:

Patient name: Mr./Mrs. Fran Foles

Length of time for the encounter (maximum time the student can be in the room—15 minutes/30 minutes/45 minutes):

Checklist time: 10 minutes

Feedback time: 10 minutes

Turnaround time: 5 minutes

Setting:

Overview of the scenario background for the patient:

(continued)

Instructions/door sign: (Information for the student to see prior to the experience includes what is to be done during the experience and ends with how many minutes the student has to complete the experience.):

Mr./Mrs. Fran Foles came to the _____ for _____.

You have _____ minutes to _____.

Opening line (What you want the patient to say at the beginning of the experience.):

Patient position at start of the scenario (sitting on table/sitting in chair):

Patient dress at start of the scenario (regular clothes/patient gown):

Challenge question (The question that the patient is to ask the student during the experience, plus the answer to the question.):

Questions during the experience (training questions) (Identify questions that the learner may ask during the experience that *require a specific answer*—List the questions below and the answers to the questions. For all other questions, the patient can "use his or her own" information.):

Please delete/change/add to the list below

What is your age? Use your own

Are you married? Use your own

Occupation? Use your own

Have you ever had anything similar in the past? Yes. I was seen in the emergency department approximately 6 months ago with the same problem.

Have you ever used any recreational drugs? No

Have you ever been hospitalized? No, or use your own if necessary (e.g., due to scar).

Have you ever had surgery? No, or use your own if necessary (e.g., due to scar)

Have you ever been pregnant? Use your own

Do you have any chronic illnesses? I have diabetes

Are you taking any medications? Insulin 70/30

How is your father? Died a few years ago from a stroke

How is your mother? Alive, has a history of knee amputation, history of diabetes

How is/are your sibling(s)? Healthy

Past health history:

Immunizations up to date?

Diet activity/exercise:

Medications:

Prescription medications—

Over the counter medications—

Medication allergies—

Seasonal allergies—

Psychosocial history:

Passing score:

Checklist items (Items used to evaluate the student during the experience. Each of these items will be marked one of the following: Done/Not Done/N/A):

Communication

1. Introduces self with name and title

2. Good eye contact (at least 50% of the time)

3. Was professional in manner

4. Speaks clearly in terms the patient can understand (three-strikes rule)

5. Active listener

6. Asked about

7. Asked about

8.

9.

10.

Physical Examination

1. Washes hands before the examination

2. Explained to me what they were doing with each step of the examination

3.

4.

5.

6.

7.

8.

9.

10.

Patient Education

1. Discussed the importance of

2. Discussed the danger signs of

3. Offered information or suggested some options for

4.

5.

6.

7.

8.

9.

10.

SP will also provide feedback—Interpersonal

Developed by Linda Wilson.

SIMULATION EVALUATION

▶ HPS SIMULATION EVALUATION

The evaluation for the HPS simulation usually includes an evaluation of a group as a team plus individual evaluations. The evaluation is developed in the form of a checklist to evaluate what the learner did or did not do during the simulation encounter. The checklist will usually include evaluation items on communication, physical examination, and patient teaching. The evaluation checklist can be as simple or complex as needed, based on the objectives of the simulation. A faculty member who observes the simulation encounter completes the checklist.

Adamson, Kardong-Edgren, and Willhaus (2013) state simulation use continues to spiral upward as an effective pedagogical method across undergraduate nursing curricula. Because of this significant surge, there is a substantial need for further development of reliable and valid measurement tools specifically designed to assess accurately student performance in the simulation environment. According to Stiller et al. (2015), it is imperative that careful consideration be given when selecting an instrument to ensure it is suitable to both the activity and the learner. "Evaluation instruments must match the scenario and be specific enough to identify the essential performance requirements in order to decrease subjectivity of the rater" (Stiller et al., 2015, p. 89).

It is equally important to continue building evidence for the use of stimulation to facilitate learning. Faculty should have an evaluation of the effectiveness of the actual simulation case created, students' subjective report of satisfaction and self-confidence levels pre- and post-simulation, and/or the educational practices at the end of the simulation. Several tools have been developed to obtain this data (Franklin, Burns, & Lee, 2014). Refer to the box titled "Evidence-Based Teaching Practice" (Franklin et al., 2014). In contrast to the skills/competencies checklist, these two scales would be completed by the student.

EVIDENCE-BASED TEACHING PRACTICE

Holland, Tiffany, Blazovich, Bambini, and Schug (2020) studied the effectiveness of a training intervention in achieving inter- and intrarater reliability among faculty who were rating students' simulation performance in high-stakes testing situations. The randomized control study of 75 pre-licensure nursing programs demonstrated that training was effective and that raters had a better inter- and intrarater reliability ratings than those without training.

▶ SP SIMULATION EVALUATION

The evaluation for the SP simulation is usually an evaluation of an individual who participated in the simulation with the SP. If there is more than one participant in the SP simulation, team evaluation can also be incorporated. The evaluation is usually developed in the form of a checklist to evaluate what the learner did or did not do during the simulation encounter (Wilson, Kane, & Price, 2018; Habibli, Ghezelieh, & Haghami, 2020). The checklist can include evaluation items on communication, physical examination, patient teaching, diagnosis, follow-up, and teamwork. The selection of evaluation items is also based on the level and type of health professions learner. The evaluation checklist can be as simple or complex as needed, based on the objectives for the simulation.

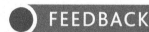

FEEDBACK

Once the standardized patient simulation encounter is done, and the evaluation checklist or post-encounter documentation has been completed, the learner and the SP will meet for the one-on-one feedback session (Wilson, Kane, & Price, 2018). During the feedback session, the SP is no longer acting, and the SP provides the learner with constructive feedback on how the learner made him or her feel like a patient, and any other specifics as determined by the faculty member prior to the encounter. The learners often comment that the feedback session is the most rewarding part of the SP simulation experience (Roberts, Oxlad, Dorstyn, & Chur-Hansen, 2020).

DEBRIEFING

Debriefing is an essential and vital learning component of simulation. Debriefing commonly takes place following an HPS simulation experience in a location near but separate from the simulation location (Wilson, Cornele, & Wittmann-Price, 2018). The time spent by the students, with faculty direction in a form of guided reflection, is the reason debriefing is a significant component of simulation. Debriefing affords the student an opportunity to analyze the events as they occurred. Students can examine the scenario from various perspectives, which will enhance their future clinical decision-making and problem-solving skills (Choi, Kim, Park, Lim, & Kim, 2021).

Essentials for the debriefing facilitator include the following:

- Formal training in debriefing
- Being present to observe the scenario to be debriefed
- Select and use a specific model for debriefing
- Facilitate guided reflection during the debriefing session

There are many different methods for debriefing, including the following:

- Structured and Supported Debriefing
- Case Study Review Debriefing (Overstreet, 2009)
- Plus/Delta Debriefing (Gardner, 2013)
- Debriefing with Good Judgement (Rudolph, Simon, Rivard, Dufresne, & Raemer, 2007)
- Promoting Excellence and Reflective Learning in Simulation: PEARLS (Eppich & Cheng, 2015)
- Debriefing for Meaningful Learning: DML (Dreifuerst, 2015)
- 3D Model of Debriefing: Defusing, Discovering, Deepening (Jigmont, 2011)

As faculty facilitators are developing their debriefing skills, they should identify which model of debriefing they find most effective. Some nursing programs may instead select a specific type of debriefing model and require that specific type of debriefing be used for all simulation activities in their program.

 ## VIRTURAL REALITY SIMULATION

Virtual reality simulation "is a technology by which computer aided stimuli create the immersive illusion of being somewhere else" (Rubin & Grey, 2020, p. 1). Through virtual reality simulation the learner becomes immersed in the experience and, in some experiences, can interact with others within the experience. With the required equipment, virtual reality experiences can be easily be created for our learners.

Serious games are interactive virtual simulations that can involve single or multiple users (Fliszar, 2018). Serious games can be used for learning purposes or evaluative purposes.

 ## REMOTE SIMULATION LEARNING EXPERIENCES

When simulation activities are not able to be completed face-to-face, many types of simulation can be done virtually, including virtual reality and serious games, as mentioned earlier. Standardized patient simulation is also very effective in a virtual environment using a virtual meeting software platform. The learners and the standardized patients can meet in the main virtual room and can then be placed into breakout rooms for individual experiences. These experiences can include history taking, interviews, patient teaching, patient assessment, and many others. The faculty can send messages to the learners in the breakout rooms to remind them of the time left for the experience as well as notification before the end of the experience. Following the individual experience, the learners can be brought back to meet with the faculty in the main meeting room to have a group discussion or focused debriefing session. This is just one example of how a virtual meeting platform can be used, and there are many other options that can be considered.

 ## SIMULATION CERTIFICATIONS

Certified Healthcare Simulation Educator (CHSE)—the CHSE certification is offered by the Society for Simulation in Healthcare (SSH). Eligibility, benefits, application process, fees, and exam prep resources can be found on the SSH website at www.ssih.org/Certification.

Certified Healthcare Simulation Educator—Advanced (CHSE-A)—the CHSE-A certification is offered by the SSH. Eligibility, benefits, application process, fees, and portfolio requirements can be found on the SSH website at www.ssih.org/Certification.

Certified Healthcare Simulation Operations Specialist (CHSOS)—CHSOS certification is offered by the SSH. Eligibility, benefits, application process, fees, and exam prep resources can be found on the SSH website at www.ssih.org/Certification.

Certified Healthcare Simulation Operations Specialist—Advanced (CHSOS-A)—The CHSOS-A certification is offered by the SSH. Eligibility, benefits, application process, fees, and portfolio requirements can be found on the SSH website at www.ssih.org/Certification.

 ## CASE STUDY

CASE STUDY 7.1

A simulation coordinator is orienting the nursing learners to the HPS for the first time. The simulation coordinator and the clinical nursing faculty members are in the simulation room with the learners. The learners start to practice vital signs on the HPS, and the clinical nursing instructor starts to tell them that they are taking the blood pressure incorrectly.

How should the simulation coordinator respond to this? Is this the purpose of the orientation session? How can difficult situations in the orientation session be prevented?

---

1. The best simulation modality to teach complex healthcare conditions on a hospitalized patient to a group of senior nursing learners is:

    A. Part-task trainers

    B. Human patient simulator

    C. Standardized (simulated) patient

    D. Role-play

2. A nurse educator requests community volunteers to be standardized patients for a group of second-semester junior nursing students. One of the volunteers has the chronic obstructive pulmonary disease. The nurse educator understands that this situation is:

    A. Legally unacceptable

    B. Difficult for junior nursing learners

    C. In need of a consent form from the standardized patient

    D. A symptomatic standardized patient

3. The novice nurse educator needs additional understanding of simulation learning when they state that an attribute of fidelity is:

    A. Realism

    B. Capabilities

    C. Complexity

    D. Risk assessment

4. The nurse educator must orientate the standardized patients (SPs) to the simulation scenario. The best method to accomplish SP orientation is:

    A. Simulation feedback

    B. Role-play

    C. Scenario review

    D. SP training

5. A nurse educator uses a rubric to score a simulation evaluative session with an advanced practice student. The student scores a passing grade of 19/22 on the simulation scenario. The simulation evaluation is worth 15% of the total course grade. What percentage should the nurse educator enter in the grade book?

    A. 11.9%

    B. 12.3%

    C. 12.5%

    D. 12.9%

1. B) Hyman patient simulator

Human patent simulator (HPS) is the formal name for manikin simulation that can be used to display complex healthcare conditions. A part-task trainer, standardized patient, or role-play is not as effective.

2. D) A symptomatic standardized patient

This is a symptomatic standardized patient and not an actor who has been trained to portray a specific type of patient or other specific role. There are no additional legal implications or consents needed than the rest of the standardized patients. Junior nursing students should be able to detect abnormal breath sounds if they have completed health assessment.

3. D) Risk assessment

Risk assessment is not an attribute associated with fidelity. Realism, capabilities, and complexity are attributes that increase fidelity.

4. D) SP training

SP training is completed with the SPs to review all the aspects of the scenario. The SPs are also given the opportunity to ask questions and clarify any questions about the scenario. Simulation feedback is the process in which they discuss how the student felt and what the student did correctly and incorrectly. Role-play is the actual enactment of the scenario. Scenario review can happen, but it is not the initial learning process.

5. D) 12.9%

19 out of 22 points is 86%. Eighty-six percent of 15% = 12.9%.

6. The best part-task trainer (PTT) for a nurse educator to choose to demonstrate basic nursing care is:

   A. Pelvis that can be used for Foley catheter insertion
   B. Pelvis that can birth a baby with complications such as bleeding
   C. An intravenous (IV) arm connected to a virtual patient
   D. Nasogastric insertion setup connected to a virtual patient

7. Following a standardized patient (SP) simulation experience, the learner has the opportunity to meet with the SP one on one for a learning session, which is called?

   A. Debriefing
   B. Evaluation
   C. Feedback
   D. Review

8. A nurse educator has chosen to use a complex a part-task trainer (PTT) to demonstrate an advanced skill. The best equipment to access for this learning session is:

   A. Patient torso with multiple lung sounds
   B. Laparoscopic trainer connected to virtual patient
   C. Intravenous cushion with multiple injection sites
   D. Pelvis with male and female genitalia

9. The best method for a new nurse educator to understand how to effectively debrief is:

   A. Observed someone else debrief
   B. Received a report of how the scenario went
   C. Select and use a specific model for debriefing
   D. Be ready to demonstrate better interventions than what was done

10. A group of students is pre-briefed on a simulation scenario. During the scenario, a student gets visibly upset and begins to cry. The best action for the nurse educator is:

    A. Continue the scenario and allow the student to continue
    B. Remove the students from the scenario
    C. Enter the scenario as a healthcare person and address the student privately
    D. Stop the scenario and debrief the group to talk about the incident

(See answers next page.)

6. A) Pelvis that can be used for Foley catheter insertion

Basic part-task trainers represent various anatomical body parts and are specifically used for practice of procedures. The hybrid use of PTT is more complicated. Pelvis that can birth a baby with complications such as bleeding is an HPS. An IV arm connected to a virtual patient and a nasogastric insertion setup connected to a virtual patient are both hybrid simulations.

7. C) Feedback

Following the standardized patient simulation experience, the learner will meet for a few minutes one on one with the standardized patient for feedback. The feedback provided during this time is usually interpersonal. Debriefing is done by faculty with a group of students. Evaluation is usually between one faculty member and one student. Review is not the correct terminology

8. B) Laparoscopic trainer connected to virtual patient

Complex task trainers are used for practice of involved procedures such as laparoscopic surgery task trainers and are usually connected to a virtual or standardized patient. A patient torso with multiple lung sounds is a PTT. An IV cushion with multiple injection sites and a pelvis with male and female genitalia are both part-task trainers.

9. C) Select and use a specific model for debriefing

A debriefer should select a specific model or method for debriefing and will use that type of debriefing on a regular basis. Observing someone else debrief is not enough—education in debriefing is needed. The debriefer does need to observe the scenario and not just receive a report. The learners should reflect on better interventions; they do not need to be ready to demonstrate them.

10. B) Remove the students from the scenario

Remove the upset student and speak with the student and, if needed, send the student to counseling. Continuing the scenario, stepping in, or stopping the scenario completely is not assisting the upset student or the other students.

REFERENCES

Adamson, K. A., Kardong-Edgren, S., & Willhaus, J. (2013). An updated review of published evaluation instruments. *Clinical Simulation in Nursing, 9*(9), e393–e400. 10.1016/j.ecns.2012.09.004

Arnold, D., & Wittmann-Price, R. (2015). Part-task trainers. In L. Wilson & R. Wittmann-Price (Eds.), *Review manual for the certified healthcare simulation educator exam.* Springer Publishing Company.

Choi, J. A., Kim, O., Park, S., Lim, H., & Kim, J. (2021). The effectiveness of peer learning in undergraduate nursing students: A meta-analysis. *Clinical Simulation in Nursing, 50,* 92–101. 10.1016/j.ecns.2020.09.002

Dreifuerst, K. T. (2015). Getting started with debriefing for meaningful learning. *Clinical Simulation in Nursing, 11*(5), 268–275.

Eppich, W., & Cheng, A. (2015). Promoting excellence and reflective learning in simulation (PEARLS). *Simulation in Healthcare, 10,* 106–115.

Fliszar, R. (2018). Virtual Reality. In L. Wilson & R. Wittmann-Price (Eds.), *Review manual for the certified healthcare simulation educator exam* (2nd ed.). Springer Publishing Company.

Franklin, A. E., Burns, P., & Lee, C. S. (2014). Psychometric testing on the NLN student satisfaction and self-confidence in learning, simulation design scale, and educational practices questionnaire using a sample of pre-licensure novice nurses. *Nurse Education Today, 34*(10), 1298–1304. 10.1016/j.nedt.2014.06.011

Galloway, S. J. (2009). Simulation techniques to bridge the gap between novice and competent healthcare professionals. *Online Journal of Nursing Issues in Nursing, 14*(2), 166–174. http://www.nursingworld.org/MainMenuCategories/ANAMarketplace/ANAPeriodicals/OJIN/TableofContents/Vol142009/No2May09/Simulation-Techniques.html?css=print

Gardner, R. (2013). Introduction to debriefing. *Seminars in Perinatology, 37*(3), 166–174. 10.1053/j.semperi.2013.02.008

Habibli, T., Ghezelieh, T. N., & Haghami, S. (2020). The effect of simulation-based education on nursing students' knowledge and performance of adult basic cardiopulmonary resuscitation: A randomized clinical trial. *Nursing Practice Today, 7*(2), 87–96.

Hardenberg, J. Rana, I, & Tori, K. (2020). As a learning modality simulation complements theory within nursing curricula. *Australian Nursing & Midwifery Journal, 27*(2), 42.

Holland, A. E., Tiffany, J., Blazovich, L., Bambini, D., Schug, V. (2020). The effect of evaluator training on inter- and intrarater reliability in high-stakes assessment in simulation. *Nursing Education Perspectives, 41*(4), 222–228. 10.1097/01.NEP.0000000000000619

Jigmont, J. J. (2011). The 3D model of debriefing: Defusing, discovering, and deepening. *Seminars in Perinatology, 35*(2), 52–58. 10.1053/j.semperi.2011.01.003

National League for Nursing. (2021). Certified Nurse Educator (CNE) 2021 candidate handbook. http://www.nln.org/docs/default-source/default-document-library/cne-handbook-2021_revised_07-01-2021.pdf?sfvrsn=2

National League for Nursing. (2021). Certified Nurse Educator Novice (CNEn) 2021 candidate handbook. http://www.nln.org/Certification-for-Nurse-Educators/cne-n/cne-n-handbook

Overstreet, M. L. (2009). *The current practice of nursing clinical simulation debriefing: A multiple case study* (Doctoral dissertation). University of Tennessee, Knoxville, TN. http://trace.tennessee.edu/utk_graddiss/627

Rubin, P., Grey, J, (2020). What is virtual reality (VR)? *The Complete WIRED Guide.* https://www.wired.com/story/wired-guide-to-virtual-reality/

Rudolph, J. W., Simon, R., Rivard, P., Dufresne, R. L., & Raemer, D. B. (2007). Debriefing with good judgement: Combining rigorous feedback with genuine inquiry. *Anesthesiology Clinics, 25,* 361–376.

Stiller, J. J., Nelson, K. A., Anderson, M., Ashe, M. J., Johnson, S. T., Sandhu, K, & LeFlore, J. (2015). Development of a valid and reliable evaluation instrument for undergraduate nursing students during simulation. *Journal of Nursing Education and Practice, 5*(7), 83–90.

Turrentine, F. E., Rose, K. M., Hanks, J. B., Lorntz, B., Owen, J. A., Brashers, V. L., & Ramsdale, E. E. (2016). Interprofessional training enhances collaboration between nursing and medical students: A pilot study. *Nurse Education Today, 40,* 33–38.

Wilson, L., Cornele, J., Wittmann-Price, R. (2018). Debriefing. In L. Wilson & R. Wittmann-Price (Eds.), *Review manual for the certified healthcare simulation educator exam* (2nd ed.). Springer Publishing Company.

Wilson, L., Kane, H. L., Price, S. (2018). Principles, practice and methodologies for SP simulation. In L. Wilson & R. Wittmann-Price (Eds.), *Review manual for the certified healthcare simulation educator exam* (2nd ed.). Springer Publishing Company.

Facilitating Learner Development and Socialization

Maryann Godshall

> *Be the change you want to see in the world.*
> —Mahatma Gandhi

▶ LEARNING OUTCOMES

This chapter addresses the Certified Nurse Educator Exam and the Certified Nurse Educator Novice exam Content Area 2: Facilitate Learner Development and Socialization. For the CNE exam it is 15% of the examination, approximately 22 questions and for the CNEn exam it is 11% of the examination or approximately 17 questions

- ■ Discuss individual learning styles
- ■ Explore the characteristics of the adult learner
- ■ Understand academic dishonesty and incivility
- ■ Recognize culturally diverse learners
- ■ Identify those with learning disabilities
- ■ Examine learning in the cognitive, affective, and psychomotor domains
- ■ Discuss socialization into nursing

● INTRODUCTION

Today, learners present educators with a wide variety of challenges in meeting their educational needs. A nurse educator must appreciate and consider the learning styles of each student. Nurse educators must understand the social determinants that affect learners such as diversity, cognitive ability, economic, culture, intellectual or developmental disabilities (ID/DD), English is an additional language (EAL) or as a second language (ESL), diverse sexual orientation and identity, and different learning styles.

Social determinants challenge faculty to incorporate diverse learning environments into their teaching and learning experiences. The incorporation of online learning, and the utilization of new technology into the classroom is paramount to make learning interactive, self-directed, engaging, collaborative, and assist socialization into the role of nursing. This challenges even the most experienced nurse educator. Integrating all these elements while also incorporating basic education principles is important so that learners not only learn but also are able to pass the National Council Licensure Examination (NCLEX®) when they graduate.

⬤ ASSESSING READINESS TO LEARN

Before learning can occur, one must determine whether learners are ready to receive the information to be learned (Table 8.1).

Readiness to learn occurs when the learner is receptive, willing, and able to participate in the learning process (Bastable, 2019). There are five major components to physical readiness that affect learning:

1. Measure of ability
2. Complexity of the task
3. Environmental effects
4. Learner's health status
5. Gender

Not only does one have to be physically ready to learn, they need to be emotionally ready as well (Bastable, 2019). Emotional or psychological readiness includes:

1. Anxiety level
2. Support systems
3. Motivation
4. Risk-taking behavior
5. Frame of mind

Table 8.1 Learner Readiness

Type of readiness	Attributes to assess to determine readiness
P = Physical readiness	▪ Measure of ability ▪ Complexity of the task ▪ Environmental effects ▪ Health status ▪ Gender
E = Emotional readiness	▪ Anxiety level ▪ Support system ▪ Motivation ▪ Risk-taking behavior ▪ Developmental age ▪ Frame of mind
E = Experiential readiness	▪ Level of aspiration ▪ Past coping mechanisms ▪ Cultural background ▪ Locus of control ▪ Orientation
K = Knowledge readiness	▪ Present knowledge base ▪ Cognitive ability ▪ Learning disabilities ▪ Learning styles

Source: Adapted from Lichtenthal (1990) in Bastable (2019, p. 132). Reprinted with permission of Jones & Bartlett Learning.

● INDIVIDUAL LEARNING STYLES

"Learning styles are cognitive, emotional, and physiological traits, as well as indicators of how learners perceive, interact, and respond to their learning environments" (Czepula et al., 2016, p. 1).

▶ CARL JUNG AND MYERS-BRIGGS TYPOLOGY

Carl Jung, a Swiss psychiatrist, developed a theory that explains personality similarities and differences by identifying attitudes of people as introverts or extroverts along with opposite mental functions, which are the ways people perceive or take in information and use it in the world around them. Isabel Myers and her mother Katherine Briggs were convinced Jung's theories had an application for increasing human understanding. According to Myers-Brigg's individuals reach conclusions about or become aware of something through a presence of judging and perceiving. By combining these different preferences, they identified 16 personality types, each which have their own strength and weakness. It is based on 4 constructs:

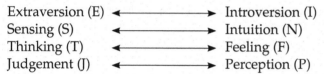

Extraversion (E) ←——————→ Introversion (I)
Sensing (S)   ←——————→ Intuition (N)
Thinking (T)   ←——————→ Feeling (F)
Judgement (J)   ←——————→ Perception (P)

These tests can be taken online so that you know your preferences of learning https://www.myersbriggs.org/my-mbti-personality-type/mbti-basics/. Table 8.2 expands on these types of learning. When looking at one's preferences in four categories, the individual's personality type is expressed as four letters.

Table 8.2 Myers-Briggs types and characteristics

Myers-Briggs Types	Characteristics
Extraversion (E)	▪ Focus on outer world ▪ Likes group work ▪ Prefers fast-paced learning, dislikes slow-paced learning ▪ Offers opinions without being asked ▪ Frequently asks questions
Sensing (S)	▪ Focuses on basic information ▪ Practical ▪ Realistic ▪ Observant ▪ Learns best from orderly sequencing of details
Thinking (T)	▪ When making decisions looks at logic and consistency ▪ Decreased need for harmony ▪ Finds ideas more interesting than people ▪ Analytical

(continued)

Table 8.2 Myers-Briggs types and characteristics

Judging (J)	■ Prefers on making solid decisions quickly ■ Organized ■ Methodical ■ Work-oriented ■ Likes to control the environment
Introversion (I)	■ Focus on inner world ■ Likes quiet space ■ Does not like interruptions ■ Desires learning that deals with thoughts and ideas ■ Offers an opinion only when asked ■ Asks questions only to facilitate their understanding of a concept or idea.
Intuition (N)	■ Prefers to interpret and add meaning when making ■ decisions ■ Always likes new things ■ Imaginative ■ Sees possibilities ■ Prefers an entire concept versus detail
Feeling (F)	■ When making decisions, looks at people and special circumstances ■ Values harmony ■ More interested in people than ideas or things ■ Sympathetic ■ Accepting
Perceiving (P)	■ Likes to stay open to new ideas or options when dealing with the outside world ■ Open-ended, fluid ■ Flexible ■ Adapts to the environment

Source: Adapted from Bastable (2019) and Myers-Briggs Foundation (2020).

Simply put, a learning style is an approach to learning that works for the individual learner. Being aware of this can help maximize student learning and facilitate educator instruction methods.

■ Learners may have more than one learning style. Learners may use multiple learning styles. Although one learning style may be dominant. Some may use different learning styles in different situations or circumstances. One's ability in less dominant styles can also be developed as well.

■ Educators must first assist learners in identifying their learning style(s) if they do not already know them, and then present information in a manner consistent with the learners' learning style(s). Educators also should use multiple modalities to present information that enhance and encompass multiple learning styles.

The four most common learning styles are defined by the acronym VARK, Visual, Auditory, Read/write (or linguistic), and Kinesthetic (Fleming and Mills, 1992). They are part of the seven learning styles listed in Table 8.3 (from Learning-Styles-online. com, 2020).

Table 8.3 VARK learning style and characteristics

Style	Characteristics
Visual (spatial)	Prefers pictures, images, spatial understanding Pictures, diagrams, flow charts, timelines, maps, and demonstrations are more effective than texts or lectures Good assignment might be concept mapping
Aural (auditory-musical)	Prefers sound and music They learn best from lectures, tapes, tutorials, group discussions, speaking, web chats, mobile phones, and talking things out loud
Verbal (linguistic or reading & writing)	Prefers words both in speech and writing; text-based input and output in all of its forms Many academics have a preference for this style of learning People with this learning style are often fond of PowerPoint presentations, the Internet, lists, dictionaries, thesaurus, quotations, and anything else featuring words
Physical (kinesthetic) or tactile learners	Prefers using your body, hands & sense of **touch** They like to think about issues while working out or exercising They like to participate, play games, role-play, act, and model experiences through practicing Learning activities tailored to this style could include simulations or real-life hands-on experiences, or videos or movies of "real things," as well as case studies, practice sessions, and applications
Logical (mathematical, analytical, or sequential)	Prefers using logic, reasoning, and systems For sequential learners, steps follow one another logically and directly, in an assigned order. These learners do not like educators who jump around from topic to topic or skip steps in a process They focus on details & facts. They like outlines or decision trees & algorithms
Social (interpersonal)	Prefers to learn in groups or with other people
Solidarity (intrapersonal)	Prefers to work alone or a self-study

EVIDENCE-BASED TEACHING PRACTICE

Ryan and Poole (2019) used virtual learning environments (VLE) to move students from passive to active learners. Active learning promotes critical thinking skills to enhance transfer of classroom acquired knowledge into the clinical environment. A randomized control trial was conducted with 40 students assigned one of two teaching sessions. Both sessions were identical in content except the second one used a VLE; the other one was solely didactic. Knowledge questionnaires were distributed 2 weeks after the experience. Qualitative data (open-ended questions) were analyzed. Virtual learning seemed to significantly improve student's engagement, satisfaction, and recall. Student learning styles seemed to have no effect on their satisfaction/engagement and ease of learning. Three key themes emerged: (1) visuals were good/helpful, (2) the talk was informative, and (3) more details/visuals were required. The key finding from this study suggests that there is a role for VLE's in the teaching of students. There is a need for introducing advanced technology into health care education such as virtual reality.

▶ MULTIMODAL/MIXTURES (M)

Multimodal learners are individuals who prefer to learn via two or more styles of learning or using a variety of methods.

- These individuals' preferred learning style may be context-specific, or they might choose a single mode to suit a certain occasion or situation.
- These individuals like to gather information from each mode and thereby often gain a deeper and broader understanding of the topic (Fleming, 2001).

EVIDENCE-BASED TEACHING PRACTICE

Yancy (2019) explored using music creatively in the teaching-learning of nursing. One strategy nurse educators might employ is using music to set the mood in a classroom, lab, or office by playing classical music as students gather to start class or playing calming music in the hallways or office area to lower stress levels and promote inspiration and concentration. Music playing while studying may also be helpful for some learners, while others may find it distracting. Personal music choice is key.

● OTHER LEARNING STYLES

In addition to the mentioned styles, there are other learning styles that include:

- Global learners
- Intuitive learners
- Reflective learners
- Accommodative learners
- Divergent learners
- Digital learners

▶ GLOBAL LEARNERS

Global learners make decisions based on their emotions and intuition.

- They are spontaneous and focus on creativity.
- A tidy environment is not important to global learners.
- These learners enjoy learning. They use humor, tell stories, and enjoy group work.
- Global learners like to participate in activities.
- These learners tend to absorb material randomly. They frequently do not see connections at first, but then suddenly "get it."
- Global learners are able to solve complex problems quickly or put things together in unique ways once they have grasped the big picture, but they may have difficulty explaining how they did it.
- These learners lack good sequential thinking abilities (Felder & Solomon, 1998; Mahoney, 2007).

▶ INTUITIVE LEARNERS

These learners like to discover the possibilities in relationships.

- Intuitive learners like solving problems using well-established methods and do not like complications or surprises.
- Intuitive learners do not like repetition.
- These learners tend to work faster and be more innovative than other learners.
- Intuitive learners hate courses that involve a lot of memorization or routine calculations and will easily become bored by them.
- Intuitive learners are prone to careless mistakes on tests because they are impatient with details and do not like repetition, such as checking math calculations (Felder & Solomon, 1998).

▶ REFLECTIVE LEARNERS

A reflective learner prefers to think about new material by reflecting quietly on it first.

- Reflective learners prefer to work alone, rather than with groups.
- These learners do not like classes that cover large amounts of material quickly.
- Reflective learners do not like to be asked simply to read and memorize material.
- These learners like to stop periodically to review what they have read and think of possible questions or applications.
- Reflective learners may find it helpful to write short summaries of readings or class notes in their own words to help them retain the material better (Felder & Solomon, 1998).

▶ ACCOMMODATIVE LEARNERS

Accommodative learners like a combination of concrete experiences and active experimentation.

- They complete tasks and are less concerned about the theories supporting their actions.
- They are risk-takers.
- They solve problems by trial and error.
- They are concerned with abstract concepts and assimilate abstract conceptualizations with reflective observations (Mahoney, 2007).

▶ DIVERGENT LEARNERS

Divergent learners have broad cultural interests and like to gather information. They are interested in people, tend to be imaginative and emotional. They like to watch instead of doing and tend to gather information and use imagination to solve problems. They are very good at viewing concrete problems from various viewpoints. They tend to be strong in the arts (McLeod, 2017). They are frequently misunderstood, and many tend to fail in academic settings.

▶ DIGITAL (ONLINE) LEARNERS

With technological advances, the millennial and generation Z students almost always use technology, smartphones, and less frequently use traditional formats such as archives, newspapers, and other print sources (Orkiszewski, Pollitt, Leonard, & Hayes-Lane, 2016). Characteristics of these learners include:

- Focus on enthusiastic and collaborative learning
- Digital literacy
- Constant connection via hand-held digital devices

EVIDENCE-BASED TEACHING PRACTICE

Shirazi and Heidari (2019) examined the relationship between critical thinking skills and learning styles and the academic achievement of nursing students. Using a cross-sectional study, 139 sophomore nursing students were chosen using random sampling. No relationship between critical thinking and academic achievement was identified. "Diverging" was the most common learning style. The highest mean level of academic achievement was earned by those students who adopted "accommodating" style of learning. A significant relationship was found between learning style and academic achievement ($p < .001$). Critically thinking skill scores were unacceptably low. Therefore, they conclude it is essential that educators pay more attention to improve critical thinking in academic lesson planning. As a significant relationship was found between learning style and academic achievement. It is suggested that educators consider the dominant style of the class and incorporate that into lesson planning and appropriate teaching methods that utilize that dominant style.

GENERATIONAL CHARACTERISTICS OF LEARNERS

When educating students, it is important to remember that characteristics of learning can be attributed to generational groups. These groups share values, attitudes towards learning, have different expectations, and may be motivated differently than one is accustomed to. To be effective as an educator, awareness is key, and then targeting teaching strategies toward the group is paramount. Table 8.4 details generations and their common characteristics.

Table 8.4 Generations and their common characteristics

Generation	Common Characteristics
Traditionalists (1922–1945)	■ Value privacy, trust, and hard work ■ Believe in hard work ■ Need details ■ Are uncomfortable with ambiguity
Baby Boomers (1945–1964)	■ Value career over personal life ■ Want to be challenged ■ Speak clearly and directly ■ Prefer face-to-face meetings

Generation X (1965–1979)	■ Value balance between career and personal life; family-focused ■ Are independent ■ Look for a leader or mentor, not a boss ■ Seek rewards based on their individual performance.
Millennials (aka Generation Y) (1980–1994)	■ Value personal life over career ■ Are highly socialized and optimistic ■ Are tech-savvy ■ Multi-task with ease ■ See education as a means to an end
Generation Z (after 1995)	■ Known characteristics of this generation are still evolving ■ Tend to be realistic, not idealistic ■ Are private about personal life ■ Are particularly tech-savvy ■ Are adept multi-taskers ■ Communicate most often via social media ■ Value virtual connectedness ■ Are passionate about learning

Information from Elliot-Yeary, S. (2020). Meet the five generations in today's workforce. Adapted from https://www.generational-guru.com/generations.

TRADITIONAL VS. NONTRADITIONAL LEARNERS

Traditional learners are typically those who enter a pre-licensure program directly after completing high school. They usually have limited life experience and work experience. Nontraditional learners can be students who are older, may be married and have a family, have previous work experience in one field, and are changing career paths, may have previous work experience but no previous academic study or degrees, and may be working full or part-time while attending school. Nontraditional students typically have additional life responsibilities and stressors that the traditional students do not. Nontraditional students are considered adult learners in that they are typically older in age. Nontraditional students' approach to learning and education is very different than their traditional counterparts. They are motivated differently and are very driven. They tend to be more vocal. They usually do not live on campus. They bring previous life experiences into the classroom. Mixing traditional and nontraditional students in the same classroom could result in challenges and needs special attention by the nurse educator to assure all needs are being met by both groups of learners.

ADULT LEARNERS

Adult learners display a variety of learning characteristics. Knowles, Houlton, and Swanson (2015) were among the first researchers to theorize how adults learn.

■ The most common reason an adult enters any learning experience is to create change. This could encompass change in their:
  ● Skills
  ● Behavior
  ● Knowledge level
  ● Attitudes about things

Barriers to adult learning include:

- Lack of time
- Lack of confidence
- Lack of information about opportunities to learn
- Scheduling problems/conflicts
- Red tape

It is important to incorporate adult learning principles into teaching to maximize learning potential for this population. Adult learners learn best when:

- Learning is related to an immediate need, problem, or deficit.
- Learning is voluntary and self-initiated.
- Learning is person-centered and problem-centered.
- Learning is self-controlled and self-directed.
- The role of the teacher is that of a facilitator.
- Information and assignments are pertinent and meaningful versus busy work as they see it.
- New material draws on past experiences and is related to something that the learner already knows. This is the best way for these learners to retain knowledge.
- The learner's perception of threats to themselves is reduced to a minimum in the educational situation.
- Learners are able to actively participate in the learning process.
- They are able to learn in groups.
- The nature of the learning activity changes frequently.
- Learning is reinforced by application and prompt feedback (Knowles et al., 2015).

LEARNERS WITH PREVIOUS EDUCATION (SECOND-DEGREE STUDENTS)

There has been a dramatic increase in accelerated nursing programs. These programs admit students with previously obtained degrees (most often bachelor's degrees) in another discipline and then have them attend an abbreviated version of the nursing curriculum. Although these students bring a broad perspective from their previous life experiences, they have a greater tendency to struggle with feeling inadequate with regard to their nursing knowledge and skills. They also have a high expectation of the faculty to be competent and professional nurses. Despite their previous experiences, faculty report that these second-degree students have a much greater need than their traditional counterparts to feel self-confident and competent (Tornwall, Tan & Bowles, 2018). These students can be challenging to the most seasoned educator. The high levels of stress they experience due to the shortened time frame of study and potential financial burdens cause them to sometimes act out and appear demanding.

Some suggestions by Christofferson (2016) are listed below to work with these students. They include:

- Abandon old teacher-centric methods in favor of active learning and by using emerging technologies such as simulation, blogging, and web-based methodologies.
- Be well-prepared and extremely organized. Do not attempt to "wing it" with this group.
- Schedule more time to meet with students frequently; collaborate; actively listen and engage them. They do not like passive listening and learning.
- Immerse students very early on into the profession both clinically and socially.
- Be aware of the uniqueness of accelerated student cohorts and use this knowledge to develop equally unique courses.
- Recognize these students begin courses with many capabilities and high motivation, acknowledge their past work and life experiences, harness these attributes, and incorporate them where possible.
- Make assignments meaningful. They hate nothing more than what they perceive as busy work.
- Be well prepared and know the material. They enjoy asking questions for clarification.

EVIDENCE-BASED TEACHING PRACTICE

In a study that examined male and female students in second-degree nursing programs in regard to key demographic, educational, and outcome variables. Male students differed from female students on many important dimensions that have relevance for teaching, research, and program planning. Overall, program and NCLEX passage rates were high for both genders. Many had plans to pursue advanced nursing education roles. Secondary analysis found these programs are a great way to entice men into the role of nursing. This will increase the diversity of nursing roles which holds great promise for the nursing profession to help alleviate the nursing shortage, enhance workforce diversity, expand nursing program capacity, and provide a potential future nursing faculty source (Spurlock, Patterson, & Colby, 2019).

CULTURALLY DIVERSE LEARNERS

The culture of the individual encompasses an individual's values, habits, attitudes, perceptions, and beliefs acquired over time in relationship to membership in a particular group. It is important for faculty to recognize that cultural diversity can influence learning ability and socializing them into the role of nurse. In addition, diversity may influence how nursing is perceived by individuals from diverse alternative cultural backgrounds. For example, a nurse who, in one culture, may be considered a "caring nurse," may be perceived by members of another culture as cold and uncaring. Perceptions and self-awareness of individuals must be considered from each individual's cultural background. It is important to remember that culture is not solely tied to an ethnicity and that some people may belong to multiple groups.

The American Association of Colleges of Nursing (AACN) issued a position statement in 1997 stating that, because the U.S. population is so culturally diverse, cultural diversity training needs to be included in nursing education, and a greater number of culturally diverse learners should be recruited into nursing schools (AACN, 2016). Despite this position statement, minorities continue to be underrepresented in nursing and nursing programs (Burruss & Popkess, 2012). Moreover, culturally diverse learners face certain barriers that may impinge on their ability to achieve success in college. The most common of these barriers are:

- The lack of ethnically diverse faculty
- Finances
- Academic preparation (Burruss & Popkess, 2012)

Culturally diverse learners may also suffer from a lack of:

- Available role models
- Academic support
- Family support
- Peer support

The culture or customs of an individual learner may, at times, may come into conflict with the values of the clinical environment This may cause their value system to be disrupted. A value represents a basic conviction about what is right, wrong, desirable, or just, and may support an individual's decision about how to act or perform in relation to what is perceived as preferable or valuable within the individual's culture.

This can contribute to forming attitudes, which are similar to values, and are learned from the individual's parents, caregivers, and family. Faculty and peers may have a significant impact on one's actions. Some learners may experience situations that differ from the values of their cultural tradition and usual behavior, therefore causing them to experience dissonance or moral distress. It is important, especially for nurse educators, to offer clear directions and rationales for decision-making for culturally diverse learners to help alleviate any sense of disharmony they might experience.

A study by Amaro, Abriam-Yago, and Yoder (2006) interviewed ethnically diverse learners who had recently completed an associate or baccalaureate nursing program, and the study identified the major themes related to educational barriers:

- **Personal needs** (lack of finances, time issues, family responsibilities and obligations, and difficulties related to language and communication)
- **Academic needs** (large or heavy workload)
- **Language needs** (difficulty reading and understanding assignments, a prejudice resulting from their accents, and verbal communication barriers)
- **Cultural needs** (expectations related to assertiveness and cultural norms, lack of diverse role models, and difficulty with communication). An important issue among culturally diverse learners is their level of knowledge of the English language, which, if inadequate, can be problematic.

ENGLISH AS AN ADDITIONAL LANGUAGE

Barriers may exist for students with English as an additional language (EAL) or previously known as English-as-a-second-language (ESL) in applying and gaining admission to nursing programs and in their ability to progress through the program, once accepted. These students may speak English but might think and process ideas in their other language. These students frequently have a difficult time understanding healthcare terminology, communicating with patients and staff, and frequently have higher attrition rates than English-speaking students. They may also have lower NCLEX pass rates (Olson, 2012). Suggestions for accommodating learners from culturally and linguistically diverse backgrounds include:

- Using nonstandardized and standardized methods of testing
- Dynamic assessments
- Nonverbal measures of ability
- Multiple methods of testing
- Testing in both the learner's native and second language
- The use of the Test of English as a Foreign Language (TOEFL) test (Overton, Fielding, & Simonsson, 2004)
- Hansen and Beaver (2012) discuss test development for EAL/ESL learners and provide the following tips:

  - Use short, simple sentences
  - Be direct when stating information; do not hide it in the sentence
  - Use questions rather than statements that need completion format
  - Highlight keywords such as *most, least, best*
  - Use common words

◎ **Critical Thinking Question**
As you teach your course each day, what concepts do you teach that might be interpreted incorrectly by a culturally diverse learner, and how might you remedy that situation?

▶ THE TOEFL EXAMINATION

The TOEFL examination measures a learner's potential ability to communicate in English in a college or university environment.

- The TOEFL score can be helpful in identifying learners who may be at risk for failure and/or may need additional support throughout a program (Educational Testing Services, 2020).
- It is important to use the TOEFL score as only one piece of admission criteria.
- Be aware that learners may be offended if they are asked to take a TOEFL examination if they have been living in the United States for many years.

Faculty commitment to the success of minority learners is crucial for the success of diverse learner populations. Minority learners need a strong learner–faculty relationship with a faculty member who is not responsible for assigning a grade to the learner.

- Learners need someone to talk to about their feelings and experiences as they move through the nursing program.
- Having a strong learner–faculty relationship will minimize learners' experiences with cognitive dissonance.
- Role models are ideal if appropriate faculty candidates are available.
- If no faculty role model is found, other faculty members must spend time with the learners to ensure their success (Burruss & Popkess, 2012).

Developing adequate support services for culturally diverse learners will increase their success in nursing or other academic programs. Reading, comprehension, and writing skills need to be developed in a nonthreatening manner to assist the diverse learner's academic success.

EVIDENCE-BASED TEACHING PRACTICE

A study by Mulready-Shick, Edwards, and Sitthisongkram (2020) concluded that non-English speakers of faculty-made, multiple-choice exam questions that had been linguistically modified promoted readability and comprehensibility; students preferred the linguistically modified versions 60% of the time. This inquiry attends to the need for greater responsiveness to student concerns about test-taking practices because of poorly written test items; language demands may negatively and unfairly impact students' exam performance and result in underperformance or failure.

● LEARNING DISABILITIES

Learning disabilities are the most common type of learner limitation found on college campuses today. Frequently, learners with a learning disability begin college before their disability has been detected.

- In nursing education, these disabilities are often noted when significant differences are noticed between a learner's classroom and clinical performance.
- Often, a learner may perform well in the clinical area but may be unable to demonstrate the same ability, skills, and competency when taking tests in the classroom.
- These learners should be referred to the appropriate academic success staff or counselors for assistance (Frank, 2012).

Learners with documented disabilities are entitled to the same access to education as traditional learners. Academic services must be available to provide learners with reading, writing, and test-taking strategy support services.

TEACHING GEM   Smith, Ooms, and Marks-Maron (2016) describe a teaching session about service users' experiences accessing and receiving health and social care that was designed and delivered by service users to first-year bachelor of science in nursing students. The aim was to enhance students' knowledge, skills, and confidence in caring for people with a learning disability. The session impacted students' knowledge and understanding of people with a learning disability. After the session, students reported that they felt more comfortable and confident interacting with people with a learning disability. In addition, they reflected on their feelings about caring for people with a learning disability.

▶ GOVERNMENT ACTS OF PROTECTION

The **No Child Left Behind (NCLB)** Act is the most significant federal education policy in a generation. This Act calls on all educators to measure all learners' performances using a set of fixed indicators, and it has tied federal monetary compensation to these performance outcomes.

It should be noted that although both these laws are aimed at elementary and secondary education, but they cannot be ignored and will have tremendous impact when learners taught under the auspices of these Acts reach college. Educators should be prepared for challenges yet to be determined that may stem from these Acts, especially NCLB (U.S. Department of Education, 2016). Students with disabilities are protected by the federal law under **the American Disabilities Act (ADA) of 1990** and the **Amendment Act of 2008**. This guarantees that persons who are qualified for admission cannot be denied access based on their disability alone, nor can they be discriminated against. Students must disclose their disability to the educational institution so that reasonable accommodations can be made.

▶ CHARACTERISTICS OF LEARNERS WITH LEARNING DISABILITIES

- Trouble with basic reading and spelling skills
- Memory difficulties
- Trouble remembering details and sequencing
- Poor handwriting
- Distractibility and difficulty concentrating
- History of poor academic performance
- Difficulty meeting deadlines
- Anxiety and low self-esteem
- Difficulty following verbal instructions
- Difficulty articulating ideas verbally
- Auditory processing deficits
- Time-management problems (Frank, 2012)

It is important for faculty to know that the nature of learning disabilities can be highly individualized and can be manifested differently through a variety of issues. Faculty should be aware that:

- These learners are usually of average or above-average intelligence (Frank, 2012).
- Employing teaching strategies that match the learners' learning styles may enhance their chances of success and may serve to minimize their learning disability.
- The skilled educator should be aware and open to employing teaching strategies to assist learning-disabled learners to achieve.

Many colleges and universities have an office that coordinates the diagnosis of learning disabilities and the accommodation and provision of support services for learners who need them.

- If a learner agrees, a faculty member can be made aware of the learner's disability, and a variety of accommodations can be made to meet his or her learning needs. One example involves giving the learner extra time to take an examination or allowing the learner to take an examination in another secured environment.

■ It is not appropriate for the faculty to discuss a student's learning disability with other faculty members unless given permission to do so by the learner (Frank, 2012).

Nurse educators must also be familiar with the accommodations made by their state for learners with disabilities. The NCLEX has accommodations for students with documented learning disabilities.

■ Accommodations must be made for students with learning disabilities in accordance with the Americans with Disabilities Act (ADA) (National Council of State Boards of Nursing).
■ It is important for educators also to be aware of learners with physical disabilities or learners with a documented or apparent physical limitation, problems with substance abuse, chemical or alcohol impairments, and/or mental health problems (Frank, 2012).

⬤ LEARNER SOCIALIZATION

Socialization of learners is where a group of individuals learn the acceptable behaviors, values, belief systems, processes, and knowledge of a professional culture, in this case becoming acclimated to the nursing profession. Socialization could be formal to include classroom lectures, assignments, working with a mentor, lab or clinical experiences, or informal activities like being part of a student nursing association. The struggle for students to take their classroom knowledge and apply it to the clinical setting can be a source of frustration. Another key for students to be adequately socialized they need to spend enough time with their mentors, preceptors, role models, or qualified senior nurses in the practice setting to provide them with adequate exposure to the nursing culture and environment (Salisu, Nayeri, Yakubu, & Ebrahimpour, 2019). This includes good role mentoring by competent nursing faculty as well as hands-on, live clinical experiences.

The transition from new graduate to professional nurse is challenging. In some cases, more than 50% of new nurses have left their position in the first year. This could be a result of inadequate socialization to the role and profession of nursing. One strategy that has been shown to yield positive results in facilitating new-graduate role transition is the nurse internship or residency program. This reduced the rate of turnover in the first year after hire when compared with traditional orientation programs (Letourneau & Fater, 2015).

Kramer's (1974) work delineates four phases of what is described as "reality shock" when a new nurse or neophyte realizes that what they learned in school does not match what is experienced in actual clinical practice.

■ The excitement of passing the licensure examination quickly fades as these new nurses struggle to move from the role of learner to the staff nurse role.
■ This reality shock leads to stress, which can cause exacerbations of symptoms that affect one's health and cause a loss of time from work (Cherry & Jacob, 2005).

Kramer's four phases of reality shock are:

1. Honeymoon
2. Shock or rejection
3. Recovery
4. Resolution

It is important to note that socialization takes place primarily through social interaction with people who are significant to an individual, usually a nursing school's faculty members (Barretti, 2004) and who are valued by the learner. Some things that might help this are:

- Positive, harmonious precepting/orientation experiences
- Social support systems of peers and departments
- Assignment congruence such as The Synergy Model put forth by the American Association of Critical Care Nurses (AACN). Where the characteristics of the patient are matched with the competencies of the nurse.

What nurse educators can do to enhance learner socialization into nursing is twofold:

1. A nurse educator should be a great role model for the profession.
2. A nurse educator should prepare nursing students for the reality of the profession by integrating socialization principles into every nursing course in the curriculum.

Also important are mentorship and a supportive learning environment. Mentors and preceptors need to be confident in their skills and teaching ability as well as knowing their learners. They need to plan learning experiences and facilitate new-graduate nurses to respond to the unexpected in the clinical environment with ease and support (Vinales, 2015). This support and mentorship are crucial in helping the novice nurse acclimate to the new role and assisting them to grow.

Today's nurse educators are shaping tomorrow's nurses. What is paramount to the successful shaping of tomorrow's nursing staff is that nurse educators not only teach nursing content but also shape the learning environment where that content is taught, including the use of appropriate clinical experiences, so that learners are fully socialized to the reality of nursing and its role. Accomplishing this will serve to reduce the chance of negative experiences and reality shock on graduation.

EVIDENCE-BASED TEACHING PRACTICE

Wildermuth, Weltin, & Simmons (2020) examined the transition experiences of nurses as students and new graduate nurses in a collaborative nurse residency program. A qualitative phenomenological study explored their lived experiences. The themes of feeling overwhelmed, supported, and confident were identified. A finding unique to this study and literature was that this nurse residency program model was a theme of overwhelming support. This nurse residency program between a hospital and college of nursing can assist others in developing nurse residency programs and can significantly reduce turnover and burnout of nurses new to the profession.

● ADDRESSING INCIVILITY

Incivility is defined as "a rude or impolite attitude or behavior" (*Merriam-Webster's Online Dictionary*, 2020).

- Incivility in the academic nursing environment may range from a variety of behaviors including groans, insulting remarks, verbal abuse, and talking when others are talking, eye-rolling, texting, shopping online, or watching non-class-related material during class. Clark (2009) defines incivility as rude and disruptive behavior that, when left unaddressed, may spiral into aggressive or violent behavior. Between 53% and 96% of nursing students report experiencing at least one uncivil incident in the academic or clinical setting (Clarke et al., 2012).

A study by Clark and Springer (2007) outlines the learner behaviors most often reported as uncivil by both learners and faculty:

- Cheating on examinations or quizzes
- Using cell phones or pagers during class
- Holding distracting conversations
- Making sarcastic remarks or gestures
- Sleeping in class
- Using computers for purposes not related to the class
- Demanding makeup examinations, extensions, or other favors
- Making disapproving groans
- Dominating class discussions
- Refusing to answer direct questions

Incivility is a symptom of a larger problem of *academic dishonesty*, which is defined as the "intentional participation in deceptive practices regarding one's academic work or the work of another" (Kolanko et al., 2006, p. 1).

EVIDENCE-BASED TEACHING PRACTICE

In an integrative review by Rose et al. (2020) examined student-to-student incivility in nursing education. They found five major points of interest: (1) *Workload and expectations* included time-consuming workloads and high academic expectations lead to incivility. (2) *Incivility occurred in degrees*. Mild acts of incivility were defined as those that do not disrupt learning but still damage working relationships. Moderate acts of incivility were defined as behaviors that disrupt the learning process and undermine academic relationships such as cheating on examinations, and severe acts included discriminating remarks, property damage, and threats of physical violence toward peers. (3) *Effects of incivility* shared that students experiencing incivility are at higher risk of developing physical, emotional, and psychological sequelae. (4) *Coping strategies* showed that students rely on a variety of coping strategies to deal with the negative consequences associated with incivility such as breathing exercises and trying to maintain a positive despite their negative feelings. (5) *Strategies to reduce incivility* included written signed civility codes, reflexive writing and reflective journaling and journal clubs via academic workshops, discussing self-care, coping strategies, and stress-reduction activities, and the use of use of web-based virtual reality simulation (VRS). In conclusion, incivility can take a tremendous toll on nursing students

> and faculty if not adequately dealt with. It can impact them personally, in their professional practice, and put patient's safety at risk. To counteract this, faculty must promote a positive learning environment and facilitate students supporting each other. Having policies and processes in place to address incivility is paramount.

- As many as 70% to 95% of learners reported having engaged in practices of academic dishonesty.
- Some have suggested that the problem of academic dishonesty is a result of a deterioration in morals, as reported over the past decade by the Josephson Institute (Kolanko et al., 2006).

Learners described the following behaviors as ineffective for deterring cheating:

- Assigning specific topics for papers
- Putting numbers on test booklets (if paper test are still used)
- Assigning seats for examinations
- Permitting only pencils to be brought into the examination room
- Not permitting anyone to leave during the course of the examination
- Leaving increased space between learners during an examination

Learners describe the following behaviors as most effective in deterring cheating:

- Having learners place their belongings in the front of the classroom
- Having a minimum of two proctors per examination to walk up and down the aisles during the examination
- Providing new examinations for each test
- Keeping each test in a locked cabinet with shredding conducted by full-time secretaries, not by student workers (if still using paper exams)
- Keep online test banks secure by not allowing recording or picture taking during exam reviews. Also, adequate proctoring of exams whether in person or remotely with computer cameras

Kolanko et al. (2006) also noted that "faculty should include opportunities within the education process for the moral development of learners in addition to their theoretical and clinical development. Learners must understand what constitutes academic integrity. Unethical behavior is ultimately responsible for the deterioration of the very fabric of the nursing profession" (p. 35).

It is also important to note that incivility can flow from the faculty member to the learner. Faculty members must always be aware of their behavior and their position as role models for learners. Unfortunately, Clark (2006) found that it is not unusual for learners to perceive faculty members as uncivil. Her study found uncivil faculty behaviors to include:

- Making demeaning and belittling comments
- Treating learners unfairly
- Pressuring learners to conform to unreasonable faculty demands

Faculty members arriving unprepared or late for class can also be considered uncivil, and any of the characteristics identified as uncivil learner behaviors can also be applied to faculty. Three themes emerged from Clark's study related to learners' emotional responses to faculty incivility:

1. Traumatization
2. Powerlessness and helplessness
3. Anger

As these studies reveal, uncivil behavior is a double-edged sword that must be examined and remedied at both ends of the learning continuum, learner and faculty.

TEACHING GEM   One of the most common topics of discussion among new nurse educators today is the increasing incidence of student incivility or classroom management of incivility resulting from changes in social norms. When a faculty member receives an affectively charged statement from a student, the worst course of action is to respond with an affectively charged response. The key is to close the communication gap. Incivility negatively affects teaching and learning outcomes. Wagner et al. (2019) compared faculty and student perceptions of incivility across disciplines at a large public university sampling 577 people. Nursing reported the highest level of perceived incivility, with all other disciplines also reporting some levels of incivility. Faculty perceived more incivility than students. With a national awareness of incivility in nursing education, this study shows that incivility does exist in other disciplines. This should serve as a starting point of discussion addressing its impact on higher education.

INCIVILITY AND BULLYING IN THE WORKPLACE

The difference between incivility and bullying is that incivility is an ambiguous, low-intensity, discourteous behavior that is intended to harm or violate the norms of respect. Bullying involves a perpetrator who continually pursues a power differential over another person (Rose et al., 2020). The most common types of incivility are lateral (nurse to nurse) and hierarchical (nurse administrator to manager to nurse, nurse to learner, faculty to learner, and physician to nurse). In July 2008, The Joint Commission (TJC) issued a **Sentinel Event Alert** that discussed intimidating and disruptive behaviors that undermine a culture of safety. In January 2009, TJC implemented leadership standards that require hospital leaders to create and maintain a culture of safety and quality. In 2012, TJC required each organization to institute a "code of conduct that defines acceptable and inappropriate behaviors. They also required the institution to "create and implement a process for managing these behaviors. In a recent study (2020), TJC reported that over half of health care works reported exposure to one of six disruptive behaviors ranging from hanging up the phone to physical violence.

TJC further noted that bullying is a contributor to healthcare errors, avoidable adverse patient outcomes, increased cost of care, as well as professional attrition. Types of abuse include verbal abuse, nonverbal abuse, sexual harassment, passive-aggressive behaviors, and bullying. Clark (2011) suggests that bullying is a threatening situation, reflective of a form of abuse that requires further consideration independent of incivility. Bullying among children is not a new concept, but its transition into adult life and professional life is an increasing concern in the workplace, the health care environment, and the nursing profession. The findings have noted that bullying can cause significant psychological and physical distress, including feelings of alienation, lack of control over working conditions, and feelings of low self-esteem and powerlessness. If these conditions are left unchecked, the victims of bullying may develop problems sleeping, exhibit signs of depression, posttraumatic stress syndrome, and low morale, and potentially suicide. These individuals may use sick time excessively and wind up leaving school or the profession (Meierdierks-Bowllan, 2015). Repeated bullying on social media is also suggested as a potential cause for attempted suicide.

The vulnerable role of nursing students and graduate nurses as they socialize to the profession of nursing can be filled with fears of incompetence and powerlessness. In addition, these new nurses experience multiple stressors such as juggling personal and work demands, financial pressures, time management difficulties, perceived lack of faculty and peer support, and potential mental health problems or personal issues—all of which can further impact students' capacity to effectively cope on a daily basis.

EVIDENCE-BASED TEACHING PRACTICE

A study examined workplace incivility in China's nursing field using "anxiety and "resilience" to analyze the effects of new nurses' job burnout caused by incivility. This study validated that workplace incivility has a significant predictive function in job burnout of new nurses in a hospital setting. Anxiety played a partial mediating role in the relationship between workplace incivility and job burnout. Resilience played a moderate role in the relationship between workplace incivility and job burnout (Shiu et al., 2018).

 ## PREVENTION IS KEY

So, what can be done to help with this situation? Prevention is the key. Some suggested solutions are the use of an organization's resources and conduct policies, to educate staff to be accountable for their own behavior, to have staff model appropriate behavior, and to not allow disruptive behavior to go unchecked (McNamara, 2012). TJC further outlined preventive strategies, including skill-based training and coaching, ongoing nonconfrontation surveillance, embedded systems to assess staff perceptions of seriousness and extent of nonprofessional behavior, and integration of policies to ensure early reporting without fear of intimidation. To prevent, one must first identify at-risk behaviors. This would incorporate a zero-tolerance policy and a nonpunitive reporting mechanism. Education and awareness are also key components (Meierdierks-Bowllan, 2015).

Within the classroom similar situations need to occur. Faculty and administration must provide programs to identify and educate against uncivil behavior. This must include policies to hold the faculty and students accountable for their actions. Role modeling, coaching, open forums for discussion, stress-reduction activities like yoga and meditation, opportunities for counseling, and communication-building activities need to be used within and outside of the classroom to change this trend.

FOSTERING LEARNER DEVELOPMENT IN THREE DOMAINS OF LEARNING

Bloom's taxonomy of learning is a way to categorize objectives according to how they relate to one another. There are three major categories: cognitive (thinking domain), affective (feeling domain), and psychomotor domain (doing or skills domain). Although they are listed separately, they are interdependent (Bastable, 2019).

▶ COGNITIVE DOMAIN

(knowledge, comprehension, application, analysis, synthesis, evaluation)
The cognitive domain, known as the thinking domain, is divided into six levels—
knowledge, where the learner can memorize or recall facts; **comprehension**, the learner
can understand what is being communicated; **application**, where the learner can use
ideas and principles and apply them to specific situations; **analysis** level, the learner
can recognize a piece of information by breaking it down into specific parts; **synthesis**
enables the learner to put together parts into a unified whole; and **evaluation**, where
the learner can analyze or judge something by applying certain criteria. Teaching in the
cognitive domain uses methods to stimulate learning, such as lecture, group discussion,
one-on-one learning, or computer-assisted instruction (Bastable, 2019).

▶ AFFECTIVE DOMAIN

(receiving, responding, valuing, origination, characterization)
The affective domain also known as the "feeling" domain uses internalization of
expressing feelings, emotions, beliefs, values, or attitudes. The levels of this domain
include **receiving,** which enables the learner to become aware of an idea. They may
admit any fears here. **Responding** allows the learner to respond to an experience. This
can enable a learner to move past the feelings of insecurity to one of confidence. **Valuing**
allows the learner to accept and integrate an idea. Receiving and responding precede
this behavior. **Origination** allows the learner to incorporate ideas by organizing,
classifying, and prioritizing values. **Characterization** level is where the learner can
show adherence to the total philosophy of a concept and show a commitment to it. For
example, showing good hand-washing technique to prevent the spread of infection
(Bastable, 2019).

▶ PSYCHOMOTOR DOMAIN

**(perception, set, guided response, mechanism, complex overt response, adaptation,
origination)**
The psychomotor domain is also known as the "skills" domain. The learner uses
fine and gross motor abilities. The levels of this domain are as follows. **Perception**
is where the learner becomes aware of the task to be performed. This may involve
reading, directions, observation of a process of a skill to be learned. The **set level** is
where the learner shows a readiness to an action adds shown by attending or favorable
body language (Bastable, 2019). For example, if a learner is shown how to hang an
intravenous fluid bag and is willing to try to accomplish that task. The **guided response
level** is where the learner performs an action under the guidance of an instructor. This
can be after or at the same time the instructor demonstrates a skill like inserting a
foley catheter on a mannequin. The **mechanism level** is where the learner can perform
steps of a certain skill repeatedly with confidence. The **complex overt response level**
is where the learner can automatically perform a complex task with independence and
correctly without hesitation. The **adaptation level** is where the learner can adapt or
modify a learned process to fit the needs of a given situation. This indicates mastery

of the process. The **origination level** is where the learner can create new motor acts to manipulate objects as a result of completely understanding a skill (Bastable, 2019). For example, after a simulation experience, a learner will be able to recognize signs and symptoms of respiratory distress like retractions and work of breathing. So, by understanding the mechanisms of good breathing, the learner distressed or abnormal breathing patterns.

ASSISTING LEARNERS TO ENGAGE IN THOUGHTFUL AND CONSTRUCTIVE SELF AND PEER EVALUATION

Whenever something is taught, it is imperative that evaluation occurs to see if actual learning has occurred. As learners move through their education programs, it is important to reflect on and evaluate their accomplishments. A self-evaluation provides the learner with the opportunity to look at themselves, critique, and explore their strengths and weaknesses. This helps with goal setting for the future. It is an excellent tool to develop professional maturity. In academia and the hospital setting, peer evaluations may be used. Peer evaluations allow learners to assess and critique each other's performance. It can assist in self-reflection as well as provide an opportunity to encounter diversity in many ways. A rubric can be used to guide both of these processes. Instructions need to be clear and relevant. Often students appreciate and assimilate feedback from their peers more readily than faculty. Learners may lack self-awareness. For example, they may perceive their demeanor as professional when others might find it cold and uncaring. This evaluation method is very valuable in the classroom and workplace.

ENCOURAGE PROFESSIONAL DEVELOPMENT OF LEARNERS

Faculty are in the perfect position to foster professional development of learners by demonstrating what the role should be. Role-modeling is a powerful tool to influence learners' attitudes, values, and morals into the profession. Many students will assimilate or become socialized into the role of the nurse by copying behaviors they see. Faculty can discuss continuing education for advanced degrees, belonging to professional organizations, engaging in professional conferences and activities. Role modeling through simulation is an excellent teaching modality to assist the learner to develop skills, values, and attitudes that will help them become successful in their careers.

CASE STUDIES

CASE STUDY 8.1

The nurse educator is working in a 12-month accelerated nursing program. As a result of the time constraints of only having the learners for 12 months, the nurse educator realizes it is essential to incorporate only the most important facts in the course. The program has successfully graduated several groups of accelerated learners. The university sends out a follow-up survey to see how these learners are doing in the clinical environment. The survey reveals comments like, "I didn't realize nursing was going to be this hard," "I wasn't really ready for the demands of working in this fast-paced environment," "I didn't think it would be this hard fitting in on the floor where I work," "no one really helps me," "I am not sure I am going to remain in nursing," "I wish I knew it was going to be like this." The nurse educator realizes that, perhaps by focusing so much on getting in all the content needed for learners to pass their licensure examinations, the university missed out on providing an important lesson. The program did not take time to "socialize" these learners to the role of nursing.

List some ideas of how you might better address the socialization of nursing learners in the future, in both your course and at the university level.

CASE STUDY 8.2

The nurse educator has been teaching in a university setting for the past 3 years. The nurse educator's class typically has 60 learners and meets in a large auditorium. The nurse educator tries to keep the learners engaged and actively involved in the learning process but frequently notices that learners are talking among themselves and texting on their cell phones while class is going on.

Is this an example of learners being uncivil? If so, what might the nurse educator do to curtail this in the classroom and engage the learner?

CASE STUDY 8.3

The nurse educator is teaching a course that has a clinical component. The nurse educator notices that a particular learner does exceptionally well in the clinical area. The learner is professional, completes excellent assessments, and interacts well with patients. However, in the classroom, this learner seems to be the last one done when taking a test and is barely passing the course.

What might the nurse educator think is going on with this learner? What should the nurse educator do to help the learner? Should the nurse educator assume this learner may have a learning disability? Answer "yes" or "no," and support your answer.

1. Which of the following would not impact a student's emotional or psychological readiness to learn?

    A. Anxiety level
    B. Support systems
    C. Motivation
    D. Lives on campus

2. The nurse educator is teaching a large class that is very culturally diverse. Which population of learners is at an increased risk for being unsuccessful?

    A. Learners who decided to pursue a second career
    B. Learners who just graduated from high school
    C. Learners who speak English as a second language
    D. Learners who transferred from another nursing program

3. Which of the following learning style describes the learner who prefers to learn by doing? They would prefer an activity that involves an actual "hands-on" learning experience.

    A. Auditory
    B. Visual
    C. Kinesthetic
    D. Reading and writing

4. Which of the following characteristics is indicative of the traditional learner versus the nontraditional learner?

    A. They typically have previous work experience
    B. They usually are working full or part-time while attending school
    C. They usually have additional life responsibilities and stressors
    D. They usually have limited life and work experience

5. Which of the following is an acceptable teaching strategy when teaching low-literacy patients?

    A. Create a professional authoritative relationship with them because you are the educator
    B. Use repetition to reinforce information
    C. Use the direct question-and-answer method
    D. Give them large amounts of information at a time as availability of a translator is limited

1. D) Lives on campus

A student's anxiety level has a big impact on whether a student is psychologically ready to learn. Undue anxiety will greatly impede learning. Having good support systems in place will help students be emotionally & psychologically ready to learn. Motivation is very important in learning. If students are being forced to learn or are not motivated, it will negatively affect their learning.

2. C) Learners who speak English as a second language

Learners who speak English as a second language are at increased risk of being unsuccessful in the program as well as on the NCLEX-RN®.

3. C) Kinesthetic

Kinesthetic learners prefer hands-on learning. They like to learn by doing. Simulation and case studies are a good learning experience for this type of learner.

4. D) They usually have limited life and work experience

The traditional learner usually has limited life and work experience as they are typically young and come to college directly after high school.

5. B) Use repetition to reinforce information

Using repetition of information will reinforce content for better learning. A trusting, open relationship is best and will facilitate learning, not an authoritative relationship. Using the direct question-and-answer method may make them uneasy and inhibit the learning session. Small bits of information should be presented at a time, as people with poor reading skills can be easily overwhelmed.

6. Which of the following best describes student learning outcomes at the highest level of the cognitive domain?

   A. A student who can describe the pathophysiology of cardiac output

   B. The student who understands that incentive spirometry is used to enhance lung function of the purpose of the incentive spirometer

   C. The student who can describe the side effects of a beta-blocker

   D. A student who develops a care plan for a patient with congestive heart failure

7. Learners are encouraged to become members of the National Student Nurses Association (NSNA). The framework of this organization indicates that the learner will gain experience in:

   A. Making decisions and being accountable for those decisions

   B. Following regulations determined by elected officers

   C. Learning how to engage in social activities while in school

   D. Discussing health information and presenting projects

8. Which of the following methods is a positive way to socialize a newly licensed nurse into the nursing profession?

   A. Invite the new nurse to go out with colleagues socially

   B. Say to the new nurse "I got your back"

   C. Invite the new nurse to attend a professional nursing conference with you

   D. Be nice to the nurse, but when you are with senior nurses, say what you really think of her abilities

9. Which of the following statements is true about learning styles?

   A. Using learning methods that are consistent with the learner is considered the best way to affect the best learning achievement

   B. Learners feel less stressed when using just one style of learning

   C. When a teacher uses a variety of teaching methods, it confuses the learner and the student learns less

   D. The educator applying learning styles theory to each learner allows the educator to recognize whether learners will process information correctly

10. The nurse educator is working in an institution and notices a new nurse and their preceptor interacting on a weekend shift. The nurse educator notices that the preceptor is in fact bullying the new nurse who quietly stands by and does not react when the preceptor embarrasses the new nurse in front of their patient. What would be the best strategy to employ to correct this behavior?

    A. Ask the patient if they are satisfied with their care

    B. Tell the nurse manager on Monday that the preceptor should not have new orientees anymore

    C. Do nothing

    D. Ask to speak with the preceptor in private, share with the preceptor the observed perceptions, and offer a suggestion as to how they might better interact with the new nurse

(See answers next page.)

6. D) A student who develops a care plan for a patient with congestive heart failure

In developing a care plan, the student must synthesize previously acquired knowledge to deliver care. This is the highest level of the cognitive domain given.

7. A) Making decisions and being accountable for those decisions

The framework for this organization is shared governance; therefore, learners will have the opportunity to discuss their opinions and make decisions. The group members are responsible for the outcome of decisions. Following regulations, engaging in social activities, and discussing information and presenting projects are not the main purposes of the NSNA.

8. C) Invite the new nurse to attend a professional nursing conference with you

This is the most positive way of including the new nurse and promoting education and growth by attending a professional conference. While inviting the new nurse to go out socially might be including them, it is done in a negative, non-coping manner. Saying "I got your back" can give mixed messages. Being nice but voicing your opinion with senior nurses is unprofessional and will not lead to an honest work relationship.

9. A) Using learning methods that are consistent with the learner is considered the best way to affect the best learning achievement

Using the teaching method that is consistent with the learning style is the best way to enhance learning. Using a variety of teaching methods makes the learner feel less stressed and enables concept understanding in that you do not know which method will work for each student. Sometimes when using only one style the learner is more stressed. This is particularly so if the teaching method being used is not congruent with the learner's individual style. Processing information and learning styles are two different things—it is important to realize that everyone processes information in different ways.

10. D) Ask to speak with the preceptor in private, share with the perceptions, and offer a suggestion as to how they might better interact with the new nurse

Ask to speak with the preceptor in private and professionally point out what was making the orientee feel embarrassed by correcting the new nurse directly in front of the patient. Gently suggest that in the future they correct the orientee in private. Do not involve the patient in the interaction. Although informing the nurse manager of concerns is not wrong, the nurse educator should intervene if someone is being bullied and embarrassed in front of a patient. Telling the manager on Monday will allow this behavior to continue all weekend. Ignoring the situation will not help the preceptee.

REFERENCES

Amaro, D., Abriam-Yago, K., & Yoder, M. (2006). Perceived barriers for ethnically diverse students in nursing programs. *Journal of Nursing Education, 45*(7), 247–254.

American Association of Colleges of Nurses. (2016). Cultural competency in nursing education. http://www.aacn.nche.edu/education-resources/cultural-competency.

Barretti, M. (2004). What do we know about the professional socialization of our students? *Journal of Social Work Education, 40*(2), 255–283.

Bastable, S. B. (2019). *Nurse as educator: Principles of teaching and learning for nursing practice* (5th ed.). Jones & Bartlett.

Benner, P. (1984). *From novice to expert: Excellence and power in clinical nursing practice.* Addison-Wesley.

Burruss, N., & Popkess, A. (2012). The diverse learning needs of students. In D. M. Billings & J. A. Halstead (Eds.), *Teaching in nursing: A guide for faculty* (4th ed., pp. 15–33). Elsevier Saunders.

Cherry, B., & Jacob, S. R. (2005). *Contemporary nursing: Issues, trends, and management.* Elsevier.

Christofferson, J. E. (2016). Teaching Accelerated Second-Degree Nursing Students: Educators from Across the United States Share Their Wisdom. *Nursing Forum, 52*(2), 111–117.

Clark, C. M. (2006). *Incivility in nursing education: Student perceptions of uncivil faculty behavior in the academic environment* (Unpublished doctoral dissertation). University of Idaho, Moscow, ID.

Clark, C. M., & Springer, P. J. (2007). Incivility in nursing education: A descriptive study of definitions and prevalence. *Journal of Nursing Education, 46*(1), 7–14.

Clark, C. M. (2009). Faculty field guide for promoting civility in the classroom. *Nurse Educator, 34*(5), 194–197.

Clark, C. M., & Kenaley, B. (2011). Faculty empowerment of students to foster civility in nursing education: A merging of two conceptual models. *Nursing Outlook, 59*, 158–165.

Clark, C., Kane, D., Rajacich, D., Lafrenier, K. (2012). Bullying in undergraduate clinical nursing education. *Journal of Nursing Education, 51*(5), 269–276.

Clark, C. M., Barbosa-Liker, C., Larecia-Money, G., & Nguyen, D. (2015). Revision and psychometric testing of the Incivility in Nursing Education (INE) survey: Introducing the INE-R. *Journal of Nursing Education, 54*(6), 306–315.

Czepula, A. I., Bottacin, W. E., Hipolito, E., Baptista, D. R., Pontarolo, R., & Correr, C. J. (2016). Predominant learning styles among pharmacy students at the Federal University of Paraná, Brazil. *Pharmacy Practice, 14*(1), 650.

Educational Testing Services. (2020). *The TOEFL® test.* https://www.ets.org/ or http://www.toeflgoanywhere.org.

Elliot-Yeary, S. (2020). Meet the five different generations in today's workforce. https://www.generationalguru.com/generations.

Felder, R. M., & Solomon, B. A. (1998). *Learning styles and strategies.* http://www4.ncsu.edu/unity/lockers/users/f/felder/public/ILSdir/styles.htm

Fleming, N. (2001). *VARK: A guide to learning styles.* http://www.vark-learn.com/english/page.asp?p=categories

Fleming, N., & Mills, C. (1992). Not another inventory, rather a catalyst for change. In D. Wulff & J. Nygist (Eds.), *To improve the academy: Resources for faculty, instructional, and organizational development* (vol. 11, pp. 137–155). New Forums.

Frank, B. (2012). Teaching students with disabilities. In D. M. Billings & J. A. Halstead (Eds.), *Teaching in nursing: A guide for faculty* (4th ed., pp. 55–75). Elsevier Saunders.

Hansen, E., & Beaver, S. (2012). Faculty support for ESL nursing students: Action plan for success. *Nursing Education Perspectives*, 33(4), 246–250.

Key, B., Woods, A., & Hanks, M. (2019). Role Modeling in Simulation as an Inductive Classroom Learning Strategy for Nursing Education, *Nursing Education Perspectives*, Advance online publication. http://ovidsp.ovid.com/ovidweb.cgi?T=JS&PAGE =reference&D=ovftu&NEWS=N&AN=00024776-900000000-99626. https://doi. org/10.1097/01.NEP.0000000000000540.

Knowles, M. S., Houlton, E. F., & Swanson, R. A. (2015). *The adult learner* (8th ed.). Taylor & Francis.

Kolanko, K. M., Clark, C. M., Heinrich, K. T., Olive, D., Serembus, J. F., & Sifford, K. S. (2006). Academic dishonesty, bullying, incivility, and violence: Difficult challenges facing nurse educators. *Nursing Education Perspectives*, 27(1), 34–43.

Kramer, M. (1974). Reality shock: Why nurses leave nursing. Mosby.

Letourneau, R., & Fater, K. H. (2015). Nurse residency programs: An integrative review of the literature. *Nursing Education Perspectives*, 36(2), 96–101. 10.5480/13–1229

Lichtenthal, C. (1990). A self-study module of readiness to learn. Unpublished manuscript re-printed in Bastable, S. (2019). *Nurse as educator: Principles of teaching and learning for nursing practice* (5th ed.). Jones & Bartlett.

Mahoney, P. (2007). *Certified nurse educator preparation course*. Villanova University.

McLeod, S. (2017). Kolb's learning styles and experiential learning cycle. Simply Psychology. https://www.simplypsychology.org/learning-kolb. html#:~:text=People%20with%20a%20diverging%20learning,be%20strong%20in%20 the%20arts.

McNamara, S. (2012). Incivility in nursing: Unsafe nurse, unsafe patients. *Association of Perioperative Registered Nurses*, 95(4), 535–540.

Meierdierks-Bowllan, N. (2015). Nursing student's experience of bullying, prevalence, impact, and interventions. *Nurse Educator*, 40(4), 194–198.

Merriam Webster Online Dictionary (2020). https://www.merriam-webster.com/ dictionary/incivility#learn-more.

Mulready-Shick, J., Edward, J., and Sitthisongkram, S. (2020). Developing Local Evidence About Faculty Written Exam Questions: Asian ESL Nursing Student Perceptions About Linguistic Modification. *Nursing Education Perspectives*, 41(2), 109–111.

Myers Briggs Foundation. (2020). https://www.myersbriggs.org/ my-mbti-personality-type/mbti-basics/.

National League for Nursing. (2021). Certified Nurse Educator (CNE) 2021 candidate handbook. http://www.nln.org/docs/default-source/default-document-library/cne-handbook-2021_revised_07-01-2021.pdf?sfvrsn=2

National League for Nursing. (2021). Certified Nurse Educator Novice (CNEn) 2021 candidate handbook. http://www.nln.org/Certification-for-Nurse-Educators/cne-n/ cne-n-handbook

Olson, M. (2012). English as a second language (ESL) nursing student success: A critical review of the literature. *Journal of Cultural Diversity, 19*(1), 26–32.

Orkiszewski, P., Pollitt, P., Leonard, P., & Hayes-Lane, S. (2016). Reaching millennials with nursing history. *Creative Nursing, 22*(1), 60–64.

Overton, T., Fielding, C., & Simonsson, M. (2004). Decision making in determining eligibility of culturally and linguistically diverse learners. *Journal of Learning Disabilities, 37*(4), 319–330.

Rose, K., Jenkins, S., Mallory, C., Asthroth, K., With, W., & Jarvill, M. (2020). An integrative review examining student-to-student incivility and effective strategies to address incivility in nursing education. *Nurse Educator, 45*(3), 165–168.

Ryan, E., & Poole, C. (2019). Impact of virtual learning environment on student satisfaction, engagement, recall, and retention. *Journal of Medical Imaging & Radiation Sciences, 50*(3), 408–415.

Salisu, W., Nayeri, N., Yakubu, I., & Ebrahimpour, F. (2019). Challenges and facilitators of professional socialization: A systematic review. *Nursing Open, 6,* 1289–1298. https://onlinelibrary.wiley.com/doi/epdf/10.1002/nop2.341, 10.1002/nop2.341.

Shiraz, F., & Heidari, S. (2019). The relationship between critical thinking skills and learning styles and academic achievement of nursing students. *Journal of Nursing Research, 27*(4), e38–e39.

Shiu, Y., Guo, H., Zhang, S, Fengzhe, X., Wang, J., Zhinan, S., Xinpeng, D., Sun,T., & Fan, L. (2018). Impact of workplace incivility against new nurses on job burn-out: a crosssectional study in China. *BMJ Open, 8,* e020461. 10.1136/bmjopen-2017-020461

Smith, P., Ooms, A., & Marks-Maran, D. (2016). Active involvement of learning disabilities service users in the development and delivery of a teaching session to pre-registration nurses: Students' perspectives. *Nurse Education in Practice, 16*(1), 111–118.

Spurlock, D., Patterson, B., & Colby, N. (2019). Gender differences and similarities in accelerated nursing education programs: Evidence of success from the new careers in nursing programs. *Nursing Education Perspectives, 40*(6), 343–351.

Tornwall, J., Tan, A., & Bowless, W. (2018). Pride and competency in accelerated nursing programs. *Nursing Education Perspectives, 39*(6), 343–349.

U.S. Department of Education. (2016). *No child left behind.* http://www2.ed.gov/nclb/landing.jhtml

Vinales, J. (2015). The learning environment and learning styles: A guide for mentors. *British Journal of Nursing, 24*(8), 454–457.

Wagner, B., Holland, C., Mainous, R., Matcham, W., Li, G., & Luiken, J. (2019). Differences in perception of incivility among disciplines in higher education. *Nurse Educator, 44*(5), 265–269.

Waltzer, T. & Dahl, A. (2023).Why do students cheat? Perceptions, evaluations, and motivations. *Ethics & Behavior, 33*(2), 130–150. 10.1080/10508422.2022.2026775

Wildermuth, M., Weltin, A. & Simmons, A. (2020). Transition experiences of nurses as students and new graduates' nurses in a collaborative nurse residency program. *Journal of Professional Nursing, 36*(1), 69–75.

Facilitating Learner Development Through Civic Engagement Experiences

Frances H. Cornelius and Maryann Godshall

The only person who is educated is the one who has learned how to learn and change.
—Carl Rogers

> ## ▶ LEARNING OUTCOMES
>
> This chapter also addresses the Certified Nurse Educator Exam and the Certified Nurse Educator Novice Exam Content Area 2: Facilitate Learner Development and Socialization
>
> - Describe the characteristics of civic engagement
> - Understand the types of civic engagement
> - Examine the benefits of civic engagement
> - Discuss methods used to operationalize civic engagement experiences
> - Analyze safety issues associated with civic engagement
> - Discuss studying abroad
> - Understand student exchange opportunities
> - Understand building cultural competence
> - Explore the use of the global classroom

⬤ INTRODUCTION

Integrating values with learning experiences can be done in a multitude of ways, including use of global classrooms, exchange programs, and civic engagement. Peterson (2015) states civic engagement is essential in higher education and maintains that "civic engagement is critical to the success of students and universities and should be enacted at all levels of educational policy and practices … it must be facilitated in a way that ensures that equity, justice, and an appreciation of diverse value systems and perspectives are included in the development of civic actors, civic learning, and shared projects of social change in local communities" (p. 17).

The American Psychological Association (APA) defines civic engagement as "individual or collective actions designed to identify and address issues of public concern, including individual voluntarism, organizational involvement and advocacy" (2020, p. 1). When integrated with the "full campus experience," civic engagement provides an opportunity for students to learn about diversity and good citizenship while developing leadership, interpersonal, and problem-solving skills.

There are four basic types of civic engagement:

1. Civic Action: participating in service learning (SL) activities or volunteering for activities that help improve a community (such as MLK Day of Service; community clean-up, or working in a soup kitchen)
2. Civic Commitment or Duty: working actively to make "positive contributions to society"
3. Civic Skills: active involvement in civil society, politics, and democratic processes.
4. Social Cohesion: building and sustaining "a sense of reciprocity, trust, and bonding to others." (Youth.gov, 2020, p. 1)

Service learning (SL) is a popular academic endeavor that integrates learning activities with voluntary, community-based activities that develop civic responsibility and engagement. SL can be provided as local, national, or global experience. According to the National Service-Learning Clearinghouse, service learning is a form of experiential education, seeks to address human and community issues and needs, creates learning opportunities through active participation in purposefully constructed service activities, includes structured reflection and debriefing to facilitate building connections between the experience and curricular content, conducted in collaboration with the community and leads to acquisition of new skills, knowledge, leadership, and a sense of caring and social responsibility.

Students who participate in SL report that they intend to "participate in community service in the future and believed that they could make a difference in their community and that contributing to their community was important ... and this finding suggests that participation in service learning may lead to an increase in civic responsibility" (Hebert & Hauf, 2015, p. 46).

SL became an educational concept in the late 1960s and has gained in popularity as a learning activity (Griffith & Clark, 2016; Carroll, Clancy, Bal, Lalani & Woo, 2018). SL is "a teaching and learning strategy that integrates meaningful community service with instruction and reflection to enrich the learning experience, teach civic responsibility, and strengthen communities" (National Service-Learning Clearinghouse, 2016, p. 1). The benefits of using SL as a learning activity are:

- It can be used to enhance cultural competence for learners in a variety of settings (Wittmann-Price, 2007)
- It can change attitudes toward homeless people
- SL can build competencies for working with diverse populations
- SL can increase nursing intervention skills
- SL fosters therapeutic communication
- It can engage learners with hands-on experiences
- SL can encourage skills and knowledge needed for real-life experiences
- SL can explore preconceived ideas and assumptions (Long, 2016)

EVIDENCE-BASED TEACHING PRACTICE

Krishnan, Richards, and Simpson (2016) studied audiology, the effect of students' (N = 12) cultural competence of participating, in a study abroad program. Data were collected qualitatively by using the Public Affairs Scale (Levesque-Bristol & Cornelius-White, 2012) and qualitative data were collected in the form of journals. The Public Affairs Scale pre- and postscores demonstrated an increase in cultural competence and journals demonstrated that students' cultural awareness increased.

 # CHARACTERISTICS OF SERVICE LEARNING

SL allows students to experience the community and forms partnerships. The students learn from the experience as they provide a needed service to humanity. SL encourages interaction, caring, cultural competence, and dialogue; an SL project can be integrated into a curriculum as an assignment.

- SL is guided by learning outcomes that include relevant content of a course.
- Learner reflection is usually incorporated as a learning and/or evaluative tool.
- SL may take place in local, community-based settings or even internationally.
- It entails recognizing the needs of the community or of a given patient population.
- SL develops cultural competency among students through reflection and through the discussion of real-life experiences.
- SL develops collaboration skills among students. A cooperative purpose is always a powerful tool in education (Wittmann-Price, Anselmi, & Espinal, 2010).

Bringle and Clayton (2012) maintain that the most effective SL design is a course or competency-based, credit-bearing educational experience in which students (a) participate in mutually identified service activities that benefit the community, and (b) reflect on the service activity in such a way as to gain further understanding of course content, a broader appreciation of the discipline, and an enhanced sense of personal values and civic responsibility (pp. 114–115).

The overall educational goal is not to practice skills but to fundamentally influence the long-term actions of students. Students stated that participating in SL made them more anxious to finish nursing school and start their careers as a nurse and will influence their future careers in that they plan to seek further mission trips and find ways to serve the underprivileged as a healthcare provider. It enriched their personal appreciation for cultural understanding and diversity (Hawkins & Vialet, 2012; Barnhardt, Sheets & Pasquesi, 2015; Curtis & Legerwood, 2018; Witkowsky & Mendez, 2018).

EVIDENCE-BASED TEACHING PRACTICE

Tapley and Patel (2016) examined the use of SL along with a precede–proceed model in physical therapy students (N = 45) and found that the combination increased students' interest, confidence, and willingness to participate in SL health–promotion programs in the community after graduation.

● STUDYING ABROAD

Study-abroad opportunities can be developed to enable students to study in another country for one course, a semester, or a year or more. This is often marketed as an opportunity for students to develop global awareness and cultural competence. Cultural competence is defined by the nursing profession as being an essential element of nursing practice in which the nurse is enabled to recognize the impact of globalization of individual health and nursing practice (Carlton, Ryan, Ali, & Kelsey, 2007; Jeffreys, 2016). Garneau and Pepin (2015) point out that awareness of cultural differences is not enough to develop cultural competence and that this "awareness" is often more likely to reinforce ethnocentric approaches to care. This presents challenges to educators who are endeavoring to build cultural competence among their learners. Cultural competence "affects the cognitive, emotional, behavioral, and environmental dimensions of a person. It involves knowledge, skills, and know-how that, when combined properly, lead to a culturally safe, congruent, and effective action" (Garneau & Pepin, 2015, p. 12). The evidence suggests that students who participate in study-abroad courses improve their knowledge of culture and global health and enjoy enhanced personal and professional development (Ruddock & Turner, 2007; Barnhardt, Sheets & Pasquesi, 2015; Tamilla & Ledgerwood, 2018). In addition, study-abroad programs and international educational opportunities have positive learning outcomes, expand personal and professional experience, can boost recruitment and retention as well as prepare students for an increasingly global workplace (Tamilla & Ledgerwood, 2018; Witkowsky & Mendez, 2018). Targeted needs assessment and focused preparation are essential for delivery of a successful study abroad program. Basic educational components and learning activities to prepare students are critical for success. Four elements of global health are prerequisite content for the pretrip educational preparation portion of the course. They are:

1. Epidemiology—causality, risk, and rates of occurrence of health and illness
2. Environmental health—environmental factors affecting health, like food and water
3. Community resources—availability and access to healthcare
4. Social welfare and the role of nursing in healthcare availability of nurses and nursing schools and the healthcare system

The final module of a study-abroad program consists of post-trip debriefing and discussion of the emotional and personal effects of the field experience. Many times, global health content is included in community health courses, exploring at greater depth the international population's health concerns and cultural factors that influence health access and disparity are needed.

These study-abroad opportunities expand on SL trips in that they enable students to gain deeper insight into culture, global health systems, and policy. They have proven to be valuable for students in developing their global health awareness and cultural competence.

As stated previously, to be successful, study-abroad experiences need a lot of preplanning—a minimum of 6 months to a year is needed. It is important to review course objectives, expectations of the student, planned clinical experiences while abroad, and to prepare the students for hardships of the trip, all of which may help to remove the "vacation" expectation some students may have of a study-abroad opportunity (Foronda & Belknap, 2012; Starr-Glass, 2018). Making expectations of the students clear prior to departure will help to promote positive outcomes and learning experiences for the students. If going to a poverty-stricken country, it is highly recommended that faculty accompany the students. Time spent abroad can be negotiated with the administration.

Palmer, Wing, Miles, Heaston, and de la Cruz (2013) suggest using graduate students and alumni as affiliate faculty members or adjuncts in study-abroad programs. In fact, this may be a resource for hiring adjunct faculty and those who are interested in nursing education. This eliminates one of the barriers to continued nursing faculty participation, which has been the personal financial cost and time investment by full-time faculty. Hiring adjunct faculty gives university backing to function as a teacher with all the inherent roles and responsibilities as well as encourages continual interest and support of the program.

There are study-abroad opportunities that may be set up with other colleges and universities for nonclinical courses, which involve classroom activity only. For these experiences students can go alone or in groups. Housing, tuition exchange, flights, and overall costs can be negotiated with the sending and receiving universities.

Studying abroad differs from SL in that the time commitment is usually longer in duration. It may or may not involve faculty members as the time commitment part of the experience, depending on whether a clinical component is involved. It also focuses on a more in-depth examination of culture, roles, policy, and experiences than providing a service of care to an underprivileged population. This experience can be as broad or narrow in scope as the faculty imagines it to be. SL differs from volunteering in that SL is a blend of learning and volunteering at the same time during the same experience.

SL and study-abroad also differ primarily in four ways. For example, much study-abroad research focuses on how international experience affects an individual's personal growth. SL, on the other hand, tends to emphasize reciprocal learning and growth for faculty and community members as well as for students. SL has longer term outcomes, with research showing that civic participation or social responsibility—the action component of connective learning—is an important SL outcome. The longer-term objective for study-abroad programs focuses on more personalized outcomes such as improved job skills or enhanced opportunities for graduate education, careers, or international travels. Cultural learning acquired through study-abroad and SL programs is also different. Study-abroad frequently emphasizes content learning about one's own and other cultures, whereas SL concentrates less on cultures per se and more on results of cultural interactions such as reduced racism or greater tolerance for diversity. Lastly, study-abroad management programs typically feature visits to for-profit organizations; SL usually involves a nonprofit organization. Study-abroad opportunities frequently include student free time that may involve interactions with international students, community, or interviews with host nationals and independent travel, whereas SL does not (Parker & Altman, 2007).

STUDENT EXCHANGE PROGRAMS

Student exchange programs involve "exchanging" a student at one university for a student at another. This can be done nationally or internationally. This is ideal in that it gives the students a chance to experience studying various topics in another learning environment or country. This can be done for credit or non-credit coursework. When done for credit, both faculty must agree on courses and content that meet both institutions' curriculum needs. Forming partnerships with nursing colleges and universities can be started with an e-mail and then followed up with site visits. Many universities have departments that assist with these processes. In fact, in some universities, the student exchange can be interdepartmental. For example, University A can send an engineering major to University B in exchange for a nursing major. The exchange can also be cross-departmental. Exchange tuition rates will need to be negotiated by the university. This is usually a very beneficial situation not only for both universities but also the relevant departments and enables more students the ability to participate in gaining intercultural competence.

 ## BUILDING INTERCULTURAL COMPETENCE

SL experiences—whether composed of on-campus diverse interactions and integrative learning or international study-abroad experiences—provide opportunities to build intercultural competence among students (Salisbury, An, & Pascarella, 2013; Stebleton, Soria, & Cherney, 2013, Tamilla & Ledgerwood, 2018; Witkowsky & Mendez, 2018; Starr-Glass, 2018). SL experiences build both hard (cognitive) and soft (social/relational) skills. Kohlbry (2016) reports that immersive international SL experiences strengthen the process of becoming culturally competent and that nurses "graduating with enhanced cultural understanding will contribute to decreased health disparities and improved patient care quality and safety" (p. 304).

The level of interest in global health among undergraduate and graduate students has grown dramatically over the past two decades (Rawthorn & Olsen, 2014; Cone & Haley, 2018; Torres-Alzate, 2019). This growth has heightened the need for interdisciplinary education and collaboration to address the complex factors impacting the health of individuals and communities worldwide. Interprofessional global health education builds global health competency and comprises both substantive content but also "non-cognitive individual and interpersonal skills, such as perseverance, openness, and ability to work as part of a team" (Rowthorn & Olsen, 2014, p. 550). International SL experiences will provide students with the opportunity to not only build intercultural competency but also build **teamwork competency**. Teamwork competency is critical and requires "the ability to work on a team" and "a broad range of skills, attitudes, and knowledge including team values, understanding relevant roles and responsibilities, and communication skills" (Rowthorn & Olsen, 2014, p. 550).

THE GLOBAL CLASSROOM

The traditional methods of teaching "lecture style" are beginning to decrease in popularity, shifting toward more integrated global-learning experiences. With the increasing growth of technology and social networking, there is an increased demand for nurses to have a more developmental learning curriculum that instructs as well as brings the students other experiences as well.

Videoconferencing has played a significant role in enhancing nursing education experiences through clinical case discussions, educational learning, and exploration of research. These conferences can be from other countries, providing a different cultural learning experience as well as enhancing the educational experience. Videoconferencing provides an innovative, active learning methodology that challenges and engages students (Amendola, Fisher, Schaffer, & Howarth, 2016).

Global learning can be done through learning collaborative classroom delivery formats or through new technologies like "FaceTime" or "Zoom." There are many new evolving classroom delivery systems that allow online courses that can be delivered in a synchronous (at the same time) or asynchronous (to be viewed later at the students' available time) teaching method. These have grown with online classroom instruction.

Thinking out of the box with courses like research and health policy enables faculty to not only conduct a conference but deliver online courses across the world. This enhances cultural diversity, student experience, and opens one's mind to new ideas and collaboration with nurses worldwide. This is a new modality and challenges faculty to explore.

FACULTY AND INSTITUTIONAL ROLES IN INTERNATIONAL SL

The Global Advisory Panel on the Future of Nursing (GAPFON) emphasizes the role of nurses and midwives in contributing to the achievement of global health goals and the role of nurse educators in preparing future generations to meet this challenge (Wilson et al., 2016). Faculty involvement in SL is critical because, in its most common form, SL is a course-driven feature of the curriculum. Therefore, it is important that the faculty become involved at an advisory-committee level in any SL initiative.

The academic organization must be committed to the SL initiative. A mechanism of support for the faculty must be in place to:

- Generate interest among the faculty in SL
- Provide the faculty with support to make the curricular changes necessary to add an SL component to a course

An overview of the faculty and institutional activities that support SL is presented in Table 9.1.

Table 9.1 **Institutional** SL **Support**

	Institution	Faculty
Planning	▣ Form a planning group of key persons ▣ Survey institutional resources and climate ▣ Attend the Campus Compact Regional Institute ▣ Develop a campus action plan for SL ▣ Form an advisory committee	▣ Survey faculty interests and SL courses that are currently offered ▣ Identify faculty for an SL planning group and advisory committee
Awareness	▣ Inform key administrators and faculty groups about SL and program development ▣ Join national organizations (e.g., Campus Compact, National Society for Experiential Education, Partnership for SL) ▣ Attend SL conferences	▣ Distribute information on SL (e.g., brochures, newsletters, and articles) ▣ Identify a faculty liaison in each academic unit
Prototype	▣ Identify and consult with exemplary programs in higher education	▣ Identify or develop prototype course(s)
Resources	▣ Obtain administrative commitments for an SL office (e.g., budget, office space, personnel) ▣ Develop a means for coordinating SL with other programs on campus (e.g., student support services, faculty development) ▣ Apply for grants	▣ Identify interested faculty and faculty mentors ▣ Maintain a syllabus file by discipline ▣ Compile a library collection on SL ▣ Secure faculty development funds for expansion ▣ Identify existing resources that can support faculty development in SL ▣ Establish a faculty award that recognizes service
Expansion	▣ Discuss SL with a broader audience of administrators and staff (e.g., deans, counselors, student affairs) ▣ Support attendance at SL conferences ▣ Collaborate with others in programming and applying for grants ▣ Arrange campus speakers and forums on SL	▣ Offer faculty development workshops ▣ Arrange one-on-one consultations ▣ Discuss SL with departments and schools ▣ Provide course development stipends and grants to support SL ▣ Focus efforts on underrepresented schools ▣ Develop faculty mentoring program ▣ Promote the development of general education and sequential and interdisciplinary SL courses

(continued)

Table 9.1 Institutional SL **Support (***Continued* **)**

	Institution	Faculty
Recognition	■ Publicize the university's SL activities to other institutions ■ Participate in conferences and workshops ■ Publish research ■ Publicize SL activities in local media	■ Publicize faculty accomplishments ■ Include SL activities on faculty annual report forms ■ Involve faculty in professional activities (e.g., publications, workshops, conferences, forums) ■ Publicize recipients of the faculty service award
Monitoring	■ Collect data within the institution (e.g., number of courses, number of faculty teaching SL courses, number of students enrolled, number of agency partnerships)	■ Collect data on faculty involvement (e.g., number of faculty involved in faculty development activities, number of faculty offering SL courses)
Evaluation	■ Compile an annual report for the SL office ■ Include SL in institutional assessments	■ Provide assessment methods and designs to faculty (e.g., peer review, portfolios) ■ Evaluate course outcomes (e.g., student satisfaction, student learning)
Research	■ Conduct research on SL within the institution and across institutions	■ Facilitate faculty research on SL ■ Conduct research on faculty involvement in SL
Institutionalization	■ Service is part of the university mission statement and SL is recognized in university publications ■ SL is an identifiable feature of general education ■ SL courses are listed in bulletins, schedules of classes, and course descriptions ■ University sponsors regional or national conferences on SL ■ Hard-line budget commitments sustain SL programs	■ SL is part of personnel decisions (e.g., hiring, annual reviews, promotion, and tenure) ■ SL is a permanent feature of course descriptions and the curriculum ■ SL is an integral part of the faculty's professional development program

FACULTY AND LEARNER SAFETY IN SL INTERNATIONAL SITUATIONS

A prime consideration for international SL is safety. Careful preparation prior to the trip will help to ensure safety. Some considerations include the following:

- Review best practice and current literature related to SL
- Understand the political conditions of the destination country
- Register at the U.S. Embassy in the destination country
- Understand the healthcare system and the role of the nurse in the destination country
- Align with an educational healthcare organization in the destination country
- Ensure faculty and learners have the proper immunizations, medications, and identifications
- Hold preparatory sessions prior to leaving to review learning outcomes and evaluation expectations as well as predeparture cultural preparation
- Understand the food preparation and water safety of the destination country
- Include learner medications that may be needed
- Have emergency contacts on standby while away (Wittmann-Price et al., 2010)
- Have opportunities for formal debriefing and reflections after the trip

---

TEACHING GEM All learners who take regular medications should carry enough with them for the entire trip, including a surplus in case the return trip is detained.

◎ **Critical Thinking Question**

What precautions should the nurse educator take when traveling to countries and places that have significantly different altitudes than the learners' place of origin?

 CASE STUDY

CASE STUDY 9.1

Two faculty members are arranging an international SL trip for six prelicensure learners to an underdeveloped country. The hostel in which their group is being housed is 90 miles from the airport in a small town.

What are some of the safety issues that must be addressed before the learners and faculty depart? What are the appropriate evaluation mechanisms to assess learning that took place while the learners were on the trip?

1. The novice nurse educator needs a better understanding of civic engagement when the nurse educator states the following are civic engagement components:

   A. Addressing areas of political concern
   B. Organizational involvement
   C. Individual volunteerism
   D. Attending department faculty meetings

2. Participating in activities to assist in improving the community, such as promoting racial equality, would be an example of what kind of civic engagement?

   A. Civic action
   B. Civic commitment or duty
   C. Civic skills
   D. Social cohesion

3. The best suggestion to provide a student who would like to get involved in civic engagement would be:

   A. Join a peer support group
   B. Become an officer for student government
   C. Participate in a fundraiser
   D. Start a peer study group for class

4. Which of the following statements indicates a student is participating in ethical and civic responsibility at their university?

   A. "I attend all class lectures and complete assignments"
   B. "I donate blood annual to the American Red Cross"
   C. "I have voted in the election for student class officers"
   D. "I do not go to clinical on Martin Luther King Day"

5. An award is being provided to a student who demonstrates a commitment to student ethical and civic responsibility in nursing. Which student would best qualify for the civic engagement award?

   A. A hardworking student who gets straight
   B. A student who forms a social group with fellow nursing students
   C. A student who excels in a study abroad opportunity
   D. A student who becomes a tutor or mentor

1. D) Attending department faculty meetings

Political concern, organizational involvement, and volunteering are all components of civic engagement. Departmental meetings are not classified as civic engagement.

2. A) Civic action

Participating in an activity that promotes racial equality would be an example of civic action.

3. B) Become an officer for student government

Becoming an officer for student government is a way to strengthening ethical and civic responsibility by becoming involved in the student governing body on campus.

4. C) "I have voted in the election for student class officers"

A student that votes in campus and local elections is demonstrating awareness and exercising their civic responsibility.

5. D) A student who becomes a tutor or mentor

A student who volunteers to tutor or become a mentor to another nursing student is an example of one who is committed to ethical and civic responsibilities in a nursing department. Excelling in school or in an extracurricular program alone does not qualify a person to receive an award, nor does bonding with fellow nursing students.

6. A nurse educator would like to recommend to a student a method to increase their social cohesion. Which of the following methods would best increase social cohesion?

   A. Study alone to get a better grade to demonstrate mastery of course content
   B. Develop long term relationships through a student nurses association
   C. Develop a blog site and provide the maintenance
   D. Enroll in a separate leadership courses to develop skills

7. A nurse educator is taking a group of students to an impoverished country on a service-learning project. Which of the following might help to build cultural competence prior to leaving?

   A. Going out to eat at a restaurant that serves that cultural food and practicing the language
   B. Watching the Netflix series about the country's government
   C. Have students find a research article about nursing in an impoverished country
   D. Facilitate a video conference with the students from the other country before leaving

8. The novice nurse educator needs additional understanding about service-learning (SL) when they state:

   A. "SL is a form of experiential education"
   B. "SL seeks to address human and community needs"
   C. "SL should include structured reflection and debriefing"
   D. "SL can be mixed with a vacation to be more effective"

9. A nurse educator is designing a service-learning (SL) experience. Which of the following would lead to an optimal service-learning experience?

   A. Instituting experiences that benefit both the student and the community
   B. Keep this experience separate from an established academic course
   C. Demand the students' complete mandatory core competencies
   D. Make sure the students remain isolated in their hotels for safety while on the trip

10. The best method to satisfy student learning outcomes related to a service-learning experience would be:

    A. Develop an international experience to observe another culture
    B. Assign students individual tasks to complete independently when on the trip
    C. Include a learner reflection piece to develop cultural awareness
    D. Assign credit, so the students take it seriously and do their best

(See answers next page.)

6. B) Develop long-term relationships through a student nurses association

A great way to promote social cohesion is to become part of a group and make life-long relationships such as can be done through a student nurses association. Social cohesion focuses on creating and sustaining a trusting environment where people feel bonded to others. Developing a blog and enrolling in separate leadership courses alone will not facilitate an environment of social cohesion. Individual mastery of course content does not factor into the social cohesion of a group.

7. D) Facilitate a video conference with the students from the other country before leaving

The best way for students and faculty to prepare for an upcoming service-learning project and develop cultural competence is to meet and talk to the nursing students and faculty in the country that will be visited. This gives experiences of the local customs and prepares all for what is expected. Although learning about the food or government may be useful while in the country, they will not necessarily build cultural competence because they do not enable the student to learn about the cultural practices of other countries. A research article about nursing in an impoverished country would most likely focus on the perspective of the nursing student without giving the student the tools to prepare them to understand a particular culture.

8. D) "SL can be mixed with a vacation to be more effective"

Service-learning is a form of experimental education that seeks to address human and community needs and should include structured reflection and debriefing. A mix of SL and vacation usually does not meet the student learning outcomes.

9. A) Instituting experiences that benefit both the student and the community

The best way to optimize a service-learning experience is to arrange and experience that benefits not only the student but helps the community where the experience is occurring. The other answer choices prevent the student from engaging in activities with the community or fail to take advantage of the SL experience.

10. C) Include a learner reflection piece to develop cultural awareness

For the experience to be rich and meaningful, the students should be given an assignment or the opportunity to reflect through a group discussion session.

● REFERENCES

Amendola, B., Fisher, K., Schaffer, D., & Howarth, K. (2016). Creating and evaluating a global classroom to teach nursing research. *Journal of Nursing Education and Practice*, 6(4), 117–121.

American Psychological Association (2020). Civic engagement and service learning, retrieved from https://www.apa.org/education/undergrad/community-service

Barnhardt, S. (2015). You expect "what?" Students' perceptions as resources in acquiring commitments and capacities for civic engagement. *Research in Higher Education*, 56(6), 622–644. https://doi.org/10.1007/s11162-014-9361-8

Bringle, R. G., & Clayton, P. H. (2012). Civic education through service learning: What, how, and why? In L. McIlraith, A. Lyons, & R. Munck (Eds.), *Higher education and civic engagement: Comparative perspectives* (pp. 101–124). Palgrave Macmillan. https://tulane.edu/cps/faculty/upload/Research-on-Service-Learning-An-Introduction.pdf

Carlton, K. H., Ryan, M., Ali, N. S., & Kelsey, B. (2007). Global health concepts. *Nursing Education Perspectives*, 28(3), 124–129.

Carroll, A. M., Clancy, T., Bal, C. K., Lalani, S. & Woo, L. (2018) Learning through partnership with communities: A transformational journey. *Journal of Professional Nursing, Volume 34*, (3), 171-175.https://doi.org/10.1016/j.profnurs.2017.09.001.

Cone, H. (2016). Mobile clinics in Haiti, part 1: Preparing for service-learning. Nurse Education in Practice, *21*, 1–8. https://doi.org/10.1016/j.nepr.2016.08.008

Foronda, C., & Belknap, R. A. (2012). Short of transformation: American ADN students' thoughts, feelings, and experiences of studying abroad in a low-income country. *International Journal of Nursing Education Scholarship*, 9(1), 1–16.

Garneau, A. B., & Pepin, J. (2015). Cultural competence: A Constructivist definition. *Journal of Transcultural Nursing*, 26(1), 9–15. https://doi.org/10.1177/1043659614541294

Generator School Network. (2016). National service-learning clearing house. https://gsn.nylc.org/clearinghouse

Griffith, T., & Clark, K. R. (2016). Teaching techniques: Service learning. *Radiologic Technology*, 87(5), 586–588.

Hawkins, J., & Vialet, C. (2012). Service learning abroad: A life-changing experience for students. *Journal of Christian Nursing*, 29(3), 173–177.

Hébert, A. & Hauf, P. (2015) Student learning through service learning: Effects on academic development, civic responsibility, interpersonal skills and practical skills, *Active Learning in Higher Education, 16*,(1), 37–49 https://doi-org.ezproxy2.library.drexel.edu/10.1177/1469787415573357

Jeffreys, M. R. (2015). Teaching cultural competence in nursing and health care, third edition: Inquiry, action, and innovation. *ProQuest Ebook Central* https://ebookcentral-proquest-com.ezproxy2.library.drexel.edu

Kohlbry, P. W. (2016). The impact of international service-learning on nursing students' cultural competency. Journal of Nursing Scholarship, *48*, 303–311. 10.1111/jnu.12209

Krishnan, L. A., Richards, K. A. R., & Simpson, J. M. (2016). Outcomes of an international audiology service-learning study-abroad program. *American Journal of Audiology*, 25(1), 1–13. 10.1044/2015_AJA-15-0054

Levesque-Bristol, C., & Cornelius-White, J. (2012). The Public Affairs Scale: Measuring the public goods mission of higher education. *Journal of Public Affairs Education, 18,* 695–716.

Long, T. (2016). Influence of international service learning on nursing students' self-efficacy towards cultural competence. *Journal of Cultural Diversity, 23*(1), 28–33.

National League for Nursing. (2021). Certified Nurse Educator (CNE) 2021 candidate handbook. http://www.nln.org/docs/default-source/default-document-library/cne-handbook-2021_revised_07-01-2021.pdf?sfvrsn=2

National League for Nursing. (2021). Certified Nurse Educator Novice (CNEn) 2021 candidate handbook. http://www.nln.org/Certification-for-Nurse-Educators/cne-n/cne-n-handbook

National Service-Learning Clearinghouse. (2018). https://gsn.nylc.org/clearinghouse

Palmer, S., Wing, D., Miles, L., Heaston, S., & de la Cruz, K. (2013). Study abroad programs: Using alumni and graduate students as affiliate faculty. *Nurse Educator, 38*(5), 198–201.

Parker, B. & Alman-Dautoff, D. (2007). Service learning and study abroad: Synergistic learning opportunities. *Michigan Journal of Service Learning, 13*(2), 40–53.

Peterson, T. H. (2015) Revising and revising the civic mission: A radical re-imagining of "civic engagement", Community-Wealth. org, Retrieved from https://community-wealth.org/content/reviving-and-revising-civic-mission-radical-re-imagining-civic-engagement

Rowthorn, V., & Olsen, J. (2014). All together now: Developing a team skills competency domain for global health education. *Journal of Law Medicine & Ethics, 42*(4), 550–563. 10.1111/jlme.12175

Ruddock, H. C., & Turner, D. S. (2007). Developing cultural sensitivity: Nursing students experiences of a study abroad programme. *Journal of Advanced Nursing, 59*(4), 361–369.

Saenz, K., & Holcomb, L. (2009). Essential tools for studying abroad in nursing courses. *Nurse Educator, 34*(4), 172–175.

Salisbury, M. H., An, B. P., & Pascarella, E. T. (2013) The effect of study abroad on intercultural competence among undergraduate college students. *Journal of Student Affairs Research and Practice, 50*(1), 1–20. http://www.tandfonline.com/doi/pdf/10.1515/jsarp-2013-0001

Source (n.d.). What is service-learning? https://source.jhu.edu/publications-and-resources/service-learning-toolkit/what-is-service-learning.html

Starr-Glass, D. (2018). Thoughtfully Preparing Business Students and Faculty for Study Abroad: Strategies for Making the Connection. *In Business Education and Ethics : Concepts, Methodologies, Tools, and Applications* (pp. 872–894).

Stebleton, M. J., Soria, K. M., & Cherney, B. (2013). The high impact of education abroad: College students' engagement in international experiences and the development of intercultural competencies. *Frontiers: Interdisciplinary Journal of Study Abroad, 22.* http://works.bepress.com/michael_stebleton/22

Tamilla, C., & Ledgerwood, J. R. (2018). Students' motivations, perceived benefits and constraints towards study abroad and other international education opportunities. *Journal of International Education in Business, 11*(1), 63–78. http://dx.doi.org.ezproxy2.library.drexel.edu/10.1108/JIEB-01-2017-0002

Tapley, H., & Patel, R. (2016). Using the precede-proceed model and service-learning to teach health promotion and wellness: An innovative approach for physical therapist professional education. *Journal of Physical Therapy Education*, 30(1), 47–59.

Wilson, L., Mendes, I. A, C., Klopper, H., Catrambone, C. & Al-Maaitah, R., Norton, M. E, & Hill, M. (2016) 'Global health' and 'global nursing': proposed definitions from The Global Advisory Panel on the Future of Nursing, *J. of Advanced Nursing* https://doi-org.ezproxy2.library.drexel.edu/10.1111/jan.12973

Witkowsky, P., & Mendez, S. L. (2018). Influence of a short-term study abroad experience on professional competencies and career aspirations of graduate students in student affairs. *Journal of College Student Development, 59*(6), 769–775. http://dx.doi.org. ezproxy2.library.drexel.edu/10.1353/csd.2018.0073

Wittmann-Price, R. A. (2007). Promoting reflection in groups of diverse nursing students. In B. Moyer & R. A. Wittmann-Price (Eds.), *Nursing education: Foundations for practice excellence*. F. A. Davis.

Wittmann-Price, R. A., Anselmi, K. K., & Espinal, F. (2010, March/April). Creating opportunities for successful international student service-learning experiences. *Holistic Nursing Practice, 24* (2),89–98.:10.1097/HNP.0b013e3181d3994a

Youth.gov (2020) Civic engagement. https://youth.gov/youth-topics/civic-engagement-and-volunteering

Using Assessment and Evaluation Strategies

Kathryn M. Shaffer

Learning without thought is labor lost.
—Confucius

▶ LEARNING OUTCOMES

This chapter addresses the Certified Nurse Educator Exam and the Certified Nurse Educator Novice Exam Content Area 3: Use Assessment and Evaluation Strategies. For the CNE it is 19% of the examination, approximately 28 questions and for the CNEn exam it is 15% or approximately 23 questions.

- Identify internal and external factors that influence admission, progression, and graduation in a nursing program
- Utilize nursing program standards related to admission and progression
- Describe the process of program evaluation to assess outcomes in a nursing curriculum
- Use a variety of strategies to assess learning in the cognitive, affective, and psychomotor domains within the context of fair testing guidelines
- Understand various frameworks and models upon which evaluation and assessment are based
- Analyze assessment and evaluation data in determining learner achievement and program outcomes
- Use assessment and evaluation data to enhance the teaching–learning process and influence program outcomes

● INTRODUCTION

This chapter focuses on the factors that influence nursing education program outcomes. The relationship of standards related to admission and progression within the parent institution in general, and in the nursing program in particular, is discussed. Methods of assessing learning and outcomes are presented to provide a mechanism for the nurse educator to determine program effectiveness and identify strategies to improve the quality of the nursing program.

● DEFINITIONS

To understand the assessment and evaluation process involved in a nursing education program, it is important to understand the terminology related to this process.

- "[A] nursing education program refers to any academic program offered in a post-secondary education institution, which results in initial licensure or advanced preparation in nursing" (Sauter, Gillespie, & Knepp, 2012, p. 467).
- Nursing programs that offer initial licensure are of three types:
  1. Baccalaureate degree—a 4-year program offered by a college or university
  2. Associate degree—a 2-year program typically offered by a community college
  3. Diploma—a 2- or 3-year program that is hospital based and offered in a school of nursing
- Nursing programs offering advanced preparation in nursing occur at the college or university level and include:
  - RN–BSN programs
  - RN–MSN programs
  - BSN–PhD programs
  - MSN degree
  - Doctorate (doctor of philosophy [PhD] or doctor of nursing practice [DNP])
- Second-degree programs or accelerated BSN or direct entry MSN degree programs deliver a baccalaureate in an accelerated format in which a student with a previous bachelor's degree in any field attends a condensed baccalaureate degree program. This can range from as little as 11 months to longer time frames but is usually less than 2 years.
- *Assessment* is a process in which information is gathered to determine whether learning has occurred. Multiple methods may be used to gather this information, analyze the information, and interpret the findings. This may result in making changes to improve learner outcomes, which is similar to formative evaluation (Billings & Halstead, 2020; Fardows, 2011; Keating, 2011).
- *Evaluation* is a systematic and continuous process in which information is gathered to determine the worth and value of the program, outcomes, and achievement of the learner. It is equated to summative evaluation, in which a judgment is made about the outcome (Billings & Halstead, 2020; Fardows, 2011; Keating, 2011).
- *Program evaluation* refers to "systematic assessment and analysis of all components of an academic program." (Billings & Halstead, 2020, p. 513).
- *Standards and guidelines* are "Statements of expectations and aspirations providing a foundation for professional nursing behaviors' of graduates of baccalaureate, master's, professional doctoral, and postgraduate APRN certificate program. Standards are developed by a consensus of professional nursing communities who have a vested interest in the education and practice of nurses" (CCNE [Commission on Collegiate Nursing Education] Accreditation Manual, 2018, p. 26). Accreditation Commission for Education in Nursing (ACEN [2017]) defines standards as "Agreed-upon rules to measure quantity, extent, value, and quality" (ACEN Manual, July 2020). CNEA (Commission on Nursing Education Accreditation) identifies their standards within their manual (NLN CNEA, 2021).
- "Key elements as defined by CCNE are designed to enable a broad interpretation of each standard in order to support institutional autonomy and encourage innovation while maintaining the quality of nursing programs and the integrity of the accreditation" (CCNE Accreditation Manual, 2018, p. 5).
- *Criteria* are "Statements that identify the variables that need to be examined in evaluation of a standard" (ACEN Manual, July 2020).

The *admission* policies of an institution are the first standards with which a learner is evaluated for admission into a nursing program. The policies must be clearly defined and published by the institution. The nursing program in an academic setting may further refine these standards and criteria to ensure the academic quality of the learners entering the program. Criteria for admission into a nursing program may include:

- Standardized testing, such as the Scholastic Aptitude Test (SAT) for undergraduate education and Graduate Record Examination (GRE) for graduate applications
- Courses taken in high school or college with a strong science and math base
  - Nursing program entry examinations such as Health Education Systems Incorporated Admission Examination (HESI A2 Exam), Educational Resources Inc. Nurse Entrance Test (NET), or the Assessment Technology Incorporated Test of Academic Skills (ATI TEAS)
- Minimum grade point average (GPA)
- Personal letter of intent
- Letters of reference
- Background checks (Farnsworth & Springer, 2006; Serembus, 2016)

Learner success on the National Council of Licensure Examination (NCLEX®) is the benchmark for all nursing programs for achieving minimum standards of competency and quality. Predictive criteria have been studied to determine the attributes of a nursing learner that are necessary for passing the NCLEX. Yin and Burger (2003) found that the following criteria were excellent predictors of which learners enrolled in an associate degree nursing program would successfully pass the NCLEX:

- College GPA before admission into the nursing program was found to be the most important predictor of success
- High GPAs in natural science courses—biology, chemistry, and anatomy and physiology
- Course grade in an introductory psychology course
- High school rank

Sayles, Shelton, and Powell (2003) found that other predictors, in addition to the aforementioned, also improved success rates of learners on the NCLEX:

- Scores on the NET Comprehensive Achievement Profiles, administered by Educational Resources, Inc.
- Pre-RN assessment scores

Carrick (2011) suggests that other factors related to learning outcomes assessment are essential to predicting NCLEX success and include the following:

- Assessment of learning outcomes on examinations using higher-level questions at the analysis and application level should be initiated after nurse educators help learners change their approach to learning.
- Nurse educators should address the underlying needs of the learner.

Personal and situational factors, such as learner anxiety and frustration, may need to be examined (p. 82). High GPAs in the natural sciences and other college courses taken prior to admission into baccalaureate nursing programs have also been predictive of learner success when taking the NCLEX. Based on this success rate, many nursing programs of all three types now require learners to complete all college requirements before admission into a nursing program. Admission into the nursing major has become very selective, based on specific criteria, as identified by the individual nursing program. In a baccalaureate program with this admission requirement, learners enter the nursing major at the junior level if they have met the strict criteria for admission into the program.

EVIDENCE-BASED TEACHING PRACTICE

Al-Alawi and Alexander (2020) completed a systematic review related to nursing education programs performing program outcome evaluations and found that most nursing educational programs only focus on program evaluation around the scheduled accreditation visits. The review also identified that most program changes were made based on descriptive outcome data rather than reliable and valid evaluation tools.

Admission criteria for graduate nursing education must be clearly developed for applicants to this program. The policies must be congruent with the institution's overall policy, but, as is seen in undergraduate education, criteria may be more selective for admission into the nursing program. Predictors of success in a graduate program have been based on the undergraduate GPA and scores on the GRE. However, Newton and Moore (2007) found that the undergraduate GPA was not always predictive of success when taking GREs and, as such, should be used with caution when making decisions related to admission into a graduate nursing program. Many nursing programs waive the standardized testing requirement if applicants have a GPA of 3.3 or 3.5 or higher. Zamanzadeh et al. (2020) also found that nursing education admission processes relied on cognitive and non-cognitive ability assessment. The cognitive abilities were assessed through standardized testing in four main areas, including mathematics, language, natural sciences, and reasoning skills. Noncognitive abilities assessment included morality, interpersonal communication skills, and psychological strength.

EVIDENCE-BASED TEACHING PRACTICE

Serembus (2016) outlined a plan to improve NCLEX-RN® pass rates and comprehensive standardized examination scores based on Deming's four phases of the continuous-improvement model (CIP): Plan, Do, Study, Act. This is a comprehensive systems approach to program evaluation. In the Plan phase of the CIP, strategies for improving NCLEX pass rates are established. Strategies are enacted in the Do phase. During the Study phase, the results of the plan are evaluated. The educator accepts or rejects the plan in the Act phase based on the outcomes. If the outcomes are successful, then the strategies are implemented and continuously assessed. If outcomes are negative, then the Plan phase is reassessed, and new approaches are identified as part of the cycle.

▶ PROGRESSION POLICIES

Progression policies within the nursing major must be congruent with the program goals and institutional standards and must be clearly identified and published. Criteria that are often included in progression policies are:

- Minimum course grades for nursing and science courses
- Minimum cumulative GPA for progression in the program
- Number of times a learner may repeat selective courses at both the undergraduate and graduate levels
- Standards in place if a learner takes a leave of absence during the program of study
- Achievement of a minimum grade on standardized achievement tests based on established benchmarks for prelicensure learners

● THE EVALUATION/ASSESSMENT PROCESS

The terms *assessment* and *evaluation* are often used interchangeably, but in reality they have different meanings.

Evaluation is the process of systematically collecting and analyzing data that has been gathered through various measurements to determine the merit, worth, and value of something and to render a judgment about the subject of the evaluation (Billings & Halstead, 2020; Fardows, 2011; Keating, 2011). Evaluation in the educational setting is conducted to determine (a) learner progress toward achieving program outcomes, (b) effectiveness of the educational process to foster learning, and (c) accomplishment of the mission of the institution to prepare nurses for entry into practice (Billings & Halstead, 2020; O'Connor, 2015).

Assessment is the process of obtaining information about learners, educators, programs, and institutions and is often used interchangeably with the term evaluation. More specific, assessment involves setting standards and criteria for learning, gathering, analyzing, and interpreting data to determine how performance matches the standards and criteria and using that information to improve learning, teaching, courses, and programs (Angelo, 1993; Billings & Halstead, 2020; Fardows, 2011; Keating, 2011).

▶ PHILOSOPHIES OF EVALUATION

The evaluation process is influenced by the evaluator's beliefs about evaluation and his or her philosophical perspective. Some examples of evaluation philosophies include:

- Practice orientation
  - Practice goals are reflected in course outcomes
  - Performance achieved at the end of the course, clinical experience, or program is the most important consideration
- Service orientation

- This perspective is based on a values approach to evaluation
- This view takes a more global or holistic view of the goals of the educational process beyond course outcomes
- This perspective includes goals that are integrated into a model of performance that represents the typical or ideal learner at a particular level of development
- With this approach, instructors view the evaluation process as a means to identify learner strengths and weaknesses in various components of performance
- This view facilitates learner progress toward model performance
- Judgment orientation
  - This perspective reflects a focus on the determination of acceptability of learner performance and the value or grade that should be assigned based on the performance
  - Instructors assign a pass/fail grade or letter or numerical grade—pass/fail is used most often in clinical grading
- Constructivist orientation
  - Assigns heaviest consideration to stakeholders who will be affected by the success or failure of the program. In nursing, the stakeholders are the employers of graduates and the recipients of the graduates' nursing care
- The evaluation process involves input from patients and staff who contribute to the assignment of the grade in the clinical setting (O'Connor, 2006)

TEACHING GEM   The best test combines aspects of both norm-referenced and criterion-referenced tests.

▶ PURPOSES OF EVALUATION

The purpose of the evaluation process must be clearly delineated for nurse educators and learners. Purposes of evaluation include:

- Promote learning
- Diagnosis of problems such as learning needs or deficits in teaching practices, courses, or the curriculum
- Decision-making related to assignment of grades, tenure, and promotion
- Improvement of products such as textbooks or course content
- Judgment of effectiveness of learner goal achievement and the meeting of standards and program outcomes (Billings & Halstead, 2020; O'Connor, 2015)

▶ FORMATIVE EVALUATION

- Refers to the evaluation of learning while it is occurring.
- Identifies a learner's readiness to learn and his or her learning needs.
- May be used to improve learner performance before the end of the course or program.
- Assigns no final grade.
- Shares the evaluation with the learner informally throughout the learning process but formally presents it in clinical courses at mid-semester (Oermann & Gaberson, 2017).

▶ SUMMATIVE EVALUATION

- Refers to the level of performance of the learner at the end of the course, program, or activity.
- Makes a judgment as to whether or not the standards and criteria have been met for the event (course, clinical, and program).
- Uses data collected throughout the learning experience as the basis for evaluation.
- Assigns a final grade (letter, number, pass/fail, and satisfactory/unsatisfactory).
- Evaluator determines evaluation and shares with the learner being evaluated while the summative period is in effect, particularly in clinical courses or activities (Oermann & Gaberson, 2017).

TEACHING GEM The learner should never be surprised to be told that they have not met course requirements in either the classroom or clinical setting. The nurse educator must keep the learner informed of their progress throughout the entire learning experience allowing for growth to occur.

▶ EVALUATION MODELS

An evaluation model is useful for explaining the process on which variables, items, or events are evaluated and provides a systematic plan or framework for evaluation. Several models are used in nursing education and should be selected based on the context, needs of the stakeholders, and the question to be evaluated. Some of the evaluation models are included here (Billings & Halstead, 2020):

Logic model

- Useful in designing program evaluations
- Helps conceptualize, plan, and communicate with others about the program
- Uses flowcharts to help clarify key elements of a program
- Inputs are resources that are needed to run the program
- Educational strategies
- Outputs are learner demographics, contact hours, assignments, and tests
- Initial outcomes–changes noted in learners in response to the learning activities
- Intermediate outcomes–longer term learner outcomes
- Ultimate outcomes–vision of what should be accomplished when learners have completed the program

Decision-oriented models: CIPP (Context, Input, Process, and Product)

- Provides information on which decisions can be made, measures strengths and weaknesses of a program, identifies target populations, and identifies options
- Uses context evaluation to identify the target population and assess needs
- Uses input evaluation to assess the capabilities of the system, uses alternative program strategies and procedural designs to implement the strategy
- Process evaluation detects defects in the design or implementation of the strategy, as well as satisfaction with the experience
- Product evaluation reflects the outcomes and results of the program

Kirkpatrick's four-level model

- Uses a variety of inputs such as students, employers, and faculty to evaluate outcomes (Billings & Halstead, 2020, p. 516)
- 4 levels: reaction, learning, behavior, results

  1. Reaction: student perspective
  2. Learning: whether it did occur
  3. Behavior: assessment of skills and application
  4. Results: students' success in translating knowledge into practice

- Provides meaning, consensus, and understanding of all involved
- Accreditation Model: Evidence-Based Evaluation
- Process used in institutions of higher learning and professional programs to determine the extent to which a program achieves its mission, goals, and outcomes
- Focus is on ongoing self-evaluation and the achievement of outcomes to support quality improvement of the program
- Three main organizations accredit nursing programs

  - ACEN (http://www.acenursing.org)
  - CCNE (www.aacn.nche.edu)
  - CNEA (https://cnea.nln.org/programs)

▶ EVALUATION METHODS

After an evaluation model has been determined, the method(s) of evaluation must be selected to assess the effectiveness of learning and the achievement of course and program outcomes in both their theoretical and clinical components. Multiple methods are often used as learning is evaluated in the three domains: cognitive (knowledge), affective (attitude), and psychomotor (skill). Using a single evaluation method does not adequately measure all three domains (see Table 10.1).

Table 10.1 Evaluation Strategies

Assessment strategy	Domain of learning assessed	Uses of assessment strategy
Papers/essays	Affective Higher cognitive levels	Demonstrates organizational skills Encourages creativity Improves critical thinking skills
Portfolios	Affective Higher cognitive levels	Measures program outcomes Shows evidence of learner progress in a specific class Advanced placement of learners within courses
Critiques	Higher cognitive levels Affective	Active learner involvement Builds critical thinking skills Reinforces expected standards

(continued)

Table 10.1 Evaluation Strategies

Assessment strategy	Domain of learning assessed	Uses of assessment strategy
Journals	Higher cognitive levels Affective	Allows for learner reflection on experiences Promotes active learning Assesses learning Enhances critical thinking skills Helps improve writing skills
Concept maps	Cognitive (all levels) Affective	Visual representation of concepts and connections Improves critical thinking Promotes understanding of complex relationships among concepts Integrates theoretical knowledge into practice
Audiotape	Cognitive (all levels) Affective	Demonstrates communication skills Demonstrates interview skills
Videotape	Higher cognitive levels Affective Psychomotor	Reviews learner performance of skills Allows learner to observe his or her performances Reflects on the experience
Role-playing	Cognitive Affective Psychomotor	Explores feelings about an experience or issue Develops problem-solving skills Reflects on the experience Effects changes in attitude, beliefs, or values
Oral presentations	Cognitive Affective	Improves communication skills Enhances critical thinking Improves organizational skills
Simulations	Cognitive Affective Psychomotor	Practice skills in a nonthreatening environment Improves critical thinking skills Improves prioritization of activities Active learning Assesses learner learning

In any case, the learner must be informed of the evaluation methods to be used to assess their learning. Grading rubrics are one method of evaluation that includes rating scales used to evaluate written work and assign a grade. Grading rubrics are usually shared with the learner before the evaluation process, so the learner is aware of the criteria. Grading rubrics are useful when evaluating:

- Tests/examinations (paper/pencil, computer)
- Written work
- Papers and essays
- Portfolios
- Critiques
- Journals
- Nursing care plans
- Concept maps
- Audiotape and videotape
- Role-playing
- Oral presentations

- Simulations
- Observations by the instructor
- Rating scales
- Skills checklists

Many nurse educators use grading rubrics to assess participation in electronic discussion boards. Rubrics range from being extremely detailed to rating scales that are more general and therefore contain some subjectivity. Table 10.2 offers an example of a grading rubric used for a journal assignment.

Table 10.2 Grading Rubric Example

Task	1 Point	2 Points	3 Points	4 Points
Identify goals and attainment	Goals not clearly identified No description of attainment of goals	Goals not clearly identified Minimal description of attainment of goals	Goals clearly identified Attainment of goals mentioned but not described completely	Goals clearly identified Attainment of goals thoroughly discussed
Score: (/4)				
Summary of interactions	Briefly summarized interactions with preceptor No identification of situations encountered	Briefly summarized interactions with preceptor Minimal identification of situations encountered	Summarized interactions with preceptor Identified situations encountered	Thoroughly summarized interactions with preceptor Identified situations encountered
Score: (/4)				
Analysis of significant events	No critical reflection evident in the analysis of the experience Minimal to no description of feelings, reactions, or responses Last journal includes little or no discussion of attainment of objectives and lessons learned	Analysis shows minimal reflection of the experience Minimal description of feelings, reactions, or responses Last journal includes minimal discussion of attainment of objectives and lessons learned	Analysis shows some critical reflection of the experience Feelings, reactions, and responses described Last journal includes discussion of attainment of objectives and lessons learned	Analysis shows critical reflection of the experience Feelings, reactions, and responses described in depth Last journal includes discussion of attainment of objectives and lessons learned

Score: (/4)					
Submission of journals		Journals submitted late		Journals submitted by due date	
Score: (/4)					
Total score: (/16) = %					

▶ ACHIEVEMENT TESTS AND ASSESSMENTS

To ensure effective evaluation, achievement tests should be related to the instruction given. The test questions should measure the achievement of the learning outcomes and should fit the learner population's learning characteristics. The results of achievement tests should be reliable and valid, and learners should benefit from the test's feedback. The results should also provide the nurse educator with feedback about content areas for which more emphasis is needed or areas that were interpreted differently than expected (Gronlund, 1993). Achievement testing can be an effective evaluative mechanism for both learner and faculty if tests are developed based on sound, evaluative principles.

▶ GUIDELINES FOR DEVELOPING CLASSROOM TESTS

According to Gronlund (1993), there are three types of evaluative mechanisms used in nursing education. Achievement tests usually denote tests that have sound psychometric reliability; many times, these are standardized tests created by an outside vendor. Norm-referenced tests are those that rank a group of learners. Someone gets the highest score, someone else receives the lowest, and the scores in between are compared to the shape of a "bell curve" for that evaluation. A *criterion-referenced test* is one that is closely aligned to an achievement test. The criteria are set, and the score is compared to a criterion, not to other scores. The specific characteristics of each type of test are listed here.

Achievement Tests
- Achievement tests should measure clearly defined learning outcomes
  - These tests are measured in terms of learner performance
  - Achievement tests should be concerned with all intended learning outcomes
  - These tests must include outcomes based on knowledge, skill, understanding, application, and complex learning
- Achievement tests should measure a representative sample of instructionally relevant learning skills
  - These tests are based on sampling
  - Instructors need to use a systematic procedure to obtain a representative sample of the test items relevant to the instruction
  - Instructors need to prepare learners for test specifications

- Achievement tests should include the types of test items that are most appropriate for measuring the intended outcomes
  - The tests need a means of determining whether the specified performance and learning have occurred
  - Key: Select the most appropriate item type and construct it to elicit the desired response
- Achievement tests should be based on plans for using the results
- Achievement tests should provide scores that are relatively free from measurement errors
- The test should provide consistent results (it should be reliable)
- The following factors increase the amount of error in test scores:
  - Ambiguous test items
  - Testing a specific skill with too few test items yields scores that are influenced by chance rather than by learner performance
  - Essay tests are subjective
  - Learners' attention, effort, fatigue, and guessing on tests

NORM-REFERENCED TESTS

- Interpreted in relation to the ranking of learners in the class
- Tell how a learner's scores compare with those of his or her peers
- Provide a wide range of scores to discriminate among levels of achievement
- Focus on a broad range of learning tasks
- Feature relatively few test items per task
- Focus on learner ranking
- Provide a percentile rank of learners from high to low achievers
- These are commonly used in national standardized tests, such as SATs and ATIs (Billings & Halstead, 2020; Gronlund, 1993; McDonald, 2007)

CRITERION-REFERENCED TESTS

- These tests are expressed in terms of the specific knowledge and skills a learner can demonstrate
- Include test items that are directly relevant to the learning outcomes regardless of the degree of difficulty
- Focus on a detailed learning domain
- Should be designed to measure the ability of a learner in a particular area
- Feature a relatively large number of test items per task
- Most are teacher made and are based on course objectives
- Items provide a detailed description of learner performance
- Scores are reported as the percentage correct based on preset standards
- Example: 100% of the learners will correctly calculate medication dosages on the calculation examination (Billings & Halstead, 2020; Gronlund, 1993; McDonald, 2007)

PLANNING THE TEST

The first step in planning a test is to determine what type of test should be given. This decision is based on the purpose of the test. The type of test given should effectively measure the learning or capability to be measured and the desired outcome of the test. Some examples of reasons why a test may be given include:

- To determine eligibility before entry into a nursing program as part of the admission criteria
- To determine appropriate academic placement
- To monitor learning progress
- To determine levels of mastery of content at the end of an instruction period

▶ IDENTIFYING AND DEFINING LEARNING OUTCOMES

The next step in planning a test is to identify and define intended learning outcomes. The use of Bloom's taxonomy of learning is one method to accomplish this step. (Refer to Chapter 2 to review Bloom's taxonomy.)

- The cognitive domain addresses areas related to intellectual abilities
- The affective domain is concerned with values and attitudes
- The psychomotor domain addresses motor skills (Table 10.3)

Table 10.3 Bloom's Taxonomy for Affective Domains

Level	Concepts	Verbs Used in Writing Objectives and Learning Outcomes, with Examples
Receiving	Awareness Willingness to receive Control of selected attention	**Verbs:** Ask, listen, focus, attend, take part, discuss, acknowledge, hear, be open to, retain, follow, concentrate, read, do, feel **Examples:** Listens to teacher or trainer, takes interest in session or learning experience, takes notes, attends; makes time for learning experience, participates passively
Responding	Acquiescence in responding Willingness to respond Satisfaction with response	**Verbs:** React, respond, seek, interpret, clarify, provide, contribute **Examples:** Participate actively in group discussion, active participation in activity, show interest in outcomes, enthusiasm for action, question, and probe ideas, suggest interpretations
Valuing	Acceptance of a value Preference for a value Commitment	**Verbs:** Argue, challenge, debate, refute, confront, justify, persuade, criticize **Examples:** Decide worth and relevance of ideas or experiences; accept or commit to particular stance or action

(continued)

Table 10.3 Bloom's Taxonomy for Affective Domains

Organization	Conceptualization of a value Organization of a value system	**Verbs:** Build, develop, formulate, defend, modify, relate, prioritize, reconcile, contrast, arrange, compare **Examples:** Qualify and quantify personal views, state personal position and reasons, state beliefs
Characterization by a value or a value complex	General set of behaviors that characterize a person Characterization of the whole person—an internal consistency	**Verbs:** Act, display, influence, solve, practice **Examples:** Self-reliant; behaves consistently with personal value set

Achievement testing is focused primarily on the cognitive domain, with the following six main areas to consider (Gronlund, 1993):

1. *Knowledge (remembering previously learned material)*
   - Intellectual abilities and skills
   - Comprehension (grasping the meaning of material)
2. *Translation (converting from one form to another)*
   - Interpretation (explaining material)
   - Extrapolation (extending the meaning beyond data)
3. *Application (using information in a concrete situation)*
4. *Analysis (breaking down material into its parts)*
   - Identify the parts
   - Identify the relationships
   - Identify the organization
5. *Synthesis (putting parts together to create a whole)*
   - Uniqueness
   - Abstract relations
6. *Evaluation (judging the value for a given purpose using specific criteria)*
   - Judgment in terms of internal evidence
   - Judgment in terms of external criteria

Another method used to plan a test is to use the NCLEX Test Plan (2019). Patient needs are the basis of the test plan and include four major areas:

1. Safe, effective care environment
2. Health promotion and maintenance
3. Psychosocial integrity
4. Physiological integrity

Each area is assigned a percentage of the number of questions on the NCLEX (Table 10.4). Most items are concerned with the application or higher levels of cognitive ability, but the examination also includes knowledge and comprehension questions.

Table 10.4 NCLEX Test Plan

CLIENT NEEDS TESTED
Safe and effective care environment
- Management of care—20%
- Safety and infection control—12%
Health promotion and maintenance—9%
Psychosocial integrity—9%
Physiological integrity
- Basic care/comfort—9%
- Pharmacological and parenteral therapies—15%
- Reduction of risk potential—12%
- Physiological adaptation—14%

Source: National Council of State Boards of Nursing (2019 NCLEX-RN® Test Plan).

▶ NEXT-GENERATION NCLEX

In 2012 the National Council of State Boards of Nursing (NCSBN®) conducted early research from practice analysis survey's on the complex decisions new to practice nurses need to make safe informed decision. Understanding that novice nurses are involved in failure to act and failure to recognize incidents most commonly in practice, a Clinical Judgment Model (CJM) offering a new approach to bedside decision-making. (Sherrill, 2019). Clinical judgment is the "observed outcome of critical thinking and decision-making. It is an iterative process that uses nurses' knowledge to observe and access presenting situation, identify a prioritized client concern, and generate the best possible evidence-based solution to deliver safe client care" (NCSBN®, 2018).

THE CLINICAL JUDGMENT MODEL

- Recognizing and Analysing Cues
- Prioritizing Hypothesis
- Generating Solutions
- Taking Action
- Evaluating Outcomes

NEXT-GENERATION TYPES OF QUESTIONS

- CLOZE
- Extended Drag and Drop—Not steps, prioritization
- Extended Multiple Choice
- Extended Hot spot/Highlight
- Extended multiple response/SATA
- Matrix

These types of questions need to start early in the program and progress of time.

▶ DETERMINING THE TYPES OF TEST QUESTIONS TO USE

Once the nurse educator has determined the purpose of the test and the plan to be used in its construction, the next step is to decide on the types of test questions to be included. This decision is based on the objectives and outcomes for the test and should include a variety of types of questions that are consistent with formats used on the NCLEX-RN exam, including the Next Generation NCLEX case study questions (NCLEX 2021), such as:

- Multiple choice
- Multiple response
- True/false
- Matching
- Fill in the blank
- Essay
- Ordered response
- Hot spots
- Multimedia, including charts, graphs, audio, sound, and tables
- Highlight (HI) text
- Highlight (HI) table
- Drag and drop cloze
- Drag and drop rationale
- Drag and drop table
- Matrix multiple choice
- Bowtie
- Trend questions

A table of specifications (test plan, test blueprint) should be used as the basis for developing achievement tests (see Table 10.5 for a test blueprint for the nursing process).

The following factors should be taken into consideration when developing a table of specifications:

- Matches the purpose of the test—be sure that the test is measuring a representative sample of the content and learning outcomes
- Relates learning outcomes to content
- Indicates the relative weight for each area based on several factors (see Table 10.5)
- How much time was spent on each area during instruction? This should be the most important consideration
- Which outcomes are most important in regard to retention and transfer value?

Table 10.5 Test Blueprint

Content Area	Assessment	Analysis	Planning	Implementation	Evaluation	Total number of items
Cardiac %						
Renal %						
Endocrine %						
Total number of items						

Table 10.6 Distribution of Test Questions

Outcomes/content	Knowledge		Comprehends principles	Applies principles	Total number of items
	Terms	Facts			
Role of nurse in decision making	4	4	3	5	16
Osteoarthritis	3	2	4	5	14
Total number of items	7	6	7	10	30

Another consideration that should be part of the table of specifications would be to determine the number of questions for each part of the content being tested based on the criteria listed earlier (see Table 10.6 for an example of the distribution of test questions by content).

▶ VALIDITY AND RELIABILITY OF TESTS

Validity refers to the appropriateness, meaningfulness, and usefulness of the inferences from the test scores (Billings & Halstead, 2020; Gronlund, 1993). A test's validity is the judgment one makes to determine whether the test measured what was intended. Approaches for testing validity include the following (Billings & Halstead, 2020; Gronlund, 1993):

- Content-related evidence
  - How well does the test measure the intended learning outcomes?
  - Did the test feature an adequate sampling of material?
  - Was the test properly constructed, administered, and scored?
- Criterion-related evidence
  - How accurately does test performance predict future performance?
  - Can one use test performance to estimate current performance on a criterion?
  - What is the degree of relationship between the test scores and the criterion—the key element?
- What was the correlation coefficient (r)?
  - Positive relationship—high or low scores on one measure are accompanied by high or low scores on another
  - Negative relationship—high scores on one measure are accompanied by low scores on another measure
- Construct-related evidence
  - How well can test performance be explained in terms of psychological characteristics?

Reliability refers to the degree of consistency of test scores. Factors that may affect reliability include insufficient test length and group variability (Billings & Halstead, 2020). Reliability is measured by a correlation coefficient. The simplest method of estimating the reliability of test scores from a single administration of a test is using the Kuder–Richardson formulas (KR-20 or KR-21). The KR-20 reflects the accuracy or power of discrimination of the test (Kehoe, 1995). Three types of information are required to determine the KR: (a) the number of items in the test, (b) the mean, and (c) the standard deviation (Gronlund, 1993). The formula for the KR-21 is shown in Exhibit 10.1.

Exhibit 10.1 KR-21 Formula

Reliability estimate $(KR\,21) = 1 - \dfrac{M(k - M)}{K(s^2)}$

K = number of items in the test
M = mean of test scores
s = standard deviation of test scores

Reported reliabilities for standardized achievement tests are .90 or better for KR formulas. Reliability coefficients for classroom tests should be between .50 and .80 (1.0 is the maximum; Kehoe, 1995).

▶ FACTORS THAT LOWER RELIABILITY OF TEST SCORES

- Too few items on the test
- Excessive numbers of very easy or very hard questions
- Inadequate testing conditions
- Items are poorly written and do not discriminate
- Scoring is subjective (remedy: prepare scoring keys and follow them carefully when scoring essay answers and performance tasks; in other words, prepare a rubric; Gronlund, 1993; Kehoe, 1995)

Exhibit 10.2 provides an example of test statistics. Try to interpret the meaning of the statistics.

▶ ITEM ANALYSIS

Item analysis is done to determine whether tests have separated the learners from the nonlearners (discrimination). Software packages can provide statistical data about the overall analysis of a test and provide a detailed analysis of each item. The following key concepts are necessary to consider when reviewing the item analysis on a classroom test.

Exhibit 10.2 Example of Test Statistics

Total possible points	50
Students in this group	17
Standard deviation	3.53
Reliability coefficient (KR-20)	0.56
Point biserial	0.18
Total group	64.71%
Upper 27% of group	80.00%
Median score	40.33
Mean score	40.35

- Item difficulty (p-value; Gronlund, 1993)
- Percentage of the group that answered the item correctly
- p = .5 (50% correct) is a good discrimination index
- Upper limit = 1.00 (100% of learners answered the question correctly)
- Lower limit depends on the number of possible responses and probability of guessing correctly
- If there are four options, then p = .25 is the lower limit or probability of guessing

See Exhibit 10.3 for a formula for calculating item difficulty.

Item Discrimination

- Differentiates between learners who knew the content from those who did not
- Measured by point-biserial correlation (measures each learner's item performance with each learner's overall test performance)
  - Questions that discriminate well have point-biserial correlations that are highly positive for the correct answer and negative for the distractors
  - Learners who knew the content answered correctly; those who did not choose the distractors
  - Indices greater than .3 are good; greater than .4 are very good
  - Item difficulty of p = .5 shows a discrimination index that is maximized. If the index is too high or too low, the index is attenuated and the item is a poor discriminator
- Distractor evaluation
  - Need to evaluate each distractor individually
  - Distractors should appeal to the nonlearner

Exhibit 10.3 Calculating Item Difficulty

EXAMPLE				
ITEM 1. ALTERNATIVES	A	B[a]	C	D
Upper 10	0	6	3	1
Lower 10	3	2	2	3
$P = \dfrac{R}{T} \times 100$				
$P = \dfrac{8}{20} \times 100 = 40\%(.40)$				

P = the percentage who answered the item correctly, R = the number who answered the item correctly, T = total number who attempted the item.

[a]B is correct answer.

- Distractors that have a point biserial of zero means learners did not select them, and they need to be revised or replaced—learners probably got the question correct by guessing.
- Negative discriminating power occurs when more learners in the lower group than in the upper group choose the correct answer. These items need to be revised or replaced.
- Compute item analysis
  1. Mean score—the average of all the learners
  2. Median—the point at which 50% are higher and 50% are lower
  3. Standard deviation—measures the variability of test scores; the degree test scores deviate from the mean

  4. D-value $= \dfrac{(R_u - R_L)}{1/2T}$

- D = index of discriminating power; R_u = number in the upper group who answered the item correctly; R_L = number in the lower group who answered the item correctly; $1/2T$ = one half of the total number of learners included in the item analysis

In other words, for a multiple-choice question to be discriminating, it should be answered correctly by the upper one-third of the class and answered incorrectly by the lower one-third of the class. See Exhibit 10.4 for a formula for calculating point biserials.

Exhibit 10.4 Formula for Calculating Point-Biserial Correlation '-'

Item 1. Alternatives	A	B[a]	C	D
Upper 10	0	6	3	1
Lower 10	3	2	2	3
D-value $= \dfrac{R_u - R_L}{1/2T}$				
$D = \dfrac{0-3}{10} = -0.3$ (for answer A)				
$D = \dfrac{6-2}{10} = 0.40$ (for answer B)				
$D = \dfrac{3-2}{10} = 0.1$ (for answer C)				
$D = \dfrac{1-3}{10} = -0.2$ (for answer D)				

[a]B is the correct answer.

Some evaluators like to purposely include one or two easy questions at the beginning of an examination to decrease learners' anxiety (Exhibit 10.5; Gronlund, 1993).

▶ ITEM REVISION

- Completed after item analysis
- Revise items with the following characteristics:
  - *p*-values that are too high or too low.
  - Correct answers with low positive or negative point biserials.
  - Distractors with highly positive point-biserial correlations.
- Items that correlate less than .15 with total test scores should be restructured. They are probably confusing or misleading to those taking the examination (Kehoe, 1995).
- The distractor was not chosen by any learner. This prevents discriminating the good learners from the poor learners (Kehoe, 1995).
- Items that all test takers get right. These questions do not discriminate among learners and should be replaced by more difficult ones.

Exhibit 10.5 Nondiscriminating Questions

(1) What do you do if you have a question that 100% of the class gets right?

$$D\text{-value} = \frac{0 - 0}{0} = 0 \text{ for the } D\text{-value or split-biserial value}$$

Is this a discriminating question?

(2) Five learners out of the top third of the class chose the correct answer on an examination question; six out of the middle third, and eight out of the lower third. Calculate the point biserial for this question as indicated in the following.

$$D\text{-value} = \frac{5 - 8}{10} = \frac{-3}{10} = -0.3 \text{ for the } D\text{-value or split-biserial value}$$

Is this a discriminating question? YES _____ NO __✓___
Rationale for answer: The question is too difficult or unclear.

(3) All learners (*n* = 10) in the upper group answered an item correctly on an examination, but none of the learners in the lower group got it correct.

$$D = \frac{10 - 0}{10} = 1.00$$

Is this a discriminating question? YES _____ NO __✓___
Rationale for answer: Question is too difficult and does not discriminate.

● COLLABORATIVE TESTING/EVALUATION

Nurses work collaboratively with other health care team members in all aspects of care for the patient. To develop cooperation and collaboration in the learning process and to foster accountability in the learner, educators often assign learners to work in groups or teams on specific assignments. Group projects can also be used in the clinical component to evaluate whether learning has occurred.

There are some important considerations that the nurse educator must take into account when developing collaborative learning assignments and evaluation of learning (Billings & Halstead, 2020):

- The assignments must be meaningful and should be designed for small groups whenever possible.
- The educator must ensure that members of the group understand the role of each person in the group.
- The groups should be structured heterogeneously with regard to gender, ethnicity, ability, experience, and so on, to increase learning.
- Enough time must be given for the group to complete and process its work.

● **TEACHING GEM** Eliminate the following from test items:

- Ethnocentrism such as "death practices in the Western culture"
- Elitism such as using words like "estate"
- Tone of language such as comments like "soul food, regatta"
- Inflammatory material as when using the issue of abortion
- Making judgments such as using "unfortunately"
- Avoid words such as never, always, and all

Also:

- Avoid "none of the above" and "all of the above"
- Randomize the correct options (Su, Osisek, Montgomery, & Pellar, 2009)

The nurse educator must also decide how the group will be evaluated or graded on the project. Some considerations for evaluation include (Gaberson & Oermann, 2018):

- All members of the group receive the same grade.
- Learners might be asked to indicate which part of the assignment they completed and receive an individual grade based on the quality of that section.
- Peer assessment of the project may be used to contribute to the grade (e.g., peer evaluation counts for 40% of the grade, educator evaluation for 60% of the grade).
- Learners can prepare a group and an individual project.
- Educators must use grading rubrics to assess group projects and assign a grade.

EVIDENCE-BASED TEACHING PRACTICE

Helms et al. (2019) studied collaborative testing on learning outcomes in a mental health nursing education course and found that collaborative testing was an excellent active teaching strategy that increased higher academic success. Additionally, collaborative testing promotes attributes that are congruent with interprofessional healthcare team cooperation.

ROLE OF STANDARDIZED TESTING IN THE CURRICULUM

To assess learning in the nursing curriculum, many programs require learners to pass standardized tests to progress through the curriculum and also as a measure to predict success of a student's passing the NCLEX-RN on the first attempt (Mee & Hallenbeck, 2015; Molsbee & Benton, 2016; Spurlock, 2013). The NLN defines using a test to predict individual student performance on the NCLEX-RN or to make decisions about progression and graduation in a program based on learner scores on standardized tests as high-stakes testing (NLN, 2012b).

The NLN created a task force to develop guidelines for the use of standardized tests as a prerequisite for learner progression in the nursing program (NLN, 2010). Outcomes of this task force included the development of a position statement on fair testing that was approved by the NLN Board of Governors (NLN, 2012b), and the development of Fair Testing Guidelines for Nursing Education (NLN, 2012a). The guidelines include the following:

- Faculty have an ethical obligation to ensure that test and decisions made based on tests are valid, supported by solid evidence, consistent across courses, and fair to all test takers.
- Faculty have the responsibility to assess students' abilities to practice nursing competently but recognize that current approaches to assessment of learning are limited.
- Multiple sources of evidence and approaches to assessment are critical to evaluating competency in knowledge and clinical abilities, especially if high-stakes decisions are based on the assessment.
- A variety of measures, including tests, are used to evaluate students' competencies, to support student learning, improve teaching, and guide program improvements.
- Standardized tests must have information available to faculty and show evidence of reliability, content, and predictive validity before faculty administer, grade, and distribute results from, or write policies related to, the use of standardized tests (NLN, 2012a, 2012b).

Standardized tests are useful in predicting success of high-performing learners in passing the NCLEX, but they are less accurate in identifying learners who will fail the NCLEX. Companies that sell standardized tests are less clear in their ability to report who will fail the NCLEX-RN (Spurlock, 2013).

When selecting standardized tests for use in a nursing curriculum or specific course(s), nurse educators need to consider the following:

- Does research support the validity and reliability of the test?
- Who are the test-item writers, and what are their qualifications as content experts?
- Does the test blueprint adhere to the NCLEX-RN blueprint?
- Does the test include key concepts and content areas that faculty want to assess?
- Are the scoring reports easy for faculty to interpret with regard to data for groups and individual learners?
- Does the item content include categories based on the requirements of accrediting agencies such as the CCNE, CNEA, ACEN, Quality and Safety in Nursing Education (QSEN), Essentials documents of the American Association of Colleges of Nursing (AACN), and the nursing process, to name a few (Mee & Hallenbeck, 2015; Eweda et al., 2020)?

◎ **Critical Thinking Question**

Should passing a standardized test be part of the course grade and, if so, what percentage should it be counted as?

 OUTCOME EVALUATION

"Educational evaluation occurs while assessing the program for its quality, currency, relevance, projections into the future, and the need for possible revisions in light of these factors" (Keating, 2006, p. 260). Program evaluation encompasses all aspects of the program, including the curriculum, learner satisfaction, congruence of the mission of the nursing program with that of the institution, faculty and staff qualifications, learner policies and development, and resources to promote achievement of the outcomes. Accreditation of nursing programs is voluntary but encouraged, as it is a public statement attesting to the quality of the program. Several accrediting bodies oversee this process:

- State Commissions of Higher Education—the entire academic institution and programs of study are evaluated by this body
- Accreditation Commission for Education in Nursing (ACEN)—evaluates diploma, baccalaureate, master's, and clinical doctorate nursing programs; also licensed practical nurse programs
- Commission on Collegiate Nursing Education (CCNE)—evaluates baccalaureate, graduate, and residency programs in nursing
- Commission for Nursing Education Accreditation (CNEA)—assesses diploma, baccalaureate, master's, and clinical doctorate nursing programs; also licensed practical nurse programs

Evaluation of the nursing program is an ongoing process. Table 10.7 gives an example of a program evaluation plan.

Table 10.7 Program Evaluation Example

Standard curriculum: The curriculum prepares learners to achieve the outcomes of the nursing education unit, including safe practice in contemporary health care environments						
Process					**Implementation**	
Component	Where documentation is found	Person responsible	Frequency of assessment	Assessment method(s).	Results and analysis of data collection and levels of achievement	Actions needed/not needed
Curriculum flows in a logical progression	Curriculum committee minutes, class, and clinical evaluation tools	Curriculum committee chairperson	Every 8 years or when revisions occur	Comparison of curriculum elements for internal consistency	Due date	Criterion met, no action required

An essential component of program evaluation is the assessment of learner outcomes. This can be achieved in several ways:

- Satisfaction surveys
  - Exit interviews—which are conducted at the conclusion of the program, before graduation
  - Employer and graduate surveys—conducted at a designated period of time, such as 9 months, 1 year, and so on. The purpose of the survey is to determine the satisfaction of the employer with the graduate nurse's ability to function effectively within the work environment. Graduates of the program are also surveyed to determine their satisfaction with the nursing program in preparing them for the responsibilities of a graduate nurse
- Graduation and retention rates of the program
- Standardized examination pass rates—NCLEX-RN, certification examinations
- Employment opportunities

A summation of program outcomes is discussed in Exhibit 10.6.

Exhibit 10.6 Summation of Program Outcomes

Evaluation of learning demonstrates that graduates have achieved identified competencies consistent with the institutional mission and professional standards and that the outcomes of the nursing education unit have been achieved.

EVIDENCE-BASED TEACHING PRACTICE

Molsbee and Benton (2016) initiated a process in an associate degree nursing program to move away from high-stakes testing to a model of comprehensive competency but still utilized standardized testing in a senior capstone course. A new course was developed consisting of theory and preceptor components. The theory component consists of review sessions in content taught by faculty experts in the content area. Faculty-made exams are given on the content. The HESI exam is required when students enter the course for diagnostic purposes to identify strengths and weaknesses. The results have shown that NCLEX-RN pass rates have remained stable, retention rates increased, and student complaints and grade appeals have decreased. These changes were implemented to ensure alignment with the NLN fair testing guidelines.

 # CASE STUDIES

CASE STUDY 10.1

The NCLEX pass rate for first-time test takers graduating from a nursing program has been 80% for the past 2 years. The program evaluation committee is charged with assessing all aspects of the nursing curriculum, including admission and progression criteria, course evaluations, and scores on standardized and classroom tests. The current admission policy into the nursing program is congruent with the university's admission policies. They include the following criteria: SAT scores of 980 or better, upper half of graduating class, minimum GPA of 2.0. Once enrolled in the nursing major, learners must maintain a minimum cumulative GPA of 2.5, and grades of C or better (75%) in the nursing and science courses. At this university, learners must meet admission and progression requirements established by the university, but individual programs may require more stringent policies for the major.

 As a member of the admission and progression committee in the nursing department, what recommendations would you make regarding admission into the nursing major? What recommendations would you make regarding progression in the nursing major through each level? What, if any, changes would you make relative to grading criteria, teacher-made tests, and the use of standardized achievement tests? Develop a program evaluation plan based on your recommendations.

CASE STUDY 10.2

The nurse educator is a member of the admission, progression, and graduation committees. There is a concern regarding declining pass rates on the NCLEX. The committee has been charged with reviewing and revising the admission and progression standards.

 What areas should the nurse educator consider priorities to address as part of the revision of the standards to improve NCLEX pass rates?

1. A nurse educator is considering a rounding policy for her course. The nurse educator develops a policy that will round only the final grade of 0.5 to the next whole number. The nurse educator's policy is placed on the course syllabus and will affect which grading aspect?

    A. The formative course grade
    B. The last class assignment
    C. The students who score a 0.45
    D. The summative course grade

2. An objective test item demonstrated the following statistics:

N = 100	A*	B	C	D
P-value	.50	.23	.10	.17
Point-biserial	0.32	−0.15	−0.23	0.22

   The correct answer is A. The nurse educator should:

    A. Discard this question because too many students got it wrong
    B. Revise distractor C because too many students choose that answer
    C. Revise distractor D because too many students choose that answer
    D. Keep the test item in its current form

3. The following grade scheme was used for an online course.

5 Discussion boards	20%
2 Care Maps	30%
4 objective tests	40%
Reflective paper	10%

   A student received the following grades on the assignments:

   5 Discussion boards = 90% .18
   2 Cap maps = 100% .3
   4 Objective tests = 87% .348
   Reflective paper 85% .085

   The student's final grade should be:

    A. (90–100%)
    B. (80–89.50%)
    C. (70–79.50%)
    D. (60–69.50%)

1. D) The summative course grade
The rounding up of a final grade from 0.5 to the next whole number effects the summative evaluation for the course. The policy does not state that students with a 0.45 final grade have the grade rounded up or down, and it does not affect the formative evaluation of one assignment specifically.

2. C) Revise distractor D because too many students choose that answer
Distractor D was chosen by learners who scored higher on this assessment, so it should be revised to make A unequivocally correct. Distractor C does not need revision because it was chosen by 23 of the learners who did not comprehend the content. Questions should rarely be discarded.

3. A) A (90–100%)
The student earned a 91.30% for the final grade.

4. The following statistics were calculated for a test item:

N = 36	A	B*	C	D
P-value	.12	.34	.12	.0
Point-biserial	−0.09	.15	−0.23	.0

The correct answer is B. The nurse educator should consider:

A. Revising distractor A
B. Revising the correct answer B
C. Revising distractor C
D. Revising distractor D

5. A group of nurse educators is evaluating the first-semester attrition rate for a baccalaureate program. The attrition rate from the first semester is 32%. The nurse educators' assessment should include analysis of:

A. Admission criteria
B. Progression criteria
C. Mid-program evaluation policy
D. Program outcomes

6. A new nurse educator is looking at the program's systematic evaluation plan for program outcomes and uses the following indicators. The new nurse educator's mentor understands that more orientation is needed due to the following indicator:

A. Licensure pass rates
B. Faculty satisfaction
C. Graduation rates
D. Employer satisfaction

7. A new baccalaureate program is reviewing trended data and should initiate a process improvement for the following area:

A. An increase diverse student population
B. An attrition rate over three years of 21%, 20%, and 23%
C. Continuous faculty vacancies
D. Licensure pass rates that are only 2% above the state average

(See answers next page.)

4. D) Revising distractor D

The nurse educator should revise distractor D because none of the student chose. All distractors should be plausible. Distractors A and C worked by distracting the lower scoring students for this assessment.

5. A) Admission criteria

The nurse educators need to first analyze admission criteria because that element will affect students in their first semester. Mid-program, progression criteria, and program outcomes affect the learning environment after the first semester.

6. B) Faculty satisfaction

Faculty satisfaction is not a typical program outcome. Student and employer's satisfaction is as well as first-time pass rates for licensure and certification. Graduation rates is a program outcome and demonstrates how effective a program is in retaining admitted students.

7. C) Continuous faculty vacancies

Continuous faculty vacancies demonstrate that the internal forces are not adequate in resource distribution to keep faculty. A diverse student population is favorable, as are attrition rates that are fairly steady or decrease. Licensure pass rates above the state average are also not a concern.

8. The following statistics were obtained in an item analysis for a multiple-choice exam

Distractor Analysis:	A	B	C*	D
Point Biserial	0	0	−0.07	0.24
Frequency	0%	0%	92%	8%

What statement is true based on this data?

A. 92 of the better learners choose the wrong answer

B. Some of the better learners read the correct answer as wrong

C. The question was clear to those learners who mastered the content

D. The learners who did not master the content did not pick the correct answer

9. The following statistics were obtained in an item analysis for a multiple-choice exam

Distractor Analysis:	A	B	C	D*
Point Biserial	−0.21	−0.01	−0.07	0.24
Frequency	32%	4%	8%	56%

The nurse educator should consider:

A. Removing the question from the examination

B. Rewording distractors A and B

C. Keep the item because it performed well

D. Remediate the class on the item content

10. A new nurse educator is reviewing an examination with a kuder-richardson (KR-20) estimate of reliability of 0.67. Fifteen students out of 100 were unsuccessful on the examination. The new nurse educator needs additional mentoring when they state:

A. "This KR-20 is good for an instructor made examination."

B. "The KR-20 demonstrates lack of homogeneity."

C. "The students who failed were outliers on this examination."

D. "This examination was too difficult."

(*See answers next page.*)

8. B) Some of the better learners read the correct answer as wrong

A negative point biserial demonstrates that more of the learners who did not score well on the examination picked the right answer as compared to the learners who scored higher on the examination.

9. C) Keep the item because it performed well

A positive point biserial demonstrates that more of the learners who scored higher on the examination picked the right answer as compared to the learners who scored lower on the examination. The item should be retained.

10. B) "The KR-20 demonstrates lack of homogeneity"

A KR-20 of 0.67 is good for an instructor-made examination and demonstrates test reliability due to homogeneity. It is not too difficult since the majority of students passed (85%).

REFERENCES

Al-Alawi, R. & Alexander, G. L. (2020). Systematic review of program evaluation in nursing programs. *Journal of Professional Nursing, 36*(4), 236–244. 10.1016/j. profnurs.2019.12.003

Accreditation Commission for Education in Nursing. (2017). Accreditation manual. http://www.acenursing.org

Angelo, T. A. (1993). Teacher's dozen: Fourteen general, research-based principles for improving higher learning in our classrooms. http://ir.atu.edu/Retention_Info/ retentionother/Thomas_Angelo's_14_Principles.pdf

Billings, D., & Halstead, J. A. (2020). *Teaching in nursing: A guide for faculty* (5th ed.). Elsevier Saunders.

Carrick, J. A. (2011). Student achievement and NCLEX-RN success: Problems that persist. *Nursing Education Perspectives, 32*(2), 78–83. 10.5480/1536-5026-32.2.78

CNEA (Commission on Nursing Education Accreditation). (2021). National League of Nursing. https://cnea.nln.org/

Commission on Collegiate Nursing Education (CCNE). (2021). *Procedures for accreditation of baccalaureate and graduate degree nursing programs.* Author. https:// www.aacnnursing.org/CCNE#

Eweda, G., Bukhary, Z. A., & Hamed, Q. (2020). Quality assurance of test blueprinting. *Journal of Professional Nursing, 36*(3), 166–170. 10.1016/j. profnurs.2019.09.001

Fardows, N. (2011). Investigating effects of evaluation and assessment on students learning outcomes at undergraduate level. *European Journal of Social Sciences, 23*(1), 34–40.

Farnsworth, J., & Springer, P. (2006). Background checks for nursing students: What are schools doing? *Nursing Education Perspectives, 27*(3), 48–53.

Gaberson, K. B., & Oermann, M. H. (2018). *Clinical teaching strategies in nursing* (5th ed.). Springer Publishing.

Gronlund, N. E. (1993). *How to make achievement tests and assessments* (5th ed.). Allyn & Bacon.

Helms, K. D., Keith, L. A., & Walker, L. P. (2019). Evaluating student learning through collaborative testing in a psychiatric mental health course. *Journal of Doctoral Nursing Practice, 12*(1), 3–9. 10.1891/2380-9418.12.1.3

Keating, S. B. (2006). *Curriculum development and evaluation in nursing.* Philadelphia, PA: Lippincott Williams & Wilkins.

Keating, S. B. (2011). *Curriculum development and evaluation in nursing* (2nd ed.). Springer Publishing Company.

Kehoe, J. (1995). Basic item analysis for multiple-choice tests. *Practical Assessment, Research & Evaluation, 4*(10). http://PAREonline.net/getvn.asp?v = 4 & n = 10

McDonald, M. E. (2007). *The nurse educator's guide to assessing learning outcomes* (2nd ed.). Jones & Bartlett Learning.

Mee, C. L., & Hallenbeck, V. J. (2015). Selecting standardized tests in nursing education. *Journal of Professional Nursing, 31*(6), 493–497.

Molsbee, C. P., & Benton, B. (2016). A move away from high-stakes testing toward comprehensive competency. *Teaching and Learning in Nursing, 11,* 4–7.

National Council of State Boards of Nursing. (2021). *NCLEX-RN examination detailed test plan.* Author. http://www.ncsbn.org

National League for Nursing. (2021). Certified Nurse Educator (CNE) 2021 candidate handbook. http://www.nln.org/docs/default-source/default-document-library/cne-handbook-2021_revised_07-01-2021.pdf?sfvrsn=2

National League for Nursing. (2021). Certified Nurse Educator Novice (CNEn) 2021 candidate handbook. http://www.nln.org/Certification-for-Nurse-Educators/cne-n/cne-n-handbook

NCSBN® (2021). Next generation NCLEX project. https://www.ncsbn.org/next-generation-nclex.htm

Newton, S. E., & Moore, G. (2007). Undergraduate grade point average and graduate record examination scores: The experience of one graduate nursing program. *Nursing Education Perspectives, 28*(6), 327–331.

O'Connor, A. B. (2015). *Clinical instruction and evaluation: A teaching resource* (3rd ed.). Jones & Bartlett.

Oermann, M. H., & Gaberson, K. (2017). *Evaluation and testing in nursing education* (5th ed.). Springer Publishing Company.

Sayles, S., Shelton, D., & Powell, H. (2003, November/December). Predictors of success in nursing education. ABNF Journal, 14(6), 116–120.

Serembus, J. F. (2016). Improving NCLEX first-time pass rates: A comprehensive program approach. *Journal of Nursing Regulation, 6*(4), 38–44.

Sherrill, K. (2020). Clinical Judgement and Next Generation NLCEX® – a positive direction for Nursing Education! *Teaching and Learning Nursing, 15*(1), 82–85.

Spurlock, D. (2013). The promise and peril of high-stakes tests in nursing education. *Journal of Nursing Regulation, 4*(1), 4–8.

Su, W. M., Osisek, P. J., Montgomery, C., & Pellar, S. (2009). Designing multiple-choice test items at higher cognitive levels. *Nurse Educator, 34*(5), 223–231.

Yin, T., & Burger, C. (2003). Predictors of NCLEX-RN success of associate degree nursing graduates. *Nurse Educator, 28,* 232–236.

Zamanzadeh, V, Ghahramanian, A., Valizadeh, L., Bagheriyeh, F., & Lynagh, M. (2020). A scoping review of admission criteria and selection methods in nursing education. *BMC Nursing, 19*(1), 1–17. 10.1186/s12912-020-00510-1

Curriculum Design and Evaluation of Program Outcomes

Marylou K. McHugh

> *The materials of instruction should be selected and organized with a view to giving the learner that development most helpful in meeting and controlling life experiences.*
> —D. E. Walker and J. Soltis (2009)

▶ LEARNING OUTCOMES

This chapter addresses the Certified Nurse Educator Exam and the Certified Nurse Educator Novice exam Content Area 4: Participate in Curriculum Design and Evaluation of Program Outcomes. For the CNE exam it is 17% of the examination, approximately 25 questions and for the CNEn exam it is 5% or approximately 8 questions.

- Discuss leadership and change behaviors that assist in curriculum development
- Analyze the process of curriculum development
- Discuss current trends in curriculum development
- Analyze evaluation methods appropriate to measuring program outcomes
- Evaluate teaching methods/strategies for classroom and clinical teaching

◗ INTRODUCTION

Curriculum development can be the most creative and satisfying part of the educational process. It is not only dynamic and vibrant but also demands the nurse educator's time. In today's educational environment, with so much content needed for thoughtful practice with an emphasis on higher level thinking, the educator is challenged even more than ever.

Curriculum is a living entity and must be reviewed regularly for its relevance to the environment in which it exists. Faculty need to consider the environmental and human factors that influence the curriculum. These factors are called "the frame" and are classified as either internal or external factors (Keating, 2017).

External frame factors consist of the elements of the environment that are outside of the parent institution that influences the curriculum. All of these elements must be considered when developing a curriculum. External frame factors include the following issues and prompt the questions that follow.

▶ FINANCIAL SUPPORT

- How will the program be financed? Are there resources available for the latest technology?
- Does the institution have available room for the program's needs?

▶ REGULATIONS AND ACCREDITATION

- What state regulations need to be considered?
- Will the program apply for national accreditation?
- Are there resources available to assist in these efforts?
- How will the program meet professional standards?

▶ NURSING PROFESSION

- Are there nursing leaders and staff nurses who will support the program and act as mentors?
- Are the professionals active in and interested in the education of future nurses?

▶ NEED FOR THE PROGRAM

- Does the community really need the program?
- Is there adequate interest in the program?
- What are the employment possibilities for the graduates?

▶ DEMOGRAPHICS

- What are the age ranges and age groups, predicted population changes, ethnic and cultural groups, and typical socioeconomic status of people in the community?
- What is the effect of globalization on the curriculum?

▶ POLITICAL CLIMATE AND THE BODY POLITIC

- Who are the individuals who exert influence within the community?
- Who are the players, and are they supportive of the program?

▶ HEALTHCARE SYSTEM AND HEALTH NEEDS OF THE POPULACE

- What are the major healthcare systems in the area?
- Can they be utilized for clinical experiences?
- What are the major healthcare problems?
- What effect has the Patient Protection and Affordable Care Act had on the healthcare system and nursing education?

▶ CHARACTERISTICS OF THE ACADEMIC SETTING

- What are the characteristics of the setting?
- Is it a private liberal arts college or a major research university?
- How will these characteristics inform the program?

Internal frame factors refer to those elements that are internal to the institution and inform the program. All of these elements must be considered when developing the curriculum. Internal frame factors and clarifying questions include (Keating, 2017) the items that follow.

▶ POTENTIAL FACULTY AND LEARNER CHARACTERISTICS

- Are there enough available, experienced nurse educators who have expertise in the various curriculum areas?
- What is the quantity and quality of the potential student body?

▶ DESCRIPTION AND ORGANIZATION OF STRUCTURE OF THE PARENT INSTITUTION

- What is the quality of the physical campus and its buildings?
- What is the role of the nursing program in the institution?

▶ RESOURCES WITHIN THE INSTITUTION AND THE NURSING PROGRAM

- Who will develop the business plan that focuses resources for program support?
- Are there endowments, financial aid programs, and/or governmental and private grants available to the program?
- Are there appropriate support services for learners and faculty, such as advising, academic help, library services, technology, and research support?

▶ INTERNAL ECONOMIC SITUATION AND ITS INFLUENCE ON THE CURRICULUM

- Is the economic status of the parent institution sound?
- Does the administration support the goals of the nursing program?

▶ MISSION OR PURPOSE, PHILOSOPHY, AND GOALS OF THE PARENT INSTITUTION

■ How will the three areas of institutional focus—research, service, and teaching—inform the nursing program and which will be prominent?
■ Will there be some attempt at balance?

◎ **Critical Thinking Question**
Have you carefully assessed your program in light of the preceding requirements that will impinge on curriculum development and the success of the program? Can you identify those external and internal factors that will be most influential in your curriculum development?

 LEADING THE PROGRAM

In any major academic endeavor, such as curriculum development, deciding on leadership is an important part of the process. What defines leadership? Where does the leader come from? Who should lead? What are the qualities that the leader will need? Leadership is the process of showing the way by going in advance, by directing the performance or activities of a group. The leader may be the dean, chair, or director in a small school or department of nursing. In a bigger institution, the leader may be a seasoned faculty member with some prior experience in curriculum development. Leaders may emerge from the group or may be appointed by the dean and set the culture of the group (Al Zemel et al., 2020).

A leader should possess knowledge of both the content and process of curriculum development as well as a caring and compassionate attitude (Yoder-Wise, 2019). Leaders emerge in the following ways:

■ Emergent leadership—The members of the group view the leader as someone who is knowledgeable and trustworthy; they recognize and accept the leader's influence to lead.
■ Imposed or organizational leadership—The leader is appointed by someone outside the group. If the group members do not have confidence in the appointed leader's abilities, they may not perform to their highest potential (Figure 11.1).

EVIDENCE-BASED TEACHING PRACTICE
Hofmeyer, Sheingold, Klopper, and Warland (2015) found that successful leaders invest time in getting to know the people they lead and help everyone to focus. Developing relationships is the first step in developing and inspiring others: A good leader promotes others at the same time, so it is not just all about them.

Figure 11.1 Leadership styles.

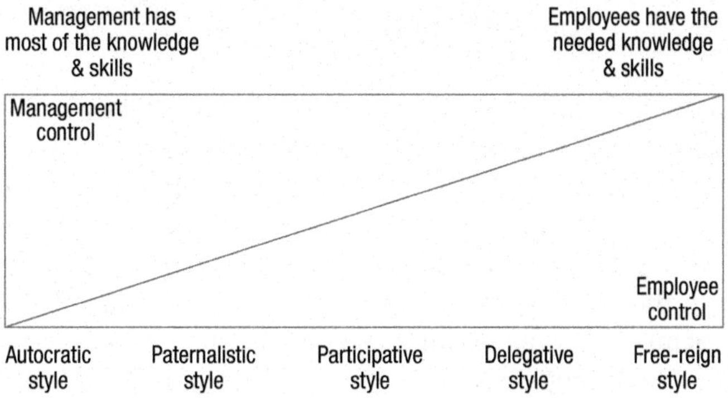

Management has most of the knowledge & skills — Employees have the needed knowledge & skills

Management control — Employee control

Autocratic style | Paternalistic style | Participative style | Delegative style | Free-reign style

Wiles and Bondi (1998) have identified the following 19 roles that a curriculum leader needs to fulfill:

Expert	Linker
Confronter	Analyzer
Instructor	Demonstrator
Counselor	Diagnostician
Trainer	Modeler
Advisor	Designer
Retriever	Advocate
Observer	Manager
Referrer	Evaluator
Data collector	

Five practices associated with exceptional leadership are (Huber, 2000) as follows:

1. Challenging the process by searching for opportunities, experimenting, and taking risks
2. Inspiring a shared vision by envisioning the future and enlisting the support of others
3. Enabling others to act by fostering collaboration and strengthening others
4. Modeling the way by setting an example and planning small successes
5. Encouraging the heart by recognizing contributions and celebrating accomplishments

Refer to Chapter 13 for a complete discussion of leadership attributes.

RESPONSIBILITIES OF FACULTY IN CURRICULUM DEVELOPMENT

Although the leader is responsible for guiding the faculty through the curriculum process, individual faculty members have their own sets of responsibilities. Many nursing leaders believe that the faculty "own" the curriculum because of their expertise in content, along with a good sense of the practice world. Because of the concept of academic freedom, faculty members may investigate new theories and ideas and express opinions in the classroom that are relevant to the course being taught (Finke, 2012). This does not mean that faculty members may develop course content in isolation; rather, they must work together to develop the plan and then follow the plan they have developed. Curriculum must build in a structured way that enables the learner to incorporate the art, science, and practice of nursing in a coherent manner. Faculty must strive to ensure that the program outcomes are achieved. The curriculum must also meet the requirements of both the state board of nursing and external accrediting bodies.

Faculty responsibilities include the following:

- Develop policies and procedures that affect learner and faculty conduct and the curriculum
- Advise administration and learners on educational issues
- Participate in administrative actions that affect the institution and community
- Ensure that content and learning experiences are sequenced toward educational outcomes
- Collect and analyze relevant information pertaining to the need for curriculum development and revision
- Prepare graduates to function in the changing and complex healthcare environment
- Develop strategies to facilitate the exchange of ideas and decision-making relevant to curriculum development and revisions (Keating, 2017)

There are certain attributes related to academic freedom, including the following three aspects, as set forth by the American Association of University Professors (1940/1970). These are:

1. Teachers are entitled to full freedom in research and in the publication of the results, subject to the adequate performance of their other academic duties, but research for pecuniary return should be based on an understanding with the authorities of the institution.

2. Teachers are entitled to freedom in the classroom in discussing their subject, but they should be careful not to introduce into their teaching controversial matter that has no relation to their subject. Limitations of academic freedom because of religious or other aims of the institution should be clearly stated in writing at the time of the appointment.

3. College and university teachers are citizens, members of a learned profession, and officers of an educational institution. When they speak or write as citizens, they should be free from institutional censorship or discipline, but their special position in the community imposes special obligations. As scholars and educational officers, they should remember that the public may judge their profession and their institution by their utterances. Therefore, they should at all times be accurate, should exercise appropriate restraint, should show respect for the opinions of others, and should make every effort to indicate that they are not speaking for the institution.

There are many factors that nurse educators have to consider in curriculum design; some of these are similar to the considerations of the total program design, as mentioned previously. These factors include:

- Institutional philosophy and mission, which provide a belief and value base for the curricular structure and content (Leddy, 2007). This operationalizes the following:
    1. Institution's reason for being, with outcome goals
    2. Program's philosophy and mission, which reflect those of the parent institutions
- Organizing framework
    1. The curriculum framework provides a way for faculty to conceptualize and organize knowledge, skills, values, and beliefs that are critical to the delivery of a coherent curriculum
    2. It facilitates the sequencing and prioritizing of knowledge in a way that is logical and internally consistent (Boland & Finke, 2012)
- Current nursing and healthcare trends
    1. Faculty should consider the economic and political issues that influence healthcare issues
    2. Issues such as bioterrorism; genetics; interdisciplinary education; an aging population; cultural illiteracy; violence; lesbian, gay, bisexual, transgender, and queer issues; quality and safety; and the use of technology such as electronic medical records, Simulation (SIM) people, and standardized patients (SPs) are important
- Community and societal needs
    1. Changes in social perceptions about ageism, sexism, gender discrimination, and racism are pertinent topics for inclusion
    2. There is a need for primary care practitioners and health educators in community settings
- Educational principles
    1. Active teaching strategies for both traditional and nontraditional learners should be considered
    2. Discussion about various educational theories should precede the actual curriculum plan
- Theory and research
    1. Evidence-based practice (EBP) is a current mandate
    2. The theory and research supporting all procedures is a priority

■ Use of technology
1. Smartphones, electronic medical records, virtual reality programs, SIM people, and SPs are a part of healthcare education
2. Faculty needs to discuss its integration into the curriculum (Keating, 2006; Leddy, 2007)

There are also standards from accrediting bodies that need to be incorporated into curriculum design. The three specialty accrediting bodies in nursing are the National League of Nursing's Commission for Nursing Education Accreditation (CNEA), American Association of Colleges of Nursing's Commission on Collegiate Nursing Education (CCNE), and the Accreditation Commission for Education in Nursing (ACEN). The standards for curriculum development are clearly stated and nurse educators systematically review curriculum to ensure that the criteria in the standard are being met. Examples from ACEN (2020) regarding curriculum include:

Standard 4—Curriculum*

The curriculum supports the achievement of the end-of-program student learning outcomes and program outcomes and is consistent with safe practice in contemporary healthcare environments.

4.1. Consistent with contemporary practice, the curriculum incorporates established professional nursing standards, guidelines, and competencies and has clearly articulated end-of-program student learning outcomes.
4.2. The end-of-program student learning outcomes are used to organize the curriculum, guide the delivery of instruction, and direct learning activities.
4.3. The curriculum is developed by the faculty and regularly reviewed to ensure integrity, rigor, and currency.
4.4. The curriculum includes general education courses that enhance professional nursing knowledge and practice.
4.5. The curriculum includes cultural, ethnic, and socially diverse concepts and may also include experiences from regional, national, or global perspectives.
4.6. The curriculum and instructional processes reflect educational theory, interprofessional collaboration, research, and current standards of practice.
4.7. Evaluation methodologies are varied, reflect established professional and practice competencies, and measure the achievement of the end-of-program student learning outcomes.
4.8. The total number of credit/quarter hours required to complete the defined nursing program of study is congruent with the attainment of the identified end-of-program student learning outcomes and program outcomes, and is consistent with the policies of the governing organization, the state, and the governing organization's accrediting agency.
4.9. Student clinical experiences and practice learning environments are evidence-based; reflect contemporary practice and nationally established patient health and safety goals; and support the achievement of the end-of-program student learning outcomes.
4.10. Written agreements for clinical practice agencies are current, specify expectations for all parties, and ensure the protection of students.
4.11. Learning activities, instructional materials, and evaluation methods are appropriate for all delivery formats and consistent with the end-of-program student learning outcomes.

*Reprinted from the 2020 Standards and Criteria, Standard 4 Curriculum, by the Accreditation Commission for Education in Nursing (ACEN) by permission of the ACEN.

◗ THEORETICAL AND CONCEPTUAL FRAMEWORKS

After completing the first step toward curriculum development, the careful review of the mission statement of both the parent institution and the nursing unit, the next step is for faculty to begin to identify the organizing framework to be used as the model for building the curriculum. All nursing programs are based on some sort of model, whether the faculty recognizes it or not (Barnum, 1998). There are many models to choose from. Remember, the framework selected for use will eventually provide learners with the basis for the conceptualization of their profession. It should be clear and practical, and faculty must be consistent in the way they use it. The nurse educator must realize that the amount of knowledge, both scientific and nursing, is increasing at a frightening rate. This necessitates nurse educators to quickly add and/or eliminate content in order to provide learners with the best and most current practice modalities. What to add and what to delete can be a real challenge. The basic goal may be to teach learners to become lifelong learners. The basic curriculum models, as well as newer models, and their characteristics include the items that follow.

▶ CURRICULUM MODEL

- Students learn the disciplines inherent to the profession
- The model may take varied forms, such as medical models
  - Courses include Medical Surgical Nursing, Pediatric Nursing, Psychiatric Mental Health Nursing, and so on
- Courses developed under the curriculum model will be very traditional. They would treat each area separately with courses such as fundamentals of nursing, Care of the Adult I, II, and III, Pediatric Nursing, and so on. The nursing process steps—assessment, diagnosis, planning, implementation, and evaluation—would be integrated into each traditional course. This model is often called the additive curriculum.

▶ INTEGRATED MODEL AND CONCEPT MODEL

- This model addresses problems such as circulatory, respiratory, and orthopedic care.
- It addresses the nursing care of patients at all developmental levels (infancy, childhood, adolescence, adulthood, and elderly).

Contrasting to the curriculum model, courses in the integrated model would be more integrated throughout the curriculum. Examples of course titles include Circulatory Problems Across the Life Cycle or Care of the Developing Family Infant would then include all of the health–illness issues associated with that topic. Many educators feel that content is often lost in this kind of model, yet for some programs, this model works extremely well.

▶ DISCIPLINE MODEL OR NURSING THEORIST MODEL

■ Curriculum is informed by a conceptual model of nursing (e.g., Levine, Orem, Neuman, or Roy)
  ● It may also be designed by the faculty from an intuited image of nursing (Barnum, 1998).
  ● The courses are specifically designed to the model (e.g., if using Levine, courses would include Issues related to Conservation of Energy, Issues related to Conservation of Structural Integrity).

Courses in the Discipline Model are integrated into the concepts of the theory used. Table 11.1 illustrates how a nursing process may be integrated into the Dorothea Orem Theoretical Model for patients who need wholly compensatory care.

TABLE 11.1 Dorothea Orem Theoretical Model

SECONDARY STEPS OF THE NURSING PROCESS	WHOLLY COMPENSATORY SYSTEM	PARTLY COMPENSATORY SYSTEM	SUPPORTIVE EDUCATIVE SYSTEM
Assessment	–	–	–
Diagnosis	–	–	–
Planning	–	–	–
Intervention	–	–	–
Evaluation	–	–	–

▶ DECONSTRUCTED, CONCEPTUAL, OR EMANCIPATOR CURRICULUM MODELS

Courses in these curricular models focus on concepts rather than on specific disease entities. Instead of teaching the same material for many populations, the concept curriculum focuses on concepts that are more useful in practice. These models promote the "development of cognitive skills necessary for knowledge transfer across contexts and the ability to transform learners into lifelong learners" (Hardin & Richardson, 2012, p. 155) and are based on brain research that demonstrates how people learn (Ignatious, 2018). They also reflect the complex nature of nursing care better than some of the other models.

Authors (Diekelmann, 2002; Forbes & Hickey, 2009; Giddens & Brady, 2007; Giddens et al., 2008; Hickey, Forbes, & Greenfield, 2010; Ironsides, 2004) have responded by supporting the concept and offering suggestions for curricular revisions. Diekelmann (2002) suggested increasing attention to the pedagogies with less attention to the content. Diekelmann stressed that reading, writing, thinking, and dialogue replace the push to include more content. Ironsides (2004) conducted a qualitative study and concluded that "challenging additive curricula and the relationship between covering content and teaching thinking by enacting new pedagogies provides teachers with ways to pursue substantive reform" (p. 11). Candela, Dalley, and Benzel-Lindley (2006) agreed that there is too much content and advocated learning-centered curricula. They offered practical suggestions for any faculty moving to a learning-centered curriculum. One of the keys to this kind of learning is conceptual learning. Giddens and Brady (2007) summarized their work by stating, "A concept based curriculum coupled with a conceptual learning approach can prepare nursing graduates who are skilled at conceptual thinking and learning; such skills are necessary to respond to a rapidly changing profession and health care environment" (p. 68). Giddens and colleagues (2008) addressed developing and implementing a new "deconstructed" curriculum along with the problems they encountered.

Some of the unique features of the curriculum included:

- A conceptual approach
- New approach to clinical education
- An innovative, web-based teaching platform has been created that is known as the "Neighborhood" (Giddens, 2007)
  - Is student-centered
  - Decreases the amount of content in the curriculum

In 2009, Forbes and Hickey summarized the literature addressing curricular reform and identified the following four themes:

- Incorporating safety and quality competencies in nursing education
- Redesigning conceptual frameworks
- Strategies to reduce content-laden curricula
- Teaching using alternative pedagogies. They called for educational research in nursing to study newer, non traditional pedagogies, such as narrative pedagogy, integrative teaching, and active learning strategies, along with their effects on student learning.

Concepts can be defined as a collection of social, cultural, and historical constructions and ideas that, over time, maintain similar form, structure, and patterns (Hardin & Richardson, 2012, p. 155).

▶ COMPONENTS OF THE CONCEPTUAL CURRICULUM

- Addressing misconceptions—all learners bring their own history and experiences to the educational setting, which must be addressed and corrected prior to learning new content.
- Building enduring understanding—when learners understand concepts, they will endure and transfer across educational and clinical contexts.
- Developing metacognition—this is the ability to understand and monitor one's own thinking (refer to Chapter 2 for a further description of metacognition).

- Teaching methods include:
  - Misconception and preconception check—may take the form of a short and simple questionnaire.
  - Discrepant event—an event that is a situation contrary to what is expected that provokes learners to search for the discrepancy.
  - Concept map—this is a diagram that links concepts to one another.
  - Approximate analogies—the nurse educator provides the first half of the analogy; the learners provide the second. For example, perfusion is to oxygenation as X is to Y. This increases creativity and is an important part of developing metacognition.
  - Check-your-knowledge quiz—a short and ungraded quiz to determine the learners' understanding of the material at one point in time (Hardin & Richardson, 2012).
  - In the conceptual curriculum, students learn about the concept of oxygenation instead of various disease entities such as asthma or pneumonia. Once they understand this concept, they can apply that knowledge to the care of patients with various respiratory disorders. By developing and linking these principles, the concept-based curriculum prepares students in the competencies outlined by the Carnegie Foundation and the IOM as essential to nursing practice (Feller, 2018).

Models that demonstrate the deconstructed curriculum include those that originate from the Institute of Medicine (IOM) or The Joint Commission. These curricular models may be based on Quality and Safety Education for Nurses (QSEN), the IOM priority areas, or Healthy People 2020 (Office of Disease Prevention and Health Promotion, 2016). In addition, concepts, such as infection, preparedness, environmental health, and community-based health, can thread through many courses. The learner focuses on thinking about connections among many healthcare problems and solves prototypes. Coaching as a teaching strategy is helpful in broadening the competency base of students (Shostrom & Schofe, 2016).

A model using the IOM's priority areas would include courses such as:

- Preventive care
- Behavioral health
- Chronic conditions
- End of life
- Children and adolescents
- Inpatient/surgical care

Nurse educators would select prototypes from Healthy People 2020 to determine specific content for each course.

A model based on QSEN would focus on the following areas. Again, nurse educators can select specific content areas from Healthy People 2020.

- Patient-centered care
- Teamwork and collaboration
- EBP
- Quality improvement
- Safety
- Informatics

EVIDENCE-BASED TEACHING PRACTICE

In 2002, The Joint Commission established its National Patient Safety Goals (NPSGs) program. The NPSGs were established to help accredited organizations address specific areas of concern in regard to patient safety (The Joint Commission, 2016).

A model based on the recommendations of The Joint Commission National Patient Safety Goals (2003) would focus on safety issues. Concepts that organize the curriculum would include:

- Improving the accuracy of patient identification
- Improving staff communication
- Improving the timely reporting of critical test results and values
- Improving the safety of using high-alert medications
- Preventing healthcare-associated infections
- Reducing the risk of patient harm resulting from falls
- Preventing healthcare-associated pressure ulcers
- Using the Universal Protocol for Preventing Wrong Site, Wrong Procedure, and Wrong Person Surgery™

Nurse educators would structure courses around prototypical health problems taken from Healthy People 2020 (Office of Disease Prevention and Health Promotion, 2016).

EVIDENCE-BASED TEACHING PRACTICE

Lewis, Stephens, and Ciak (2016) threaded the concepts of QSEN throughout the curriculum using classroom, clinical, and simulation strategies. A qualitative analysis of preceptors' perceptions after a year demonstrated an increase in student's and faculty's ability to meet QSEN competencies.

▶ THE CARNEGIE FOUNDATION FOR THE ADVANCEMENT OF TEACHING

In the spring of 2009, the Carnegie Foundation for the Advancement of Teaching (2013) released its study of nursing education. The purpose of this study was to understand the demands of learning to be a nurse and the most effective strategies for teaching nursing. The Preparation for the Professions Program (PPP) took a comparative perspective to the issues of teaching, learning, assessment, and curriculum in nursing education. The PPP has identified three dimensions of apprenticeships for professional education. In nursing education, these are high-end apprenticeships and include:

- Intellectual training to learn the academic knowledge base and have the capacity to think in ways important to the profession
- A skill-based apprenticeship of practice, including clinical judgment
- An apprenticeship to the ethical standards, ethical comportment, social roles, and responsibilities of the profession through which the novice is introduced to the meaning of an integrated practice of all dimensions of the profession, grounded in the profession's fundamental purposes

Benner, Sutphen, Leonard, and Day (2009) have authored a book explaining the findings of the PPP and offer suggestions for nursing education. Highlights follow; you can also go to the Carnegie Foundation website for more information. The key PPP findings are:

- Major gap in practice versus education
- Radical separation of classroom and clinical teaching
- Faculty development needed for classroom teaching

There are three cross-professional frames for the five Carnegie Foundation studies of professional education (they are in the process of releasing their findings on medical education).

FIRST FRAMEWORK

- Civic professionalism rather than technical professionalism: Focus is on civic responsibilities to the client and society rather than solely on technology. It emphasizes autonomy and control over professional knowledge development and professional participation.

SECOND FRAMEWORK

Cognitive apprenticeship: Knowledge of science, theory, and principles required for practice

- Practice apprenticeship: Clinical reasoning and decision-making
- Formation and ethical comportment apprenticeship: Learning to embody and enact upstanding professional practice

THIRD FRAMEWORK

Experiential teaching and learning

- Situated cognition or learning how to think in action
- Situated teaching and learning or readiness to respond to a situation

- Reflection on particular cases and situations in relation to patient outcomes
- Development of ethical comportment or doing the right thing

◎ **Critical Thinking Question**
How would you include the Carnagie Foundation's suggestions into your curriculum? What other institutional departments would you include as you implement these suggestions?

Table 11.2 illustrates a curriculum grid for incorporating the nursing health–illness concerns into the integrated model approach.

Whatever curricular model is chosen, time for including the process of debriefing should be included as faculty develop the curriculum. The NLN (2015), in collaboration with the International Nursing Association for Clinical Simulation and Learning (INACSL), concluded that it is critical for nurse educators to have a chosen theory-based method, formal training, and ongoing assessment of competencies. They also believe that "integrating debriefing across the curriculum not just in simulation has the potential to transform nursing education" (p. 2).

TABLE 11.2 Integrated Model Approach

DOMINANT NURSING PROBLEM COMPONENTS						
SECONDARY DEVELOP- MENTAL LEVELS	CIRCULATORY HEALTH TO ILLNESS	RESPIRA- TORY HEALTH TO ILLNESS	NEURO- LOGIC HEALTH TO ILLNESS	ENDOCRINE HEALTH TO ILLNESS	GASTRO- INTESTINAL HEALTH TO ILLNESS	RENAL HEALTH TO ILLNESS
Infancy	–	–	–	–	–	–
Childhood	–	–	–	–	–	–
Young adult	–	–	–	–	–	–
Middle-aged adult	–	–	–	–	–	–
Elderly	–	–	–	–	–	–

◎ **Critical Thinking Question**
What kind of curriculum model do you feel is most appropriate for your unit, faculty, and learners, and why? How will you choose which concepts to teach?

 # MULTICULTURALISM IN NURSING EDUCATION

Significant changes are taking place in the population demographics of the United States, with shifts occurring in both ethnic and minority groups. A diverse population can refer to a population that differs in ethnicity, age, gender, sexual orientation, ability, or life experiences. Because of these changes, nurse educators must adapt and adjust both curricula and teaching methods to assist these diverse populations. The five dimensions of multicultural education are (Banks & Banks, 2010):

1. Content integration
2. Knowledge construction

3. Equity pedagogy
4. Prejudice reduction
5. Empowering school and social culture

Lou (1994) identified three prerequisites for equity in teaching a diverse population:
1. Attitude—the nurse educator is open to making changes in classroom teaching, using active rather than passive methods
2. Personal perception—the nurse educator gains an insight into his or her own cultural perspective that might be brought into the classroom
3. Knowledge—the nurse educator must be knowledgeable about the learning styles of students

Multicultural teaching and teaching for cultural competency include:

- Understanding one's own cultural values
- Assisting learners to understand their cultural values
- Taking cultural considerations into all stages of course development
- Delivering instruction that is free from bias
- Encouraging group activity and involvement
- Assessing knowledge of cultural competency (Rowles, 2012)

◎ **Critical Thinking Question**
What are your biases? Do they affect your behavior when dealing with students? Do they affect your behavior when dealing with peers?

 ## THE ANTI RACIST CURRICULUM

Contrasting with multicultural education is anti-racist education. Anti-racist education is defined as educational policies aimed at eliminating the practice of labeling people according to the color of their skin or racial identity. This definition infers that racism exists and that beliefs, actions, movements, and policies need to be adopted or developed to oppose racism. Narin, Hardy, Paruinal, and Williams (2004) stated that the curriculum should identify racism and promote anti-racist teaching. If anti-racism is clear in the curriculum, it makes teachers more aware of the skills necessary to suppress racism in the classroom (Hassouneh, 2006).

◎ **Critical Thinking Question**
Are you including both anti-racist and multicultural content in your curriculum?

 ## VIOLENCE IN THE NURSING CURRICULUM

The statistics on domestic violence indicate the magnitude of this problem; as a result of this significant issue, many nursing organizations have addressed the role of nursing in this public health problem. The American Association of Colleges of Nursing (AACN) has developed a position statement and suggested content that nurse educators should consider for inclusion in the curriculum.

"Because of the prevalence of physical and psychological violence in our society, nurses frequently care for the victims, the perpetrators, and the witnesses of physical and psychological violence. In addition, nurses also may be at risk for experiencing violence in the workplace. As members of the largest group of healthcare providers, nurses should be aware of assessment methods and nursing interventions that will interrupt and prevent the cycle of violence.

In particular, the AACN recognizes domestic violence as a special form of violence with a high incidence and prevalence that requires healthcare interventions. AACN recommends that faculty in educational institutions preparing nurses in baccalaureate and higher degree programs ensure that the curricula contain opportunities for all learners to gain factual information and clinical experience regarding domestic violence (Table 11.3). The content should include:

- Acknowledgment of the scope of the problem
- Assessment skills to identify and document abuse and its health effects
- Interventions to reduce vulnerability and increase safety, especially of women, children, and elders
- Competence in recognizing how cultural factors influence the patterns of and responses to domestic violence to individuals, families, and communities
- Legal and ethical issues in treating and reporting domestic violence
- Activities to prevent domestic violence (American Association of Colleges of Nursing, 2016a, 2016b)

Many nurse educators today are sensitized to the importance of including content on violence and victim/survivor care in various nursing education programs. Although a survey of Ontario's schools of nursing in Canada revealed a considerable number of hours devoted to this topic, the approach is largely incidental, depending heavily on individual faculty interests. To achieve this goal and avoid pitfalls such as an "add-on" approach to curriculum revision, nurse educators' needs in Ontario were addressed in a series of workshops involving collaboration among faculty, clinical preceptors, and community-based experts in victim/survivor care (Hoff, 1995).The majority of university schools of nursing provided experiential instruction in the area of violence, but the other types of schools of nursing provided very little such instruction. Findings revealed sensitivity to the importance of including content on violence in nursing curricula; however, the approach to this content is largely incidental and heavily dependent on individual faculty interests. Implications of this study point to the need for the systematic inclusion of violence-related content and the sharing of resources among schools of nursing(Connor, Nouer, Speck, Mackey, & Tipton, 2013; Ross, Hoff, & Coutu-Wakulczyk, 1998).

In addition to issues such as domestic violence and bullying, faculty need to include content addressing natural disasters and terrorist attacks.

TABLE 11.3 Content and Activities for Inclusion

CONTENT	ACTIVITIES
Screening and assessment	Didactic content Physical assessment course work Screening with valid and reliable tools All clinical settings are appropriate for these activities
Intervention and documentation	Clinical experiences in all settings using skills obtained in course and college laboratory Early case finding Appropriate referrals
Ethical, legal, and cultural issues	Didactic content in sociology, ethics, and nursing courses Know state and local regulations
Prevention activities	Participate in health fairs, public awareness activities

INTERPROFESSIONAL CURRICULUM

In 2011, the AACN was part of group that developed competencies for interprofessional learning. The goal of interprofessional learning is to prepare all health professions students for deliberatively working together with the common goal of building a safer and better patient-centered and community/population-oriented U.S. healthcare system. Interprofessional education (IPE) occurs when two or more professions learn about, from, and with each other to enable effective collaboration and improve health outcomes. Collaborative practice in healthcare occurs when multiple health workers from different professional backgrounds provide comprehensive services by working with patients, their families, careers, and communities to deliver the highest quality of care across settings. Practice includes both clinical and nonclinical health-related work, such as diagnosis, treatment, surveillance; health communications; management; and sanitation engineering. Health and education systems consist of all the organizations, people, and actions whose primary intent is to promote, restore, or maintain health and facilitate learning, respectively (Inter-Professional Education Collaboration Expert Panel, 2011). While in its infancy, this panel began to develop core competencies to guide curriculum development. The core competencies developed include:

- Create a coordinated effort across the health professions to embed essential content in all health professions education curricula
- Guide professional and institutional curricular development of learning approaches and assessment strategies to achieve productive outcomes
- Provide the foundation for a learning continuum in interprofessional competency development across the professions and the lifelong learning trajectory
- Acknowledge that evaluation and research work will strengthen the scholarship in this area
- Prompt dialogue to evaluate the "fit" between educationally identified core competencies for interprofessional collaborative practice and practice needs/demands

- Find opportunities to integrate essential IPE content consistent with current accreditation expectations for each health professions education program
- Offer information to accreditors of educational programs across the health professions that they can use to set common accreditation standards for IPE, and so they know where to look in institutional settings for examples of implementation of those standards
- Inform professional licensing and credentialing bodies on how to define potential testing content for interprofessional collaborative practice (Exhibit 11.1)

Exhibit 11.1 The Core Competencies of IPE

Interprofessional Education (IPE) is necessary for all health professional education programs. The Association of American Colleges of Nursing (2011) describes IPE in terms of:

- Values and ethics
- Roles and responsibilities
- Interprofessional communication
- Teams and teamwork

Each component of IPE concentrates on the fundamental principles of teamwork, which include building respect; understanding each other's roles and communicating with patients, families, and each other clearly; and building team relationships that enhance the concept of working together for a common patient care goal.

◎ Critical Thinking Question

What teaching and learning strategies would you include in an IPE course and clinical experience?

 PROGRAM GOALS, OBJECTIVES, AND OUTCOMES

The next stage of curriculum development is to identify the program goals, outcomes, and terminal objectives of the program and to identify how one will measure these outcomes to determine whether they were achieved. The science of writing objectives was discussed in Chapter 2. This section discusses how to articulate a program's outcomes and develop the objectives for each level of learning. These are called **level objectives** and are used to guide the shaping of course selection and content throughout the years (or levels) through which the learners progress. These statements must be specific and must reflect the institution's and the program's mission statements. Faculty should discuss the following questions:

1. What exactly should the graduating students look like?
2. What characteristics and competencies does the student need to possess upon completion of the program?
3. How do these objectives address the mission and terminal objectives of the program?

The development of specific program outcomes and goal objectives will flow from the answers derived from the discussion of these three pertinent and important questions. Leveling a program is an important concept in curriculum development; it orchestrates where to place course materials and what can be expected from learners in the clinical area.

> **TEACHING GEM** The curriculum has moved from being politically correct to being theoretically pluralistic; it now incorporates caring and humanitarianism as core values rather than being dominated by technology; and the centrality of the student–teacher relationship is now prized over esoteric scholarship (NLN, 1993).

● LEVEL OBJECTIVES

The next task pertaining to leveling and course placement is to develop level objectives that delineate what skills the learner will need to develop if they are to achieve the program outcomes. Level objectives are meant to guide course design while feeding into the program outcomes.

Level objectives can be teased out to reflect specific program objectives, course objectives, and clinical objectives. Table 11.4 illustrates how program, course, and clinical objectives for each level lead to the final outcomes of a program.

- Level One: Learners begin to identify the ethical issues that may affect the care of their patients.
- Level Two: Building on level one, the learners apply these concepts.
- Level Three: Learners are required to analyze the effects of the legal–ethical system on the care of patients, families, and communities.
- By the end of the program, learners are expected to be able to integrate these concepts into their patient care.

> **TEACHING GEM** Program objectives and level objectives for the program reflect program outcomes and plan for the sequential development of the knowledge and competencies necessary to achieve those outcomes. The objectives address the same core competencies but at different levels of sophistication and with different populations. The related course objectives mirror the program and level objectives, but express how the objective is achieved within the content and related clinical experiences learners cover in the course (O'Connor, 2006).

On the basis of the program outcomes and the level objectives, faculty will develop courses that will lead to the learners' achievement of the goals. Competencies at the course level are much more specific and lead the faculty to prepare content, learning activities, and clinical experiences.

Table 11.4 Level Objectives

LEVEL ONE	LEVEL TWO	LEVEL THREE	LEVEL FOUR
Identify legal and ethical issues that affect the professional nurse's delivery of care to patients and their families.	Apply ethical and legal concepts to the care of patients and their families.	Analyze the effect of legal and ethical issues to the care of patients, families, and communities.	Integrate ethical/legal concepts and principles, the Code of Ethics for Nurses, and professional standards into practice within professional, academic, and community settings.
COURSE OBJECTIVES			
LEVEL ONE	LEVEL TWO	LEVEL THREE	LEVEL FOUR
Discuss the content inherent in the ANA's Code of Ethics for Nurses.	Apply legal/ethical content to case studies involving patients and families.	Develop care plans based on criteria found in the Standards of Practice of the American Nurses Association and the Code for Nurses.	Compare and contrast the appropriate Standards of Practice and Code of Ethics to various practice situations.
CLINICAL OBJECTIVES			
LEVEL ONE	LEVEL TWO	LEVEL THREE	LEVEL FOUR
Using the Code of Ethics for Nurses, identify one issue that has impinged on your nursing care of a patient and/or the family.	Apply legal/ethical principles in caring for your patient and family.	Analyze the effects of the Health Insurance Portability and Accountability Act (HIPAA) on the care of your patient and family.	Consciously practice using the Code of Ethics for Nurses and the appropriate Standards of Practice when caring for patients, families, or communities.

 # MAPPING THE CURRICULUM

As faculty develop curriculum, they may participate in curriculum mapping, an evidence-based approach to curriculum design that promotes faculty collaboration and quality assurance in nursing education. It enables faculty to identify gaps in the curriculum, spot redundancies, and improve transparency across the program curricula. Concept mapping helps:

- Create a curriculum roadmap for meeting nursing education accreditation standards and national guidelines.
- Encourage faculty discussion of teaching methodology and lesson planning.
- Reveal gaps in curriculum content, instructional design, or student assessment measures.
- Establish a written representation or blueprint for course information.

Align program outcomes with course outcomes throughout the nursing curricula (Neville, Norton, & Cantwell, 2019).

BACCALAUREATE OUTCOMES OF THE AACN AND NLN

In July 2021, the American Association of College of Nursing (AACN) revised the Essentials or the criteria on which nursing education should be based. Many of the revisions were made to bring the Essentials up to date and conform to the United States Department of Education (DOE) requirements that mandated more emphasis on interprofessional education, the integration and use of technology in healthcare, and changing population needs. A primary intent of the developed Essentials is to create more consistency in graduate outcomes, influenced by the robustness of the learning experiences and demonstration of competencies. By emphasizing the attainment of competencies within an academic program, employers will have a clear expectation of knowledge and skill sets of nursing graduates.

In order to structure the curriculum, AACN has identified four Spheres of Care:

1. Systems based practice—communication across settings which include local, national, and global which all contribute to healthcare.

2. Information and Technology—basic competency and basic information fundamental to nursing practice.

3. Engagement and Experience—inclusive and ongoing relationship to enhance a positive experience for clients.

Academic/Practice Partnerships – to enhance mutual research, leadership, and shared commitment to redesign practice environments (CCNE, 2021).

AACN has further defined Domains that are areas of competence that when considered in the aggregate, constitute a descriptive framework for nursing practice (AACN, 2021). These domains also provide a framework for competency-based nursing education. The ten domains are:

Domain 1: Knowledge for Nursing Practice
Domain 2: Person-Centered Care
Domain 3: Population Health
Domain 4: Scholarship for Nursing Practice
Domain 5: Quality and Safety
Domain 6: Interprofessional Partnerships
Domain 7: Systems-Based Practice
Domain 8: Information and Healthcare Technologies
Domain 9: Professionalism
Domain 10: Personal, Professional, and Leadership Development

In addition to domains, there are featured concepts associated with professional nursing practice that are integrated within the Essentials. A concept is an organizing idea or a mental abstraction that represents important areas of knowledge (AACN, 2021).

The featured concepts are:
- Clinical Judgement
- Communication
- Compassionate Care
- Diversity, Equity, and Inclusion
- Ethics
- Evidence Based Practice
- Health Policy
- Social Determinants of Health

The first Competency for both Entry-Level Professional Nursing Education and Advance Level Nursing Education asks that the student "Demonstrate an understanding of the discipline of nursing's distinct perspective and where shared perspectives exist with other disciplines". In order to address that competency faculty may include the theories and science that guide practice into the undergraduate content. The graduate student, on the other hand, would be expected to translate and apply those theories and the science into practice. This content could address the first Domain: Knowledge for Nursing Practice as well as the concept of Evidence Based Practice.

The Essentials offer concrete example of how faculties can synthesize these domains and concepts into a coherent curriculum that will prepare both undergraduate and graduate nurses to participate in interprofessional practice. Faculty members will need to carefully study the document as they revitalize their curricula.

◎ Critical Thinking Question
How will your faculty begin the process of changing your curriculum to competency based?

In 2010, the NLN developed outcomes and competencies for graduates of practical/vocational, diploma, associate degree, baccalaureate, master's, practice doctorate, and research doctorate programs in nursing. The NLN stated that nursing educators must prepare individuals who

- Are grounded in values and ethics
- Understand that knowledge is continually evolving
- Are able to evaluate that knowledge
- Apply it in situations where nurses touch the lives of others

Graduates of any program should have several things in common. All nurses should be able to:

- Provide safe care that is culturally and developmentally appropriate and that is centered on building and sustaining positive, healthful relations with individuals, families, groups, and communities
- Practice within a legal, ethical, and professional scope that is guided by accepted standards of practice
- Continually learn and grow as professionals whose practice is supported by evidence
- Advocate for access to and quality of healthcare (NLN, 2016a, p. 9)

In addition, the NLN has defined program outcomes as

[T]he expected culmination of all learning experiences occurring during the program, including the mastery of essential core nursing practice competencies, built upon the seven core values and the six integrating concepts. Course outcomes are the expected culmination of all learning experiences for a particular course within the nursing program, including the mastery of essential core competencies relevant to that course. Courses should be designed to promote synergy and consistency across the curriculum and lead to the attainment of program outcomes. (NLN, 2016a, p. 32)

The NLN's competencies model consists of the following elements:

1. Core values
   - Caring
   - Diversity
   - Excellence
   - Holism
   - Integrity
   - Patient centeredness
2. Integrating concepts
   - Context and environment
   - Knowledge and science
   - Personal and professional development
   - Quality and safety
   - Relationship-centered care
   - Teamwork
3. Program outcomes
   - Enhance human flourishing
   - Show sound nursing judgment
   - Develop professional identity
   - Approach all issues and problems in a spirit of inquiry
4. Nursing practice
   - Unbounded by any closed structures, the four program outcomes converge into nursing practice depending on the program type

Competencies for graduates of baccalaureate programs are provided as an example in Table 11.5.

◎ Critical Thinking Question

How do you measure the outcomes of your curriculum to determine if goals and objectives are truly being met?

Table 11.5 Competencies for Graduates of Baccalaureate Programs

OUTCOME	COMPETENCY
Human flourishing	Incorporate the knowledge and skills learned in didactic and clinical courses to help patients, families, and communities continually progress toward fulfilment of human capacities
Nursing judgment	Make judgments in practice, substantiated with evidence, that synthesize nursing science and knowledge from other disciplines in the provision of safe, quality care, and promote the health of patients, families, and communities
Professional identity	Express one's identity as a nurse through actions that reflect integrity, a commitment to EBP; caring; advocacy; and safe, quality care for diverse patients, families, and communities; and a willingness to provide leadership in improving care
Spirit of inquiry	Act as an evolving scholar who contributes to the development of the science of nursing practice by identifying questions in need of study, critiquing published research, and using available evidence as a foundation to propose creative, innovative, or evidence-based solutions to clinical practice problems

When building curricular models, nurse educators must realize that there are many ways to conceptualize the curricula. The goal is to develop curricula so that the entire faculty are in agreement and are willing to keep the model clear and simple enough so that the learners develop an understanding of the practice of nursing as a whole, not just of discrete parts of a medical model.

CHANGING OR REVISING THE CURRICULUM

Changing an existing curriculum is sometimes more difficult than developing a curriculum from scratch because faculty members have a history with the outgoing curriculum. A contemplated change process must be used to change an existing curriculum effectively. When leaders or managers are planning to manage change, there are six key principles that need to be kept in mind:

1. Different people react differently to change
2. Everyone has fundamental needs that must be met
3. Change often involves a loss, and people go through the "loss curve"
4. Expectations need to be managed realistically
5. Fears have to be dealt with
6. There should be a good reason for the change

Here are some tips for applying the above principles when managing change.

■ Give people information—be open and honest about the facts but do not give into overly optimistic speculation. Meet people's openness needs but in a way that does not set unrealistic expectations.

■ For large groups, produce a communication strategy that ensures that information is disseminated efficiently and comprehensively to everyone (do not let the grapevine take over). Tell everyone at the same time. However, follow this up with individual interviews to produce a personal strategy for dealing with the change. This helps to recognize and deal appropriately with the individual reactions to change.

■ Give people choices and be honest about the possible consequences of those choices. Meet their control and inclusion needs.

■ Give people time to express their views and support their decision-making. Provide coaching, counseling, or information as appropriate to help them through the loss curve.

■ Where the changes involve a loss, identify what will or might replace that loss—loss is easier to cope with if there is something to replace it. This will help assuage potential fears.

■ When it is possible to do so, give individuals the opportunity to express their concerns and provide reassurances—this also helps to assuage potential fears.

■ Maintain good management practices, such as making time for informal discussions and feedback. Even though the pressure might make it seem that it is reasonable to let such things slip, during difficult change such practices are even more important (Team Technology, 2008).

Treat change as a project. Do this by applying all the rigors of project management to the change process: produce plans, allocate resources, appoint a steering board and /or project sponsor, and so on. The six principles listed earlier should form part of the project objectives (Team Technology, 2008).

CHANGE THEORIES

▶ FIRST-ORDER AND SECOND-ORDER CHANGES

■ First-order change does not challenge or contradict the established context of an organization. This type of change does not usually threaten people, either personally or collectively.

■ The bigger changes that frustrate leaders and threaten followers are planned second-order changes. These changes intentionally challenge widely shared assumptions, disintegrate the context of "organization," and, in general, reframe the social system. This, in turn, generates widespread ambiguity, discontinuity, anxiety, frustration, confusion, paranoia, cynicism, and anger as well as temporary dysfunction.

The varieties of change theories often used in nursing are reviewed in Chapter 14. To provide a theoretical example that could be used in changing a curriculum, Lewin's force-field analysis model is used to illustrate elements of change and resistance to change. A force field relates to all the behaviors of a group in its environment during a given period of time.

According to this model, pressing for change tends to threaten stability and thus increases the power of those forces maintaining the system. Therefore, the most effective way to bring about change is to *reduce the forces of resistance*. The major concepts of the model are outlined in the following list (Goad & Hough, 1993):

- Driving forces—the past, present, and future elements, along with hopes, aspirations, and emotional investments that tend to affect a social event in a positive direction
- Restraining forces—the past, present, and future elements, along with hopes, aspirations, and emotional investments that tend to affect a social event in a negative direction
- Status quo—a dynamic equilibrium composed of a balance between the driving and restraining forces
- Motivators—the initial stimuli that convince the concerned parties there is a need for change
- Confirmation of non-accomplishment—information that confirms the fact that the desired job is not being accomplished
- Confirmation of lack of obtainment—information that confirms the fact that what is wanted, needed, or expected is not being obtained
- Confirmation of lack of growth or maturation—information that confirms the fact that growth or maturation is not being achieved

▶ STAGES

- Unfreezing—the stage in the change process during which the change agents create dissatisfaction, followed by inspiring the motivation to accept some type of change
- Moving—a cognitive redefinition by the participants of attitude and behavior toward the planned change
- Refreezing—the new behaviors are practiced and reinforced
- Change agent—the responsible person who moves those to be affected by change through the stages of change in a logical manner

Curriculum development and curriculum change are complex endeavors that require nursing education expertise, leadership, and vision. These processes should be done often and systematically to meet the goals of today's healthcare systems.

● PLANNING LEARNING WITHIN THE CURRICULUM

Planning learning activities require considerable faculty preparation time. Activities should be planned to enhance critical thinking and can be very important for enhancing students' learning. Planning learning activities involves the following six steps:

1. Developing the learning outcomes for the specific learning session
2. Creating an anticipatory set

3. Selecting a teaching strategy (refer to Chapter 3 for classroom teaching strategies)
4. Considering implementation issues
5. Designing closure for the session
6. Designing formative and summative evaluation strategies (Scheckel, 2012, p. 205)

 ## CASE STUDIES

CASE STUDY 11.1

A seasoned nursing faculty member at a major university has been asked by the dean to serve as the curriculum coordinator and as mentor to a new faculty member. The new faculty member is also on the curriculum committee and comes to the university with 8 years of teaching experience at a midsized university.

Discuss the mentor–mentee relationship in this situation. What are some of the assets they can both bring to the curriculum committee? How should curriculum chair approach this responsibility? What are the key elements of mentorship that they should be certain to address? What is a new faculty member's responsibility in this relationship?

CASE STUDY 11.2

An area nurse educator is chosen to lead the curriculum committee in its efforts to update the school's curriculum from a medical model to a conceptually based curriculum.

What would be the initial process to accomplish this task? Consideration needs to include change theory, conceptual base, concepts to include, and teaching strategies.

1. When developing a curriculum for a new nursing program, which statement the faculty member makes is most indicative of the potential success of the program?

   A. "I have obtained both state board and external accreditation requirements"
   B. "I am not sure the clinical agencies will approve of this curriculum"
   C. "Why do we need community support and interest?"
   D. "The college has made budget cuts that may impact us"

2. The faculty view the dean of the program as someone who is knowledgeable and trustworthy and are anxious to work with the dean on the new curriculum. This leader is known as which kind of leader?

   A. Imposed
   B. Manager
   C. Emergent
   D. Advisor

3. The dean enables the faculty by fostering collaboration and strengthening others. This is part of the criteria of a(an)

   A. Faculty counselor
   B. Exceptional leader
   C. Team observer
   D. Inspiring person

4. The nurse faculty member who teaches psychiatric nursing inserts her political biases about an upcoming election into her lecture. This is in violation of which of the following organization's regulations?

   A. The Affordable Care Act (ACA)
   B. The Health Insurance Portability and Accountability Act (HIPPA)
   C. The American Association of University Professors (AAUP)
   D. The U.S. Department of Education Rules and Regulations

5. The novice nurse educator needs additional mentoring when they include the following social topic in their course:

   A. LGBTQIA+ issues
   B. Anti-racist issues
   C. Standardized Participants
   D. Violence

1. A) "I have obtained both state board and external accreditation requirements"

Faculty need to develop their programs so that they can achieve the appropriate accreditation. Worries about the alternate comments are a sign of inappropriate support.

2. C) Emergent

The skills of the emergent leader are such that the faculty will accept his/her leadership as they develop the program. The other options will not lead to a successful endeavor.

3. B) Exceptional leader

The skills of the exceptional leader include fostering faculty collaboration.

4. C) The American Association of University Professors (AAUP)

AAUP regulations state that teachers are entitled to freedom in the classroom in discussing their subject, but they should be careful not to introduce controversial matter that has no relation to their subject into their teaching.

5. C) Standardized Participants

The use of Standardized Participants is not a social issue, while the others are.

6. Which of the following is inherent in an organizing framework for a nursing curriculum?

   A. Considers the economic and political issues
   B. Facilitates the sequencing of knowledge
   C. Changes in social perception
   D. The institution's reason for being

7. The courses in the _____ model include Medical Surgical Nursing, Pediatric Nursing, Obstetrical Nursing, and Psychiatric Nursing.

   A. Curriculum
   B. Integrated
   C. Discipline
   D. Conceptual

8. The faculty has included content addressing ethical standards, ethical components, social roles, and responsibilities of the profession into the curriculum so that the novice is introduced to all dimensions of the profession. These concepts are fostered by which organization?

   A. National League for Nursing
   B. American Association of Collegiate Educators
   C. American Nurses Association
   D. Carnegie Foundation for the Advancement of Teaching

9. The student nurse states, "I am a visual learner. I like to look at graphs, pictures, and videos." The nurse educator plans a lesson including these teaching aids/strategies. This shows that the educator is knowledgeable about:

   A. The need for variety in her teaching methods
   B. The need to listen the wants of a student
   C. Understanding the variety of learning styles of students
   D. Using various technologies and programs

10. Which strategy does the Carnegie Foundation Report believe has the potential to transform nursing education?

    A. Simulation
    B. Reflection
    C. Debriefing
    D. Listening

(See answers next page.)

6. B) Facilitates the sequencing of knowledge
The organizing framework guides the sequencing of content and knowledge.

7. A) Curriculum
The curriculum model is more traditional, with courses addressing the original areas of nursing. The integrated model addresses problems such as circulatory and respiratory care across the lifespan. The discipline model focuses on models of nursing such as Levine and Orem. The conceptual model focuses on concepts and new approaches rather than on specific disease entities.

8. D) Carnegie Foundation for the Advancement of Teaching
The Carnegie foundation studied nursing education and in 2013 published a report addressing the dimensions of apprenticeships for professional education, which included ethical standards.

9. C) Understanding the variety of learning styles of students
It is important to include various teaching strategies in order to address the various learning styles—visual, auditory, kinesthetic.

10. C) Debriefing
Debriefing is the process which includes reflection and promotes higher level thinking. Debriefing encompasses reflection and listening. Simulation is a modality.

⬤ REFERENCES

American Association of College of Nursing. (2021). *The essentials: Core competencies for professional nursing practice.* American Association of College of Nursing. Washington, D.C. https://www.aacnnursing.org/AACN-Essentials

Al Zamel, L. G., Lim, A. K., Chan, C. M., & Piaw, C. Y. (2020). Factors Influencing Nurses' Intention to Leave and Intention to Stay: An Integrative Review. *Home Health Care Management & Practice, 32*(4), 218–228. 10.1177/1084822320931363

American Association of Colleges of Nursing. (2008). *The essentials of baccalaureate education for professional nursing practice.* Author.

American Association of Colleges of Nursing. (2011). Core competencies for intercollaborative practice. http://www.aacn.nche.edu/education-resources/ipecreport.pdf

American Association of Colleges of Nursing. (2016a). *Position statement on violence as a public health problem.* Report of the AACN Task Force on Violence as a public health problem. http://www.aacn.nche.edu/publications/position/violence-problem

American Association of Colleges of Nursing. (2016b). *Commission on collegiate nursing education (CCNE).* http://www.aacn.nche.edu/ccne-accreditation

American Association of University Professors. (1970). *Statement of principles on academic freedom and tenure with interpretive comments.* http://www.aaup.org/statement/Redbook/1940 stat.htm (Original work published 1914)

Banks, J. A., & Banks, C. A. M. (2010). *Multicultural education: Issues and perspectives* (7th ed.). Wiley.

Barnum, B. J. (1998). The advanced nurse practitioner: Struggling toward a conceptual framework. *Nursing Leadership Forum, 3*(1), 14–17.

Benner, P., Sutphen, M., Leonard, V., & Day, L. (2009). *Educating nurses: A call for radical reform.* Jossey-Bass/Carnegie Foundation for the Advancement of Teaching.

Boland, L., & Finke, L. (2012). Curriculum designs. In D. M. Billings & J. A. Halstead (Eds.), *Teaching in nursing: A guide for faculty* (4th ed., pp. 119–137). Elsevier Saunders.

Candela, L., Dalley, K., & Benzel-Lindley, J. (2006). A case for learning-centered curricula. *Journal of Nursing Education, 43*(2), 59–65.

Carnegie Foundation for the Advancement of Teaching. (2013). https://www.carnegiefoundation.org/resources/publications

Diekelmann, N. (2002). "Too much content".... epistemologies' grasp and nursing education. *Journal of Nursing Education, 41*(11), 469–470.

Finke, L. M. (2012). Teaching in nursing: The faculty role. In D. M. Billings & J. A. Halstead (Eds.), *Teaching in nursing: A guide for faculty* (4th ed., pp. 1–14). Elsevier Saunders.

Forbes, M., & Hickey, M. (2009). Curricular reform in baccalaureate nursing education: Review of the literature. *International Journal of Nursing Education Scholarship, 6,* 27.

Feller, F. (2018). Transforming nursing education: A call for a conceptual approach. *Nursing Education Perspectives, 39*(2), 105–110. 10.1097/01.NEP.0000000000000187

Giddens, J. (2007). The neighborhood: A web-based platform to support conceptual teaching and learning. *Nursing Education Perspectives, 28*(5), 251–256.

Giddens, J., & Brady, D. (2007). Rescuing nursing education from content saturation: The case for a concept-based curriculum. *Journal of Nursing Education, 46*(26), 5–12.

Giddens, J., Brady, D., Brow, P., Wright, M., Smith, D., & Harris, J. (2008). A new curriculum for a new era of nursing education. *Nursing Education Perspectives, 29*(4), 2000–2004.

Goad, S., & Hough, L. (1993). Lewin's field theory with emphasis on change. In S. Zeigler (Ed.), *Theory-directed nursing practice* (pp. 183–192). Springer Publishing.

Hardin, P., & Richardson, S. (2012). Teaching the concept curricula: Theory and method. *Journal of Nursing Education, 51*(3), 155–159. 10.3928/014834-20120127-01

Hassuouneh, D. (2006). *Anti-racist pedagogy.* Challenges faced by faculty of color in predominantly white schools of nursing. *Journal of Nursing Education, 45*(7), 255–62. 2039275027.

Hickey, M., Forbes, M., & Greenfield, S. (2010). Integrating the institute of medicine competencies in a baccalaureate curricular revision: Process and strategies. *Journal of Professional Nursing, 26*(4), 214–222.

Hoff, L. A. (1995). Violence content in nursing curricula: Strategic issues and implementation. *Journal of Advanced Nursing, 21*(1), 137–142.

Hofmeyer, A., Sheingold, B., Klopper, H. C., & Warland, J. (2015). Leadership in learning and teaching in higher education: Perspectives of academics in non-formal leadership roles. *Contemporary Issues in Education Research, 8,* 181–192.

Huber, D. (2000). *Leadership and nursing care management* (2nd ed.). W. B. Saunders.

Ignatious, D. (2018). *Teaching and learning in a concept based curriculum: A how to best practice approach.* Jones & Bartlett Learning.

Interprofessional Education Collaboration Expert Panel. (2011). *Core competencies for expert practice in collaboration: Report of an expert panel.* Interprofessional Collaborative.

Ironsides, P. (2004). "Covering content" and teaching thinking: Deconstructing the additive curriculum. *Journal of Nursing Education, 43*(4), 5–12.

Keating, S. (2017). *Curriculum development and evaluation in nursing* (4th ed.). Lippincott Williams & Wilkins.

Leddy, S. (2007). Curriculum development in nursing education. In B. Moyer & R. A. Wittmann-Price (Eds.), *Foundations of practice excellence* (pp. 66–81). F. A. Davis.

Lewis, D. Y., Stephens, K. P., & Ciak, A. D. (2016). QSEN: Curriculum integration and bridging the gap to practice. *Nursing Education Perspectives, 37*(2), 97–100. 10.5480/14-1323

Lou, R. (1994). Teaching all students equally. In H. Roberts, J. C. Gonzales, & O. Scott (Eds.), *Teaching from a cultural perspective* (pp. 28–44). Sage.

Morris, W. (Ed.). (1970). *American Heritage dictionary of the English language* (3rd ed.). American Heritage Publishing Company.

Nairn, S., Hardy, C., Parumal, L., & Williams, (2004). Multicultural or anti-racist teaching in nurse education: A critical appraisal. *Nurse Education Today, 24,* 188–195.

National League for Nursing. (2021). Certified Nurse Educator (CNE) 2021 candidate handbook. http://www.nln.org/docs/default-source/default-document-library/cne-handbook-2021_revised_07-01-2021.pdf?sfvrsn=2

National League for Nursing. (2021). Certified Nurse Educator Novice (CNEn) 2021 candidate handbook. http://www.nln.org/Certification-for-Nurse-Educators/cne-n/cne-n-handbook.

Neville, M. Norton, B. & Cantwell, (2019). Curriculum mapping in nursing education: A case study for collaborative curriculum design and program quality assurance. *Teaching and Learning in Nursing, 14*(2) A1-A8. https://doi.org/10.1016/j.teln.2018.12.001Get r

O'Connor, A. (2006). *Clinical instruction and evaluation: A resource guide* (2nd ed.).: Jones & Bartlett.

Office of Disease Prevention and Health Promotion. (2016). *Healthy people 2020: Improving the health of America.* http://www.healthypeople.gov

Ross, M. M., Hoff, L. A., & Coutu-Wakulczyk, G. (1998). Nursing curricula and violence issues. *Journal of Nursing Education, 2,* 53–60.

Rowles, C. J. (2012). Strategies to promote critical thinking and active learning. In D. M. Billings & J. A. Halstead (Eds.), *Teaching in nursing: A guide for faculty* (4th ed., pp. 258–284). Elsevier Saunders.

Scheckel, M. (2012). Selecting learning activities to achieve curriculum outcomes. In D. M. Billings & J. A. Halstead (Eds.), Teaching in nursing: A guide for faculty (4th ed., pp. 170–187). Elsevier Saunders.

Shostrom, B., & Schofer, K. (2016). A case-based curriculum with nurse as coach. *Journal of Nursing Education, 55*(5), 292–296.

Team Technology. (2008). *MMDI™ personality test.* Retrieved from http://www.teamtechnology.co.uk

The Joint Commission. (2016). *Performance measurement.* https://www.jointcommission.org/performance_measurement.aspx

The Joint Commission National Patient Safety Goals. (2003). TIPS, *10*(1), 4–6.

Walker, D. E., & Soltis, J. (2009). *Curriculum and aims* (5th ed.). Teachers College Press.

Wiles, J., & Bondi, J. (1998). *Curriculum development: A guide to practice* (5th ed.). W. B. Saunders.

Yoder-Wise, P. S. (2019). *Leading and managing in nursing* (7th ed.). Elsevier.

Pursuing Systematic Self-Evaluation and Improvement in the Academic Nurse Educator Role

Linda Wilson and Frances H. Cornelius

*If you don't know where you are going,
any road will take you there.*
—Lewis Carroll, *Alice in Wonderland*

▶ Learning Outcomes

This chapter addresses the Certified Nurse Educator Exam Content Area 5: Pursue Systematic Self Evaluation and Improvement in the Academic Nurse Educator Role. For the CNE exam it is 12% of the examination, approximately 18 questions and for the CNEn exam it is Content Area 6 and 8% of the exam or approximately 12 questions

- Identify activities that promote one's socialization to the nurse educator role
- Discuss the importance of a mentor across the career trajectory
- Discuss the importance of a commitment to lifelong learning
- Discuss the importance of membership and active participation in professional organizations
- Identify professional development opportunities that increase one's effectiveness in the nursing role
- Identify sources of feedback to improve role effectiveness

● INTRODUCTION

The National League for Nursing (NLN) states that "academic nurse educators engage in a number of roles and functions, each of which reflects the core competencies of nursing faculty. The extent to which a specific nurse educator implements these competencies varies according to many factors, including the mission of the nurse educator's institution, the nurse educator's rank, the nurse educator's academic preparation, and the type of program in which the nurse educator teaches" (NLN, 2020, p. 2).

To pursue systematic self-evaluation and improvement in the nurse educator role, it is necessary that they

- "Engage[s] in activities that promote one's socialization to the role
- Maintain[s] membership in professional organizations
- Participate[s] actively in professional organizations
- Demonstrate[s] a commitment to lifelong learning
- Participate[s] in professional development opportunities that increase one's effectiveness in the role
- Manage[s] the teaching, scholarship, and service demands as influenced by the requirements of the institution
- Use[s] feedback gained from self, peer, student, and administrative evaluation to improve role effectiveness
- Practice[s] according to legal and ethical standards relevant to higher education and nursing education
- Mentor[s] and support[s] faculty colleagues in the role of an academic nurse educator
- Engage[s] in self-reflection to improve teaching practices" (NLN, 2020, p. 8)

This chapter focuses on the essential elements required in the pursuit of systematic self-evaluation and continuous improvement. These include:

1. Socialization to the faculty role
2. Role of mentorship across the career continuum
3. Active membership in professional organizations
4. Commitment to lifelong learning
5. Balancing teaching, scholarship, and service
6. Practice within legal and ethical standards
7. Self-reflection to promote professional development

● SOCIALIZATION TO THE EDUCATOR ROLE

The role of a new academic nurse educator can be both exciting and challenging. One of the most important support systems for a new educator is appropriate mentoring (NLN, 2006). An orientation program should include:

1. Introduction to key personnel
2. Introduction to other faculty members
3. A review of available resources within the department and organization
4. A review of courses and their related content (curriculum matrix)
5. A review of job benefits (done by the human resource department)
6. A review of administrative and governance structures (chain of command)
7. An introduction to the culture and political environment (full university faculty meetings and voting procedures for university committees)
8. Presentations on key aspects of the curriculum (what is emphasized in the curriculum has to do with the educational unit's core values)
9. A review of expectations for teaching, research, and service (for promotion and tenure—see Chapters 15 and 16 for further explanation)
10. Assignment of a faculty mentor

Many nurse educator orientation programs are completed one on one with a mentor. Some larger schools of nursing have developed extensive faculty orientation programs.

MENTOR AND SUPPORT FACULTY COLLEAGUES

Academic nurse educators have many roles and responsibilities, including the responsibility of mentoring. Nursing faculty have a responsibility to mentor colleagues, assisting them in their development as both educators and scholars (Billings & Halstead, 2019; Nowell, Norris, Mrklas, & White, 2017). Faculty mentorship includes guiding, coaching, and supporting faculty as they advance in their careers. Mentoring is extremely important, particularly for novices, because graduate school often provides little preparation for the academic nurse educator role. Mentoring is also important throughout all career stages.

Mentorship can be either formal or informal. Generally, formal mentorship relationships are most effective because they offer structured and clear expectations. (Hundey, Ansltey, Cruickshank, & Watson, 2020) Mentorship arrangements or types can vary across settings. Hurley et al. (2020) identify ten mentorship arrangements in Exhibit 12.1.

Exhibit 12.1 Types of Mentorship Arrangements

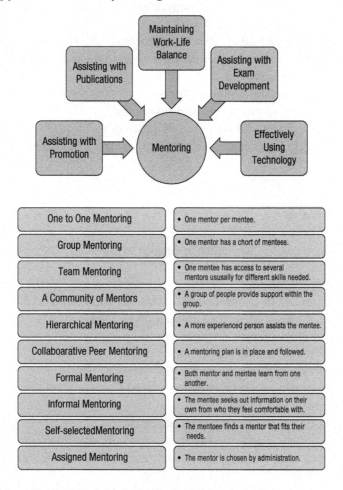

Source: Adapted from Hundey, Ansltey, Cruickshank, & Watson, 2020.

■ Bruner goes on to recommend that because of the diversity of roles of the contemporary nursing faculty, a gap analysis must first be conducted to identify mentorship needs. These gaps can be utilized to customize the mentorship program for the faculty (Nick et al., 2012). Phillips and Dennison (2015) identify specific areas in which all new faculty need mentor guidance:

- They need to feel connected with others and the larger community
- They need help with time management
- They need help with prioritizing
- They need advice with balancing teaching and research
- They need advice with balancing work and life outside the university
- They need editorial help with their writing (particularly if English is their second language) (p. 7)

MENTORING THROUGHOUT THE CAREER CONTINUUM

The NLN's (2008) position paper regarding mentoring of nurse faculty highlights key mentoring activities beneficial at various stages of a nurse educator's career. These include:

■ Early-career faculty members: Mentorship targets the faculty member who is new to both the educator role and the institution
■ Mentoring helps the uninitiated learn the complexities of the faculty role
■ Mentoring provides information about the knowledge, skills, behaviors, and values that comprise the faculty role
■ Formal orientation programs often include:
- An introduction to key personnel and resources
- A review of the courses and curricula being taught
- An overview of job benefits and administrative and governance structures
- An introduction to the culture and political environment of the institution
■ Throughout the entire first year, an assigned mentor should:
- Answer questions
- Interpret situations
- Provide direct help
- Share a similar schedule to ensure optimum availability
- Be friendly and caring
■ Midcareer faculty members: Mentorship supports faculty as they identify and test innovative pedagogies, propose new solutions to problems, and evolve as educators or scholars in local, regional, and national arenas. Mentoring is:
- Eclectic, varied in its content and process
- Directed more by the mentee than by the mentor
- Involves reciprocal sharing, learning, and growth
- Individually focused and takes time to evolve
■ Faculty may select a mentor for:
- Formal and informal mentoring relationships
- Shared interests inside and outside their academic communities
- Development of specific aspects in teaching, evaluation of learning, curriculum design, scholarship, service, and leadership
- Guidance in transitioning into academic leadership positions

- Faculty may develop "multiple mentoring partnerships, where each mentor assists them to grow in a particular area, such as grant-writing or conducting research on a particular topic" or a mentor can "provide guidance in selecting and transitioning into academic leadership positions" (NLN, 2008, p. 6).
- Late-career faculty members: The foundation of mentorship at this level is the responsibility to "identify new faculty members who show potential as leaders in nursing and nursing education and enter into mentor–protégé relationships with them, relationships that extend over long periods of time" (NLN, 2006, p. 4). The mentoring relationship at this level:

  - Is a source of satisfaction derived from guiding another in attaining self-clarity, personal growth, and as the educator continues to develop his or her skills
  - Cultivates a relationship that is situated in common interests and is built upon mutual respect for one another's knowledge and talents
  - Is "characterized by the investment of time, effort, and caring; the identification of mutual goals; and regular, ongoing dialogue designed to ensure the accomplishment of those goals" (NLN, 2006, pp. 7–8).

In the mentor–protégé relationship, the mentor shares her/his wisdom, knowledge, and expertise; builds connections in multiple communities by introducing personal networks; and keeps open a future of possibilities for someone who is expected to make significant contributions to the profession. Through an extended relationship, the mentor nurtures leadership in the protégé (NLN, 2006, p. 4).

- The most important factor in a successful mentorship relationship is for the mentor openness and caring. New faculty "overwhelmingly report that the most important aspect of the relationship is that someone actually cares about them and their success" (Phillips & Dennison, 2015, p. 6).
- It is important to note that mentorship is not limited to a relationship between two faculty members.
- Constellation mentoring is a group mentoring approach in which new faculty are provided with more than 1 mentor giving them the "opportunity to work and learn from a variety of experienced academics" (Webber, Vaughn-Deneen & Anthony, 2020, p. 211).
- Mentoring, in an ideal sense, involves the entire academic community. Everyone within the organization bears a responsibility to provide a supportive and welcoming environment and to foster a sense of belonging.
- An ongoing commitment to the practice of mentoring requires support from administrators and the entire nursing faculty. "Establishing a healthful work environment where collaborative peer and co-mentoring are an expectation, rather than a possibility, is the responsibility of all involved in nursing education" (Wasburn, 2007, p. 4).

During economic downturns and nursing faculty shortages, mentoring is a retention strategy (Jakubik, 2016). Faculty turnover is costly for educational organizations and disrupts the education process within the program.

Additional information on choosing a mentor in relation to career development is discussed in Chapter 15. Mentorship is so important that it can make or break a person's transition into a role and is crucial for new faculty success (Goode, 2012; Cole, Zehler, & Arter, 2020).

The NLN recommendations for mentoring at all levels are outlined in Exhibit 12.2.

EVIDENCE-BASED TEACHING PRACTICE

Jakubik (2016) is writing a leadership series about faculty mentoring. The researcher's literature review reveals that mentoring does help retention of faulty, but specifics about best practices are lacking.

Ideally, "the teaching of nursing must be evidence-based, with research informing what is taught, how learning is facilitated and evaluated, and how curricula/programs are designed" (NLN, 2002, p. 3). Kalb, O'Conner-Von, Brockway, Rierson, and Sendelbach (2015) report that although evidence-based teaching practice (EBTP) is deemed a professional standard, and most nurse educators are familiar with evidence-based practice, "many were not aware of EBTP or the need to use evidence in their teaching and faculty responsibilities. This lack of aware-ness has significant implications for the preparation of new nurse faculty and the professional development of current faculty" (p. 217).

Exhibit 12.2 The NLN Levels of Mentoring

For nursing faculty
- Contribute to the development of a mentoring program at your institution by identifying the needs of new faculty members and the resources required to meet those needs.
- Actively participate in mentoring relationships.
- Make the teaching done by experienced faculty members more visible to new faculty.
- Be open and friendly to new faculty and identify opportunities to be a "one-minute mentor" through brief, supportive interactions (Oermann, 2001).
- Become sensitive to existing and potential academic community practices that exclude new faculty members.
- Spend time together as a nurse faculty community, talking and listening to one another, and include the new faculty members.
- Attend professional development workshops and seminars on mentoring.
- Collaborate with the dean/director/chairperson to establish a mentoring program.
- Include content on mentoring in undergraduate and graduate curricula, including how to identify and select caring colleagues with whom to work closely and how to collaborate with colleagues.

For deans/directors/chairpersons
- Initiate and provide support for mentoring initiatives at your institution.
- Engage new, mid-career, and seasoned faculty in developing mentoring initiatives at your institution.
- Incorporate innovative strategies for mentoring new faculty members, such as the use of retired nurse educators (Bellack, 2004).
- Value the mentor role and reward faculty who actively serve in mentoring roles.
- Support the development of faculty mentors.
- Model mentoring.

For the NLN
- Support research on mentoring in the academic environment.
- Offer workshops and seminars on mentoring.
- Develop a mentoring toolkit (NLN, 2008).

◎ **Critical Thinking Question**

Mentoring is a voluntary activity and can extend over a long period of time (Jakubik, 2016). What types of expectations should the mentor have of the protégé?

EVIDENCE-BASED TEACHING PRACTICE

Stamps, Cockerell, and Opton (2021) studied new nurse faculty mentoring and identified three main components for success. The components needs are: (1) an extensive orientation, (2) mentorship, and (3) ongoing faculty development.

Kalb et al. (2015) identify several areas in which faculty can use evidence for teaching:

1. To revise courses
2. To design curriculum
3. To develop course content
4. To guide teaching
5. To answer questions about educational practices
6. To evaluate the effectiveness of teaching
7. To select teaching methods
8. To evaluate the quality of student learning
9. To critique evidence to inform teaching
10. To select evaluation methods

Kalb et al. (2015) emphasize that in order to support EBTP, a deliberate, structured, and sustained approach is required at institutional, administrative, and collegial levels to promote faculty effectiveness and student learning.

MEMBERSHIP IN PROFESSIONAL ORGANIZATIONS

It is important for academic nurse educators to be members of professional organizations. These organizations include, but are not limited to, the following:

- American Nurses Association (ANA)
- State nursing organizations
- National League for Nursing (NLN)
- Sigma Theta Tau International (STTI) Honor Society for Nursing
- Specialty nursing organizations (American Society of Perianesthesia Nurses, Association of Perioperative Registered Nurses, National Association of Orthopaedic Nurses, Oncology Nursing Society, American Association of Critical Care Nurses, etc.)
- Other related professional organizations (American Pain Society, Society for Critical Care Medicine, American Medical Informatics Association, etc.)

Membership in professional organizations provides the opportunity for knowledge enhancement, networking, and professional activities.

ACTIVE PARTICIPATION IN PROFESSIONAL ORGANIZATIONS

Professional organizational membership and leadership activities are an excellent mechanism for taking an active role in determining the future of nursing. These activities are also important in satisfying the service requirements for nurse educators who can:

- Participate on a committee
- Participate in a special interest group
- Serve as chair of a committee
- Serve as chair of a special interest group
- Run for office or a role on the board of directors at the local, state, or national level
- Participate in a task force
- Volunteer to work on specific initiatives for the organization
- Participate in a strategic work team

COMMITMENT TO LIFELONG LEARNING/ FACULTY DEVELOPMENT

According to the ANA's *Scope and Standards for Nursing Professional Development* (2019), the following are some of the beliefs that guided the development of the standards:

- "Lifelong learning is the responsibility of the nurse and is essential to maintain and increase competence in nursing practice" (p. 1).
- "Continuing professional nursing competence is essential to the provision of safe, quality health care to all members of society" (p. 1).
- "The public has a right to expect continuing professional nursing competence throughout the career of the nurse" (p. 1).
- "Self-directed learning is an integral part of continuing education, staff development, and academic education" (p. 2).

The *Scope and Standards* (ANA, 2019) also states that the lifelong professional development of a nurse requires participation in learning activities to assist in the development and maintenance of competence, enhancement of practice, and support for the attainment of career goals. The academic nurse educator has a personal and professional responsibility to:

- Seek continuing-education activities to maintain competency
- Expand knowledge and expertise in a nursing specialty

The NLN's (2001) position statement regarding lifelong learning acknowledges that the "concept of lifelong learning for nursing faculty (or faculty development) is complex and multi-faceted" (p. 1), and that learning starts in a master's and/or doctoral study program, but continues beyond formal education as a lifelong pursuit. Lifelong learning continues "through self-study and a constant inquisitiveness about the role and all its dimensions" (p. 1). In addition, the NLN (2018) stresses that concepts of lifelong learning should also be integrated through interprofessional collaborations.

PRACTICE WITHIN LEGAL AND ETHICAL STANDARDS

Nursing educators must be cognizant of the established legal and ethical standards in higher education.

▶ FAMILY EDUCATIONAL RIGHTS AND PRIVACY ACT

An important legal standard is the Family Educational Rights and Privacy Act (FERPA). FERPA is a "federal law that protects the privacy of students' education records. Educational agencies and institutions that receive funds under a program administered by the U.S. Department of Education (ED) must comply with FERPA. FERPA does apply to virtually every postsecondary institution in the United States" [U.S. Department of Education (USDOE), January 23, 2020, p. 2]. FERPA guarantees eligible students specific rights. Specifically, students have the right:

- To inspect and review the student's education records maintained by the school;
- To request amendment of any education records that they believe to be inaccurate or misleading; and
- To consent to the disclosure of personally identifiable information (PII) from the student's education record to third parties, subject to certain exceptions (USDOE, January 23, 2020, p. 4).

It is important for you to remember that student education records are considered private and your access to any student information is solely based upon your role and responsibilities as faculty (USDOE, January 23, 2020). Under FERPA, faculty:

- Has the legal obligation to protect the confidentiality of student education records in their possession
- Has access to student information only for legitimate use in the completion of your responsibilities
- Cannot share or "release lists or files with student information to any third party outside your college or departmental unit…without written consent of the student. Student information stored in electronic format must be secure and available only to those entitled to access that information" (USDOE, January 23, 2020).

Under FERPA, educational records include records "containing information directly related to a student that are maintained by an educational agency or institution (or by a party acting for the agency or institution). Education records may be in any form (handwritten, printed or saved on computer media, video or audio tape or film, microfilm or microfiche)" (USDOE, January 23, 2020). Faculty are not permitted to share student information about academic progress without written permission from the student. In addition, faculty should not include information from educational records in letters of recommendation.

▶ ETHICAL CONSIDERATIONS

The nurse educator's behavior is guided by the "norms, standards, and professional responsibilities members of a profession have toward others. Members of a profession are socialized into the role, either through formal education or by observing the behavior, conduct, and actions of senior members and by adhering to professional guidelines established by professional or licensing organizations" (Smith, 2012, p. 333).

Smith (2012) identifies key ethical implications for nurse educators as follows:

- Senior faculty should educate and assist junior faculty members to recognize and respond to issues involving ethical dilemmas.
- Faculty must socialize students to the ethical dimensions of professional practice.
- Faculty must be honest, professional, caring, and considerate in interactions and endeavors with others.
- All students should be respected and treated equally and fairly.
- All Colleagues should be treated in a collegial manner and assisted in professional development (pp. 333-4).

Furthermore, ethical considerations for nurse educators in respect to the roles of teaching, research and service must include:

- adequate preparation for teaching, from developing the syllabus to assigning the final grade
- protecting research participants, reporting fair and accurate results, and adhering to publishing guidelines
- balancing service activities to prevent interference with academic responsibilities (Smith, 2012, p. 333)

● PARTICIPATION IN PROFESSIONAL OPPORTUNITIES TO ENHANCE ONGOING DEVELOPMENT

To maintain high-quality nursing education programs, it is imperative that all faculty remain not only proficient with basic principles but also current with emerging technology and pedagogical trends. There are many different types of professional development opportunities in which the academic nurse educator can participate.

- Provider directed, provider paced educational activity

1. The provider-directed, provider-paced educational opportunity is "an activity in which the provider controls all aspects of the learning activity" (American Nurses Credentialing Center [ANCC], 2015, p. 47).
2. Examples of provider-directed, provider-paced educational opportunities include seminars, national conferences, and live webcasts.

■ Provider directed, learner paced educational activity

1. A provider-directed, learner-paced educational opportunity is "an activity in which the provider controls the content of the learning activity, including the learning outcomes based on a needs assessment, and chooses the content of the learning activity, the method by which it is presented, and the evaluation methods. Learners determine the pace at which they engage in the activity" (ANCC, 2015, p. 47)
2. Examples of provider-directed, learner-paced educational activities include continuing-education journal articles and online continuing-education modules

■ Learner-directed, learner-paced educational activity

1. A learner-directed, learner-paced activity is,

"a learning activity in which the learner takes the initiative in identifying his or her learning needs, formulating learning goals, identifying human and material resources for learning, choosing and implementing appropriate learning strategies, and evaluating learning outcomes. The learner also determines the pace at which they engage in the learning activity. Learner-directed activities may be developed with or without the help of others, but they are undertaken on an individual basis" (ANCC, 2015, p. 46).

Although similarities in learning needs exist, the elements of lifelong learning for the nurse educator vary according to:

■ Type of faculty appointment
■ Full-time, part time, or adjunct
■ Tenure track or nontenure track
■ Academic or service setting
■ Career stages
■ Novice faculty
■ Mid-stage faculty
■ Senior faculty
■ "The mission of a university affects the nature of expectations for the (NLN, 2001, p. 1):
  ● Scope of the role of faculty
  ● The educator role"

The NLN (2001) maintains that faculty development programs should be individualized and adaptable and should offer a wide range of topics in multiple modalities. Topics relevant to nurse educators include but are not limited to:

■ Classroom management
■ Student advisement
■ Student incivility
■ Cultural competency
■ Informatics competency
■ Clinical teaching
■ Clinical evaluation
■ Test construction

- Developing goal statements and learning objectives
- Outcomes assessment
- Teaching/learning technologies
- Curriculum development and modification
- The accreditation process
- The faculty role as leaders in the university community
- Creative teaching strategies
- Strategies to promote critical thinking
- Strategies to integrate informatics within the curriculum

It is important to note that "no single program or approach will meet the needs of everyone, and even the most senior tenured full professor must never think that she/ he has nothing new to learn" (NLN, 2001, p. 2).

 ## CASE STUDIES

CASE STUDY 13.1

Professor Unruh, a novice nurse educator, is teaching a senior-level nursing course. The professor's enthusiastic and is committed to ensuring that all students are successful. Professor Unruh has noticed that several students are struggling with some key concepts, so the professor decided to meet individually with each of these students. To prepare for these meetings, the professor wants to review all student information, including previous coursework and grades, so he can identify areas of weakness for targeted student support.

What guidance would you give the novice nurse educator about this plan? What recommendations would you give to the professor?

CASE STUDY 13.2

A nurse educator is mentoring a novice faculty member who was hired to teach the maternal–child health course. The learners in the course are a mixed group of prelicensure students. Fifty percent are traditional and 50% are second-degree learners.

What preparation tips would you give to the novice nurse educator about the learners in the class? What strategies to engage these learners would you recommend? How would you instruct the novice nurse educator to conduct test reviews?

1. A majority of faculty have identified a need for mentorship to accomplish which of the following priorities:

    A. Maintain classroom teaching
    B. Establish a work–life balance
    C. Prepare for social integration
    D. Identifying venues for community involvement

2. Mentoring a late-career faculty member may include:

    A. Encouraging and supporting the faculty to identify and test innovative pedagogies
    B. Providing guidance in transitioning into program chair or leadership position.
    C. Encouraging the faculty to identify new faculty members who show potential as leaders in nursing and nursing education
    D. Encouraging faculty to propose new solutions to problems and to evolve as educators and scholars in local, regional, and national arenas

3. Early-career faculty need mentorship in the following area:

    A. Identifying and testing innovative pedagogies
    B. Developing as an academic leader
    C. Navigating political and administrative environment
    D. Evolving as scholars in the national arena

4. The novice nurse educator needs additional mentoring about student boundaries established when they tell the mentor that they:

    A. Share personal stories that emphasize a content point
    B. Demonstrate a positive attitude with students
    C. Show enthusiasm for students learning new techniques
    D. Discuss personal life challenges

5. Nurse educators understand that one of the main consequences of lack of mentorship is a decrease in:

    A. Curricular revision
    B. Socialization into the role
    C. Dissatisfaction of faculty
    D. Attrition of faculty

1. B) Establish a work–life balance

The majority of faculty have identified a need for mentorship to obtain work–life balance; mentors can help with this and it can help prevent burnout. Mentors can also help faculty identify venues for professional involvement but should assist with professional integration, improve classroom teaching, and assist with professional organization involvement.

2. C) Encouraging the faculty to identify new faculty members who show potential as leaders in nursing and nursing education

Encouraging faculty to identify new faculty members who show potential as leaders in nursing and nursing education is appropriate for a late-career faculty member. After identifying a faculty member who shows potential, the late-career faculty can enter into a mentorship relationship to support this individual's professional development.

3. C) Navigating political and administrative environment

Early-career faculty need mentorship and guidance in navigating the political and administrative environment of their new institution. Identifying and testing innovative pedagogies and evolving as scholars in the national arena is addressed during the mid-career. Developing as an academic leader occurs later in their career.

4. D) Discuss personal life challenges

The novice nurse educator needs additional mentoring about student boundaries established when they tell their mentor that they discussed personal life challenges with a student. Sharing personal stories that emphasize a content point is OK as long as the storytelling is appropriate and relevant. Demonstrating a positive attitude with students and showing enthusiasm for students learning new techniques are also appropriate.

5. B) Socialization into the role

One of the main consequences of lack of mentorship is a decrease in socialization into the faculty role. Curricular revision is not the main consequence of last of mentorship. Lack of mentorship increases faculty dissatisfaction and attrition.

6. A new faculty member is constantly comparing the current teaching methods of the faculty to methods used by faculty at her previous educational unit. The mentor's best response would be to:

   A. Encourage the new faculty member to return to the previous position
   B. Ask the faculty member to stop complaining and assess
   C. Have the faculty member do a review of the literature on teaching methods.
   D. Explain to the new faculty member that there are many methods that work well

7. The director of the educational unit asks a seasoned faculty to mentor a new hire, and the seasoned faculty member objects. The best way to handle this situation would be to:

   A. Document the situation and find someone who is willing
   B. Insist that the faculty mentor take the responsibility
   C. Terminate the faculty mentor who refuses
   D. Tell the faculty mentor that it is a requirement of the position

8. A faculty member tells another faculty member in the hallway that their skills are outdated because they no longer practice clinically. The director of the educational unit would best respond to this comment by telling:

   A. The faculty member who made the comment that it is uncivil
   B. The faculty member who does not work clinically that it would be a good idea
   C. Both faculty members to take their conflict behind closed doors
   D. Both faculty members that competency is based on many different aspects

9. The novice nurse educator understands that faculty role expectations include:

   A. Completing a terminal degree
   B. Concentrating on teaching rather than service
   C. Attending conferences in the future
   D. Incorporating ethical and legal principles into teaching practice

10. An important orientation activity for nurse educators is:

    A. Developing a curriculum matrix to follow
    B. Attending departmental meetings
    C. Conducting a university-wide survey
    D. Socializing with other faculty

(See answers next page.)

6. D) Explain to the new faculty member that there are many methods that work well

When a new faculty member is constantly comparing the current teaching methods of the faculty to methods used by faculty at her previous educational unit. The mentor's best response would be to explain to the new faculty member that there are many methods that work well. Encouraging the new faculty member to return to their previous position does not help with team-building, and asking them to stop complaining may be viewed as non-supportive.

7. A) Document the situation and find someone who is willing

The best way to handle this situation would be to document the situation and find someone who is willing. There is no reason to want to force the seasoned faculty member to do this, as it will not encourage a supportive mentor–mentee relationship. However, this should be discussed at evaluation time because it is an expected professional obligation. Insisting that the mentor take responsibility or telling that it is a requirement of the position will not encourage a supportive mentor–protégé relationship. Terminating the mentor is not a good idea with a faculty shortage.

8. D) Both faculty members that competency is based on many different aspects

The director of the educational unit would best respond to this comment by telling both faculty members that competency is based on many different aspects of the academic role. Telling the faculty member who made the comment that it is uncivil will set up further conflict. Telling the faculty member who does not work clinically that it would be a good idea is not necessary. Telling both faculty members to take their conflict behind closed doors may not resolve the issue.

9. D) Incorporating ethical and legal principles into teaching practice

The faculty role expectations include incorporating ethical and legal principles into teaching practice. Completing a terminal degree depends on the type of education unit they are employed in. All areas need to be addressed, so focusing on teaching and not service is not appropriate. Attending conferences in the future is not expected, though they are helpful.

10. B) Attending departmental meetings

An important orientation activity for nurse educators is attending departmental meetings as this is an important learning experience and will help the faculty socialize to the faculty role. Developing a curriculum matrix is done by the curriculum committee members. Socializing with faculty is more helpful than conducting a university-wide survey, but it is not the initial priority.

⬤ REFERENCES

American Nurses Association. (2019). *Nursing Professional Development Scope and Standards of Practice* (3rd ed.). Author.

American Nurses Credentialing Center. (2015). 2015 *ANCC primary accreditation provider application manual*. Author.

Bellack, J. P. (2004). Seasoned faculty: To retire or not? One solution to the faculty shortage—Begin at the end. *Journal of Nursing Education, 43*(6), 243–244.

Billings, D. M., & Halstead, J. A. (2019). *Teaching in nursing: A guide for faculty* (6th ed.). Elsevier Saunders.

Bruner, D. W., Dunbar, S., Higgins, M., & Martyn, K. (2016). Benchmarking and gap analysis of faculty mentorship priorities and how well they are met. *Nursing Outlook*, 321–331. 10.1016/j.outlook.2016.02.008

Cole, B., Zehler, A., & Arter, S. (2020) Role-reversal mentoring: Case study of an active approach to faculty growth. *Journal of Nursing Education, 59*(11), 627–630. https://doi.org/10.3928/01484834-20201020-05

Foster, C. W. (2012). Institute of medicine the future of nursing report, lifelong learning, and certification. *Medsurg Nursing, 21*(2), 115-6. http://ezproxy2.library. drexel.edu/login?url=https://www-proquest-com.ezproxy2.library.drexel. edu/scholarly-journals/institute-medicine-future-nursing-report-lifelong/ docview/1008665087/se-2?accountid=10559

Goode, M. L. (2012). The role of the mentor: A critical analysis. *Journal of Community Nursing, 26*(3), 33–35.

Hundey, B., Anstey, L., Cruickshank, H. & Watson, G. P. L. (2020). Mentoring faculty online: A literature review and recommendations for web-based programs, *International Journal for Academic Development, 25*(3), 232–246. 10.1080/1360144X.2020.1731815

Jakubik, L. D. (2016). Leadership series: "How to" for mentoring. *Part 1: An overview of mentoring practices and mentoring benefits. Pediatric Nursing, 42*(1), 37–38.

Kalb, K. A., O'Conner-Von, S. K., Brockway, C., Rierson, C. L., & Sendelbach, S. (2015) Evidence-based teaching practice in nursing education: Faculty perspectives and practices *Nursing Education Perspectives, 36*(4), 212–219.

Modi Owied, A. M. (2019). Self-directed and lifelong learning: A framework for improving nursing students' learning skills in the clinical context. International Journal of Nursing Education Scholarship, (1) http://dx.doi.org.ezproxy2.library. drexel.edu/10.1515/ijnes-2018-0079

National League for Nursing. (2001). Position statement: Lifelong learning for nursing faculty. http://www.nln.org/docs/default-source/about/ archivedposition-statements/lifelong-learning-for-nursing-faculty-pdf. pdf?sfvrsn=8

National League for Nursing. (2002). The preparation of nurse educators [Position statement]. http://www.nln.org/docs/default-source/about/nln-vision-series-(position-statements)/nlnvision_6.pdf

National League for Nursing. (2006). Position statement: Mentoring of nurse faculty. *Nursing Education Perspectives, 27*(2), 110–113.

National League for Nursing. (2008). Position statement: Preparing the next generation of nurses to practice in a technology-rich environment: An informatics agenda. http://www.nln.org/docs/default-source/professional-development-programs/preparing-the-next-generation-of-nurses.pdf?sfvrsn=6

National League for Nursing. (2018). Certified nurse educator (CNE) 2018 Candidate handbook. http://www.nln.org/docs/default-source/professional-development-programs/certified-nurse-educator-(cne)-examination-candidate-handbook.pdf?sfvrsn=2

National League for Nursing. (2016b). NLN research priorities in nursing education 2015–2019. http://www.nln.org/docs/default-source/professional-development-programs/nln-research-priorities-in-nursing-education-single-pages.pdf?sfvrsn=2

Nick, J. M., Delahoyde, T. M., Del Prato, D., Mitchell, C., Ortiz, J., Ottley, C., … Siktberg, L. (2012). Best practices in academic mentoring: A model for excellence. *Nursing Research and Practice*, 2012, Article ID 937906. 1155/2012/937906

Nowell, L., Norris, J. M., Mrklas, K., & White, D. E. (2017) A literature review of mentorship programs in academic nursing, *Journal of Professional Nursing*, 33(5), 334–344, https://doi.org/10.1016/j.profnurs.2017.02.007

Oermann, M. H. (2001). One-minute mentor. *Nursing Management*, 32(4), 12–13.

Phillips, S. L., & Dennison, S. T. (2015). Faculty mentoring: A practical manual for mentors, mentees, administrators, and faculty developers. ProQuest Ebook Central https://ebookcentral-proquest-com.ezproxy2.library.drexel.edu

Smith, M. H. (2012). *The legal, professional, and ethical dimensions of higher education* (2nd ed.). Lippincott, Williams & White.

Stamps, A., Cockerell, K., & Opton, L. (2021). A modern take on facilitating transition into the academic nurse educator role. *Teaching & Learning in Nursing*, 16(1), 92–94. 10.1016/j.teln.2020.04.002

U.S. Department of Education (January 23, 2020) FERPA 101: For Colleges & Universities, https://studentprivacy.ed.gov/training/ferpa-101-colleges-universities

Wasburn, M. H. (2007). Mentoring women faculty: An instrumental case study of strategic collaboration. *Mentoring & Tutoring: Partnership in Learning*, 15(1), 57–72.

Webber, V. (2020). Three-generation academic mentoring teams: A new approach to faculty mentoring in nursing. *Nurse Educator*, 45(4), 210–213. https://org/10.1097/NNE.0000000000000777

Functioning as a Change Agent and Leader

Frances H. Cornelius

Leadership: the art of getting someone else to do something you want done because he wants to do it.
—Dwight D. Eisenhower (1890–1969; former president of the United States)

> ▶ **LEARNING OUTCOMES**
>
> This chapter addresses the Certified Nurse Educator Exam Content Area 6A: Function as a Change Agent and Leader. For the CNE exam Content Area 6 includes 6A, 6B, and 6C, and makes up 15% of the examination, approximately 22 questions for the CNEn exam it is Content Area 5 and makes up 7% of the exam or approximately 11 questions
>
> ■ Discuss the importance of cultural sensitivity when advocating for change
> ■ Discuss the effect of organizational culture on the climate of innovation within nursing education
> ■ Identify strategies to support a climate of creativity and innovation within nursing education
> ■ Identify measures to evaluate organizational effectiveness in nursing education
> ■ Analyze the nurse educator's leadership role with respect to creating an environment of innovation
> ■ Analyze strategies that drive organizational change
> ■ Elaborate on strategies for integrating a long-term, innovative, and creative perspective into the nurse educator role

INTRODUCTION

This chapter focuses on the nurse educator's role as a leader who interfaces with the larger academic community and administration, the role of the nurse educator within the larger system, and becoming a change agent within a variety of systems.

THE NURSE EDUCATOR'S ROLE AS A LEADER AND CHANGE AGENT

Giddens and Thompson (2018) state that the essential qualities of an academic nurse leader include having competence, confidence, courage, creativity, collaboration, and therapeutic communication skills. Academic nursing leaders must create and communicate a clear vision to strategically mobilize to educational solutions not only to prepare future generations for nurses but also to prepare "recruit, develop, and retain a new generation of nursing faculty and mentor the next generation of academic leaders" (Giddens & Thompson, 2018, p. 73). In addition, nursing administrators, educators, and clinicians have a responsibility to keep abreast of the rapidly changing environment in higher education, healthcare, and technology and to make changes proactively (Prut & Thompson, 2018). In order for nurse educators to create or influence change, they must be aware of the key issues affecting the nursing profession. In the current environment, academic institutions must pursue transformation in order to remain viable and relevant therefore strategic competencies such as being a visionary and open-minded about change are essential (Ma Regina, Caringal-Go & Magsaysay, 2018). This makes it all the more critical that academic nurse leaders develop openness to new ideas as a key leadership skill. Academic nursing leaders must be "open" to consider non-traditional educational models to meet the needs of changes that are occurring in higher education and healthcare.

Opportunities are abound for nurses to lead, but few are born leaders; most nurses must learn effective leadership skills. Effective leadership is enhanced by paying attention, having followers, moving in the right direction, and continually acting and questioning what can be done to make a difference (Dickenson-Hazard, 2004; Weber, Ward, & Walsh, 2015; Hechanova, 2018)). Rohrich and Durand (2020) note that leaders often have a "complementary role being a group mentor or role model" as well as identify the most important characteristic is the "unique selfless trait of motivating an organization or a group of people with a diverse background to advance a common role or function" (p. 1099).

The functions of a nurse leader include:

1. Acting as a role model for others
2. Providing expert nursing care based on theory and research findings
3. Demonstrating knowledge about organizational theory to support and influence organizational policies
4. Collaborating with others to provide optimum healthcare
5. Assuming responsibility for providing information and support to patients
6. Using advocacy to help effect changes that will benefit patients and the healthcare organization
7. Using the nursing codes of ethics and standards of practice as guidelines for individual and professional accountability (Grant & Massey, 1999, as cited in Mahoney, 2001, p. 270)

The American Nurses Association (ANA) outlines essential leadership competencies, and they are:

- Collaboration
- Communication
- Education
- Environmental Health
- Ethics
- Evidence-based Practice
- Leadership
- Professional Practice Evaluation
- Quality of Practice
- Resource Utilization (ANA, 2018).

Although leadership is often used interchangeably with management skills, it is important to note that there is a difference between leadership and management skills. A classic differentiating statement is that "leaders have followers" and "managers have subordinates" (Clyatt, 2017; Arruda, 2016). In today's complex environment, the lines between these two roles blur, and often the blending of these two provides benefits for influencing and motivating while overseeing operations and processes (Clyatt, 2017).

SKILLS AND ATTRIBUTES OF A LEADER

Carroll's (2005) study comparing the perceptions of female leaders and nurse executives about what skills and attributes would be needed to succeed in the 21st century remains relevant today. The six factors identified included:

1. Personal integrity—includes adherence to ethical standards, trustworthiness, and credibility
2. Strategic vision/action orientation—related to creating and articulating a vision of a preferred future, managing change, seeing possibilities instead of obstacles, exhibiting a determination to succeed and a commitment to action, being proactive, evaluating, being resilient, promoting excellence, and seeing the big picture
3. Team building/communication—skills used to build coalitions, make effective oral presentations, debate and discuss important issues, build a team, and build consensus
4. Management and technical competence—ability to make decisions, think critically, solve problems, plan, direct, organize, control, and be technically competent in a field, profession, or discipline
5. People skills—ability to empower others, network, value diversity, and work collaboratively
6. Personal survival skills/attributes—political sensitivity, self-direction, self-reliance, courage, a competitive and entrepreneurial spirit, and candor

▶ LEADERSHIP PROTOCOLS

Rubino (2011) discusses the responsibility of the leader to serve as a role model for the organization. He identifies a list of "protocols" that describe certain key behaviors that are essential for effective leaders. These include:

1. Professionalism
2. Reciprocal trust and respect
3. Being confident, optimistic, and passionate
4. Being visible
5. Being an open communicator
6. Taking risks/entrepreneur
7. Admitting fault

▶ QUALITIES OF A LEADER

Qualities of an effective and successful leader have been studied extensively. The impact these qualities can have on the success of an organization or academic institution is significant (Olanrewaju & Okorie, 2019). While the lists vary among researchers, upon review, one will note that the overall essence of the lists is quite similar. King (2011) identifies key qualities of a leader, which include:

- Ambition—having an objective/goal to work toward
- Knowledge of the business—a solid understanding of the history and operations of the organization
- Consistency—consistent behavior inspires trust and is the foundation for integrity; this is possible only through consistency of thought and action
- Good listening skills—essential to build trust and effective working relationships; effective listening contributes to the knowledge and understanding of the leader and provides critical information for decision-making
- Creativity—a leader will adapt quickly to new information and have the creativity and vision to handle change
- Ability to own up to mistakes—a leader who accepts responsibility for his or her mistakes and does not scapegoat others; builds trust among his or her subordinates
- Decision-making skills—a strong business leader is decisive and has the courage to stand by the decision taken
- Hossain (2015) identified the following as critical qualities of an effective 21st-century leader: (1) honesty, (2) vision, (3) inspiration, (4) communication, (5) delegation, (6) decision, (7) courage, (8) fairness, (9) kindness, (10) magnanimity, (11) forward-thinking, (12) knowledge, (13) competency, (14) confidence, (15) commitment, (16) gentle, (17) accountability, (18) creativity, (19) sense of humor, (20) intuition, (21) focus, (22) assertiveness, (23) optimism, and (24) balance. These are not ranked in order of importance.
- Muteswa (2015) identified the nine qualities of a good leader as "1) confidence, 2) toughness and inspiration, 3) ability to communicate the vision and values, 4) ability to establish the right culture in the organization, 5) displays honesty, integrity and transparency, 6) humble, 7) learns from failure and bad experiences, 8) commitment, and 9) ability to identify and attract talent" (p. 136).
- Olanrewaju1 and Okorie (2019) identified the primary qualities of a good leader to be: "1) accessibility and dedication, 2) neutrality and modesty, 3) aspiration and attentiveness, 4) believe and aptitude, 5) dignity and amiability, 6) insight and confidence, 7) vitality and concentration, 8) originality and honesty, 9) responsibility and team spirit, 10) decency and self-assurance, 11) charitable, 12) comical and maintenance culture, and 13) reliability" (p. 142).

▶ LEADERSHIP ACTIVITIES OF SENIOR NURSES

Senior nurses, at all levels and in all settings, should adopt a supportive leadership style and work to develop others by providing opportunities for them to apply theoretical frameworks to practice, encourage risk taking in a safe, supportive environment in order to support leadership development as a continuous process. "This approach incorporates mentorship, coaching, and supervision as core values" (Frankel, 2011; Pesut & Thompson, 2018; Giddens & Thompson, 2018).

▶ LEADERSHIP STYLES

There is extensive literature on leadership styles. The leadership styles that are most common include:

1. Democratic—decisions are made with input from each team member.
2. Autocratic (authoritarian)—leader makes decisions without input from team members or without any consideration of the impact on the team.
3. Laissez-Faire—a leader gives up decision-making authority to the team.
4. Strategic—leader is able to communicate a vision for the organization that motivates/persuades others to share and work towards that vision.
5. Transformational—a leader is empathetic and creates an environment that is intellectually stimulating, inspiring, and challenging to support subordinates' development and maximize performance outcomes.
6. Transactional—a leader who uses a transactional leadership style communicates effectively, particularly in clarifying instructions. This leader will also establish a contractual reward or punishment system for performance outcomes.
7. Affiliative—a leader using an affiliative approach to leadership already has a staff who is highly motivated, so the objective is to create a friendly workplace and minimize conflict or friction.
8. Coach-style—a leader who uses a coaching leadership style is interested in the professional development of his or her subordinates and strives to establish a team-spirit atmosphere in the work setting. This leader focuses on identifying and developing the individual strengths of each member of the team.
9. Servant—a leader characterized by a concern for others (e.g., team members and employees) within the organization/community with a focus on others' needs and interests.
10. Bureaucratic—a leader who makes decisions that "fit" with company policy or is congruent with established practices (Sims, 2009; Becker, 2020; Pullen, 2016; Eva, Robin, Sendjaya, van Dierendonck, & Liden, 2019).

Anderson and Sun (2017) observed that the dominant leadership paradigm is that of transformational/transactional leadership styles. The literature abounds with exemplars of leadership skills and practices associated with the transformational leader. Key transformational leadership practices include:

- Inspiring a shared vision—envisioning the future by imagining exciting and ennobling possibilities; enlisting others in a common vision by appealing to shared aspirations
- Challenging the process—being creative and innovative, searching for opportunities by seeking new ways to change, grow, and improve; experimenting and taking risks; generating small wins; and learning from mistakes
- Enabling others to act—fostering collaboration by promoting cooperative goals and building trust and strengthening others by sharing power and discretion along the way
- Encouraging the heart—recognizing individual contributions, showing appreciation for excellence, and celebrating victories by creating a spirit of community
- Modeling the way—finding voice and clarifying personal values by setting an example and aligning actions with the shared values of the team (Ross, Fitzpatrick, Click, Krouse, & Clavelle, 2014; Snow, 2019).

Snow (2019) points out that the top two transformational leadership practices are "enabling others to act" and "modeling the way." It is important to note that most effective leaders use a variety of leadership styles—modifying their approach to the context of the situation. An important skill of an effective leader is to be flexible and attuned to the need to adjust one's approach.

Meyer and Meijers (2017) propose that effective leaders must be agile and able to move easily between different leadership styles in order to be effective in a variety of circumstances. The authors identify 10 leadership styles that have a corresponding counterpart on the other end of the spectrum. Specifically, they discuss various leadership styles on a continuum where given the situation, the leader may be "leaning" more toward one end of the continuum. For example, in a situation when immediate decisive action is warranted, an effective leader will shift on the continuum towards the autocratic leadership style rather than on the democratic leadership style.

EVIDENCE-BASED TEACHING PRACTICE

Delgado and Mitchell (2016) conducted a cross-sectional, online survey to identify nurse faculty leadership qualities that are currently valued and relevant and found the qualities to be integrity, communication clarity, and problem-solving ability.

▶ COMPETENCIES ASSOCIATED WITH LEADERSHIP

Weber, Ward, and Walsh (2015) noted that it is essential that key competencies are identified and nurtured within a nursing leadership structure to ensure optimal succession planning. These competencies include:

- Influence
- Emotional intelligence
- Driving for results
- Facilitating change
- High-impact communication
- Business acumen

- Aligning performance for success
- Building a successful team
- Leading through vision and values
- Building trust
- Making decisions/problem solving (p. 48)

Snow (2019) maintains that in order for organizations to remain viable, competitive, and adaptive to change creativity and innovation are essential competencies required for nurse leaders. Effective nurse leaders should encourage creative thinking to inspire new ways of "knowing something" and building "new connections" to what has been previously learned. The role of the nurse educator in this endeavor is critical. Snow states that to "achieve a more innovative culture, nurse leaders will need to role model, teach, and foster competencies necessary for a creative workforce" (p. 311).

Giddens (2015) also believes that innovation and creativity are highly valued competencies for nurse educators and states that not all nurse educators have the aptitude for innovation, however, all faculty share a responsibility to promote innovation in nursing education by maintaining a culture of openness to diverse ideas and developing strategies that encourage innovation.

Many believe that creativity and innovativeness are skills that can be learned. Snow (2019) identifies the following strategies that can be used to accomplish this type of learning:

- Educate on the value of creative problem-solving and innovation for the organization.
- Educate on the science and evidence in support of creative "play" at work as serious business for new idea generation.
- Express a personal value for creativity, risk-taking, and use of unconventional methods to create innovations that improve practice.
- Role model use of creative problem-solving practices.
- Demonstrate design thinking by reaching out to social, political, and economic sciences as well as business and humanities fields to better inform policy and create work environments that foster a collaborative and innovative spirit.
- Recognize and celebrate risk-taking even when it does not result in the desired change; and, especially when it does (p. 311).

THE NURSE EDUCATOR AS A CHANGE AGENT

ANA's position is that nurse leaders must possess change management competencies to "facilitate organizational change initiatives and overcome resistance to change" (2018, p. 8). Essential behaviors associated with these competencies include:

- Leads change by example
- Adapts plans as necessary
- Takes into account people's concerns during change
- Effectively involves key people in the design and implementation of change
- Adjusts management style to changing situations
- Effectively manages others'' resistance to organizational change
- Adapts to the changing external pressures facing the organization

- Is straightforward with individuals about consequences of an expected action or decision
- Accepts change as positive

Higher education is in the midst of a major transformation that requires leaders possess competencies such as being visionary and open-minded about change in order to strategically pursue change. Thompson and Miller (2018) observe that disruptions in traditional approaches to higher education have resulted in "changes that are affecting the lives of students, faculty, staff and alumni of universities and colleges. Regardless of the size of student bodies or sources of operating revenue and financial support, academic institutions are rapidly adapting to innovations required for growth and sustainability" (p. 92). Hechanova, Caringal-Go, and Magsaysay (2018) point out that it is important for leaders to be cognizant of the nuances of organizational context to determine the best way to manage change and foster commitment to the change.

Giddens (2015), a nurse educator, points out that academia is not often receptive to innovation and change but acknowledges that one significant barrier is that often there is a lack of evidence that the innovation/method/process is better. Innovators/change agents may encounter resistance which Giddens describes as the "paradoxical challenge is that there is rarely robust evidence for innovative ideas initially, yet faculty are expected to base their practice on evidence, and it takes time for clear evidence to emerge." Dr. Giddens urges nurse educators to develop a strategy to obtain objective, non-biased outcome measurements to demonstrate efficacy.

Green (2006) also identifies several critical competencies for nurse educators that relate to the role ofchange agent and leader. These include:

- Collaboration
  - Teamwork—an essential component of the nurse educator's role
  - Developing networks and partnerships to improve nursing's influence within the community
  - Working with faculty and students to support progress toward the achievement of realistic and optimal learning goals
  - Conferring with nursing leadership to make recommendations and develop educational interventions
- Systems thinking
  - Involving the ability of the nurse educator to incorporate the body of knowledge, resources, and tools available within and outside the healthcare system to optimize learning experiences and teaching opportunities
  - Focusing on interrelationships and how these impact the process of change and are, in turn, affected by this process
  - Identifying the social, economic, political, and institutional forces influencing nursing education
- Advocacy/moral agency
  - Monitoring legal and ethical issues relevant to higher education and nursing education, and act to influence, plan, and implement policies and procedures
  - Guiding decisions and actions with ethical principles grounded in an appreciation of cultural diversity and individual rights

Nelson, Godfrey, and Purdy (2004) studied hospital mentoring programs. They found that hospitals that used a mentorship program spent less and realized great benefits. It was a successful way to recruit and retain the brightest graduate nurses. Hospital-based mentorship programs increase recruitment and retention and are cost-effective (Nelson et al., 2004). Mentors are nurses who facilitate learning and model leadership skills.

EVIDENCE-BASED TEACHING PRACTICE

Getha-Taylor, Fowles, Silvia, and Merritt (2015) analyzed data from a local government leadership development program to examine how time affects conceptual and interpersonal leadership skill education and found that skills decline over time. The study indicates a need for consistent and continuous skill reinforcement.

There are three theoretical perspectives that explain how a person can become a leader:

1. Trait Theory—a "natural-born" leader possesses natural leadership traits that lead him or her into leadership roles.
2. Great Events Theory—an ordinary person responds to a crisis or disastrous event and emerges a leader.
3. Transformational Leadership—a person chooses to become a leader by seeking opportunities to develop leadership skills (Clark, 2008).

To develop leadership skills, a nurse educator must assume the responsibility of seeking out opportunities for professional development. It is essential to take the initiative to obtain an accurate assessment of one's current leadership skills and performance.

- This process can be started by creating a list of strengths and weaknesses.
- Typically, it is fairly easy to identify one's strengths, but most people find it difficult to identify their weaknesses.
- The nurse educator must seek out opportunities to develop leadership skills, link with potential leadership mentors and coaches, and actively solicit very specific feedback from a variety of sources.
- It is essential to be receptive to feedback and reflect on it throughout the process.

© Critical Thinking Question

Veenema and colleagues (2015) put out a call-for-action paper for nurses as leaders in disaster preparedness and response. What type of leadership style would you assume in a disaster response situation?

▶ ESSENTIAL LEADERSHIP SKILLS

Sources of influence—creative and innovative leaders must embody the following traits and abilities:

- "Organizational understanding" and political skills
- Creative thinking skills for idea evaluation
- Self-awareness

- Adaptability is needed in changing environments and to compensate when there are areas that need improvement
- Collaborative thinking—creative work frequently involves collaboration with other disciplines, as well as with non-traditional partners; looking for partnerships outside one's usual circles can lead to successful, win–win partnerships (Glasgow & Cornelius, 2005)
- Integration minded—leaders are more effective when using an integrative style that permits them to orchestrate expertise, people, and relationships in such a way as to bring new ideas into being; there are three critical elements to this integrative style of leadership:
  - Idea generation—stresses the role of the leader in facilitating others' idea generation
  - Idea structuring—refers to guidance with respect to the technical and organizational merits of the work, setting output expectations, and identifying and integrating the projects to be pursued
  - Idea promotion—involves gathering support from the broader organization for the creative enterprise as a whole as well as implementation of a specific idea or project (Mumford, Scott, Gaddis, & Strange, 2002, pp. 738–739)

In other words, making sure resources are available (time, staff, funds, etc.) to complete the project.

 ## EVALUATING ORGANIZATIONAL EFFECTIVENESS

Research has called for organizations to be more flexible, adaptive, entrepreneurial, and innovative to meet the changing demands of today's environment more effectively (Snow, 2019). Additional research has found that organizational performance is linked to participative leadership and an innovative organizational culture (Casida, 2008; Ogbonna & Harris, 2000; Shahzad, Luqman, Khan, & Shabbir, 2012; Pillay & Morris, 2016; Snow, 2019).

Thibodeaux and Favilla (1996) define organizational effectiveness as the "extent to which an organization, by the use of certain resources, fulfills its objectives without depleting its resources and without placing undue strain on its members and/or society" (p. 21). There are a number of models that facilitate the evaluation of organizational effectiveness. For the most part, the first step in all approaches to evaluate organizational effectiveness is to identify the criteria for evaluation. Generally, the model selected to approach the organizational assessment will determine which criteria will be utilized, and the model selected is dictated by the type of organization being evaluated. Traditional organizational assessment models include:

1. Goal Model
2. Systems Model
3. Process Model
4. Strategic Constituencies Model
5. Competing Values Framework
6. Baldrige National Quality Program (Martz, 2008)

Many of the models of organizational effectiveness have similar attributes/criteria that demonstrate organizational effectiveness. These include:

- Clear goals that are well communicated
- Resources allocated to innovation and change
- Members (faculty) who are satisfied
- Success is marketed
- Education is rewarded
- A plan for the future exists (Cheng, 1996)

Martz (2008) states that regardless of the organization type, any organization can be assessed by "incorporating an explicit focus on the common functionality innate to all organizations regardless of the organization size, type, structure, design or purpose" (p. 19).

Martz (2010) identifies six steps to use in assessing an organization's effectiveness:

1. Establish the boundaries of the evaluation
2. Conduct a performance needs assessment
3. Define the criteria of merit
4. Plan and implement the evaluation
5. Synthesize performance data with values
6. Communicate and report evaluation findings

▶ OUTCOMES

Donabedian (2005) conceptualizes evaluation into three dimensions: structure, processes, and outcomes. The outcome of medical care, in terms of recovery, restoration of function, and of survival, has been frequently used as an indicator of the quality of medical care. The most common effectiveness measurements are difficult to define and measure; therefore, a frequent problem is ambiguity and measurement error.

▶ PROCESSES

Leaders understand that outcome is the focus and that micromanagement of the process can lead to limited productivity. They understand that the difference between process and outcome and process management includes:

- Look at "how things are done" versus the outcome.
- Measure work quantity or quality.
- Substituting process criteria for outcome criteria can compromise service. In order for an organization to be effective, the following criteria should be evaluated (Exhibit 13.1).

Exhibit 13.1 Outline of the Organizational Effectiveness Checklist

1. Establish the boundaries of the evaluation.
    1.1 Identify the evaluation client, primary liaison, and power brokers.
    1.2 Clarify the organizational domain to be evaluated.
    1.3 Clarify why the evaluation is being requested.
    1.4 Clarify the timeframe to be employed.
    1.5 Clarify the resources available for the evaluation.
    1.6 Identify the primary beneficiaries and organizational participants.
    1.7 Conduct an evaluability assessment.

2. Conduct a performance needs assessment.
    2.1 Clarify the purpose of the organization.
    2.2 Assess internal knowledge needs.
    2.3 Scan the external environment.
    2.4 Conduct a strength, weakness, opportunity, and threat (SWOT) analysis.
    2.5 Identify the performance-level needs of the organization.

3. Define the criteria to be used for the evaluation.
    3.1 Review the universal criteria of merit for organizational effectiveness.
    3.2 Add contextual criteria identified in the performance needs assessment.
    3.3 Determine the importance ratings for each criterion.
    3.4 Identify performance measures for each criterion.
    3.5 Identify performance standards for each criterion.
    3.6 Create performance matrices for each criterion.

4. Plan and implement the evaluation.
    4.1 Identify data sources.
    4.2 Identify data-collection methods.
    4.3 Collect and analyze data.

5. Synthesize performance data with values.
    5.1 Create a performance profile for each criterion.
    5.2 Create a profile of organizational effectiveness.
    5.3 Identify organizational strengths and weaknesses.

6. Communicate and report evaluation activities.
    6.1 Distribute regular communications about the evaluation progress.
    6.2 Deliver a draft of the written report to client for review and comment.
    6.3 Edit report to include points of clarification or reaction statements.
    6.4 Present written and oral reports to client.
    6.5 Provide follow-on support as requested by client.

Source: Martz (2010).

▶ STRUCTURES

- "Concerned with such things as the adequacy of facilities and equipment; the qualifications of medical staff and their organization; the administrative structure and operations of programs and institutions providing care; fiscal organization and the like" (Donabedian, 2005, p. 695).

- Indicators include:
  - Organizational features (equipment age or type)
  - Participant characteristics (degree attained, licensing, etc.)

● ESTABLISHING A CULTURE OF CHANGE

Pullen (2016) states that the "change process is best accomplished using the servant, transformational, and democratic leadership approaches. These three styles often result in people who are motivated through inspiration" (p. 28).

Magsaysay and Hechanova (2017) identify the five dimensions of ideal change leaders:

- Strategic/technical competence
- Execution competence
- Social competence
- Character
- Resilience

An organization's climate and culture have a significant impact on the creativity and innovation displayed within it.

- **Climate** is defined as "people's perceptions of organizational interactions and characteristics" (Mumford et al., 2002, p. 732).
- **Culture** is defined as the "normative expectations for desirable behavior," which determines, to a large extent, how people act within that organization (Mumford et al., 2002, p. 732).

The predominant view is that organizational culture cannot be "managed"; however, there are key events/interventions that can leverage the opportunity to "manage" organizational culture (Willcoxson & Millett, 2000). These include:

- Recruitment, selection, and replacement—culture management can be affected by ensuring that appointments strengthen the existing culture(s) or support a culture shift.
- Removal and replacement may be used to dramatically change the culture.
- Socialization—induction and subsequent development and training can provide for acculturation to an existing or new culture and also for improved interpersonal communication and teamwork, which is especially critical in fragmented organizational cultures.
- Performance management/reward systems can be used to highlight and encourage desired behaviors, which may (or may not) in turn lead to changed values.
- Leadership and modeling are needed from executives, managers, and supervisors who can reinforce or assist in the overturning of existing myths, symbols, behavior, and values and demonstrate the universality and integrity of vision, mission, or value statements.

- Participation of all organization members in cultural reconstruction or maintenance activities and associated input, decision-making, and development activities are essential if long-term change in values, and not just behaviors, is to be achieved.
- Interpersonal communication satisfying interpersonal relationships does much to support an existing organizational culture and to integrate members into a culture; effective teamwork supports either change or development in and communication of culture.
- Structures, policies, procedures, and allocation of resources need to be congruent with organizational strategy and culture and objectives.

Change may be initiated by a crisis or a shift in leadership, but there are other sources of influence that can drive change. Effective change agents influence and drive change by using several different strategies at the same time. By combining multiple strategies or sources of influence, they increase the likelihood of success and producing substantial, sustainable change (Grenny, Maxfield, & Shimberg, 2008; Hechanova, 2018). Grenny and colleagues specifically identify six sources of influence that a nurse educator can utilize to influence change. Those sources are divided into motivation and ability under the realms of personal, social, and structural influences. The sources of influence under *motivation* include (a) linking to mission and values, (b) harnessing peer pressure, and (c) aligning rewards and assuring accountability. The sources of influence under *ability* include (a) overinvesting in skill building, (b) creating social support, and (c) changing the environment.

An example of personal motivation to change occurs when the change is valued and the ability for personal change comes with education. Social motivation to change may come in the form of peer pressure, but the social ability to change uses a supportive environment. Structural motivators to change may come in the form of incentives, and the ability to change is found in organizational structures that support change. Nurse educators can effect change if they reflect on the motivational aspects of change and the ability to change within the personal, social, and structural systems in which they function. Influencing healthcare policy is a primary method to effect change (Exhibit 13.2).

Exhibit 13.2 Healthcare Policy, Finance, and Regulatory Environments

Rationale:

Healthcare policies, including financial and regulatory policies, directly and indirectly influence nursing practice and the nature and functioning of the healthcare system.

These policies shape responses to organizational, local, national, and global issues of equity, access, affordability, and social justice in healthcare. Also, healthcare policies are central to any discussion about quality and safety in the practice environment.

The baccalaureate-educated graduate will have a solid understanding of the broader context of healthcare, including how patient care services are organized and financed, and how reimbursement is structured. Regulatory agencies define boundaries of nursing practice, and graduates need to understand the scope and role of these agencies.

Baccalaureate graduates will also understand how healthcare issues are identified, how healthcare policy is both developed and changed, and how that process can be influenced through the efforts of nurses and other healthcare professionals, as well as lay and special advocacy groups.

Healthcare policy shapes the nature, quality, and safety of the practice environment, and all professional nurses have the responsibility to participate in the political process and advocate for patients, families, communities, the nursing profession, and changes in the healthcare system, as needed. Advocacy for vulnerable populations with the goal of promoting social justice is also recognized as a moral and ethical responsibility of the nurse.

A baccalaureate program prepares a graduate to:
1. Demonstrate basic knowledge of healthcare policy, finance, and regulatory environments, including local, state, national, and global healthcare trends.
2. Describe how healthcare is organized and financed, including the implications of business principles, such as patient and system cost factors.
3. Compare the benefits and limitations of the major forms of reimbursement on the delivery of healthcare services.
4. Examine legislative and regulatory processes relevant to the provision of healthcare.
5. Describe state and national statutes, rules, and regulations that authorize and define professional nursing practice.
6. Explore the impact of sociocultural, economic, legal, and political factors influencing healthcare delivery and practice.
7. Examine the roles and responsibilities of the regulatory agencies and their effect on patient care quality, workplace safety, and the scope of nursing and other health professionals' practice.
8. Discuss the implications of healthcare policy on issues of access, equity, affordability, and social justice in healthcare delivery.
9. Use an ethical framework to evaluate the impact of social policies on healthcare, especially for vulnerable populations.
10. Articulate, through a nursing perspective, issues concerning healthcare delivery to decision-makers within healthcare organizations and other policy arenas. Participate as a nursing professional in political processes and grassroots legislative efforts to influence healthcare policy.
11. Advocate for consumers and the nursing profession.

Sample Content:
- Policy development and the legislative process
- Policy development and the regulatory process
- Licensure and regulation of nursing practice
- Social policy/public policy
- Policy analysis and evaluation
- Healthcare financing and reimbursement
- Economics of healthcare
- Consumerism and advocacy
- Political activism and professional organizations
- Disparities in the healthcare system
- The impact of social trends, such as genetics and genomics, childhood obesity, and aging, on health policy
- Role of nurse as patient advocate
- Ethical and legal issues
- Professional organizations' roles in healthcare policy, finance, and regulatory environments
- Scope of practice and policy perspectives of other health professionals
- Negligence, malpractice, and risk management
- Nurse Practice Act

Many studies have identified interactional factors that foster an environment of creativity and innovation (Cooper & Jayatilaka, 2006; Denti, 2016; Faber, 2016; Isaksen, 2009; Pillay & Morris, 2016; Rowlings, 2016; Sandeen, 2010; Snow, 2019; Vaidyanathan, 2012). These factors include:

1. Challenge/involvement
2. Freedom
3. Trust/openness
4. Time to brainstorm ideas
5. Playfulness/humor
6. Conflict
7. Idea support
8. Debate
9. Risk taking

The presence of these interacting factors influences the individual's perception of the organization's openness to creativity, and consequently affects his or her willingness to engage in creative efforts and will serve as a catalyst for innovation (Denti, 2016; Faber, 2016; Isaksen, Aerts, & Isaksen, 2009; Isaksen & Akkermans, 2007; Rowlings, 2016; Hechanova, 2018; Snow, 2019).

THE PROCESS OF CHANGE

Nauheimer (2005) states that sustained change requires transformation on three levels: individual, team/unit, and organization or larger system. Successful change can be better understood and facilitated through the lens of change theory.

- In this process, the nurse educator can assist in the identification of positive opportunities for change and strategies to effectively manage change, whether planned or unplanned.
- The nurse educator must not only have skill in applying change theory but also have a keen understanding of which interventions will affect, encourage, and manage the change process.
- It is essential to keep in mind that not all change is improvement, but all improvement is change (White, 2004).

▶ THE NURSE LEADER AS A CHANGE AGENT

Nurses, by virtue of their training and education, are well prepared to serve as change agents in a variety of settings and working at all levels (Craig, 2019; Green, 2019; Eads & Maruzella, 2016). Essential role functions of a nurse require "require being good communicators and listeners, … be agile, focused, and detailed oriented in order to care for their patients" and be critical thinkers in order to "judge situations and make appropriate decisions" (Craig, 2019, p. 4). These skills are the foundation for being an effective change agent. However, acquiring and incorporating the skill sets of effective change agents can help nurse leaders to implement any change successfully. These skills include the ability to:

- Combine ideas from unconnected sources
- Energize others by keeping the interest level up and by demonstrating a high personal energy level
- Develop skill in human relations, such as well-developed interpersonal communication skills, group management, and problem-solving skills
- Retain a big-picture focus while dealing with each part of the system
- Be flexible and willing to modify ideas if the modification will improve the change, but resist nonproductive tampering with the implementation
- Be confident and avoid the tendency to be easily discouraged
- Think realistically regarding how quickly staff will accept and perform new processes competently
- Be trustworthy, with a track record of integrity and success through other systemic changes
- Articulate a vision through insights and versatile thinking to instill confidence in others
- Be able to handle resistance to a new process (White, 2004)

▶ CHANGE THEORIES

The predominant models of change include:
1. Lewin's Three-Step Change Theory
2. Lippitt's Phases of Change Theory
3. Havelock's Six Phases of Change
4. Prochaska and DiClemente's Change Theory
5. Social Cognitive Theory
6. Theory of Reasoned Action
7. Theory of Planned Behavior
8. Diffusion of Innovation
9. Davis's Technology Acceptance Model

▶ CHARACTERISTICS OF VARIOUS CHANGE THEORIES

Lewin's Three-Step Change Theory

Lewin's Three-Step Change Theory (unfreeze, change, refreeze) sees change as a dynamic balance of forces working in opposing directions.

- Driving forces:
  - Facilitate change
  - Push individuals/organizations in the desired direction for change

- Restraining forces:
  - Hinder change
  - Push individuals/organizations in the opposite direction of the desired change
  - Forces must be analyzed and manipulated to shift the balance in the direction of the planned change

Lewin's model is very rational and goal- and plan-oriented. It does not take into account personal factors that can affect change.

Lippitt's Phases of Change Theory

- Lippitt's Phases of Change Theory is an extension of Lewin's Three-Step Change Theory and focuses on the *change agent*, rather than the change itself (Udod & Wagner, 2018).
- Lippitt's theory includes seven steps:
  1. Diagnose the problem.
  2. Assess the motivation and capacity for change.
  3. Assess the resources and motivation of the change agent. This includes the change agent's commitment to change, power, and stamina.
  4. Choose progressive change objects. In this step, action plans are developed, and strategies are established.
  5. The role of the change agents should be selected and clearly understood by all parties so that expectations are clear. Examples of roles are cheerleader, facilitator, and expert.
  6. Maintain the change. Communication, feedback, and group coordination are essential elements in this step of the change process.
  7. Gradually withdraw from the helping relationship. "The change agent should gradually withdraw from their role over time. This will occur when the change becomes part of the organizational culture" (Lippitt, Watson, & Westley, 1960, pp. 58–59, as cited in Kritsonis, 2004–2005).

Havelock's Six Phases of Change

Havelock also modified Lewin's change theory focusing on creating a process for "change agents to organize their work and implement innovation," by approaching the change process as "cycles of action that are repeated as change advances," which the change agent must pay close attention to as the change moves through six distinct steps (White, 2021, p. 62). These steps are:

1. "Building a relationship. Havelock regarded the first step as a stage of "pre-contemplation" where a need for change in the system is determined.
2. Diagnosing the problem. During this contemplation phase, the change agent must decide whether or not change is needed or desired. On occasion, the change process can end because the change agent decides that change is either not needed or not worth the effort.
3. Acquire resources for change. At this step, the need for change is understood and the process of developing solutions begins as the change agent gathers as much information as possible relevant to the situation that requires change.
4. Selecting a pathway for the solution. A pathway of change is selected from available options and then implemented.
5. Establish and accept change. Individuals and organizations are often resistant to change, so careful attention must be given to making sure that the change becomes part of new routine behaviour. Effective communication strategies, staff response strategies, education, and support systems must be included during implementation.

6. Maintenance and separation. The change agent should monitor the affected system to ensure the change is successfully stabilized and maintained. Guiding the client system in self renewal – the ability to change" (Udod & Wagner, 2018, p. 15).

Prochaska and DiClemente's Change Theory

Prochaska and DiClemente's Change Theory considers change from the perspective that a person moves through stages of change. The stages are

1. Precontemplation
2. Contemplation
3. Preparation
4. Action
5. Maintenance

Prochaska and DiClemente's model is cyclical, not linear. It takes relapses or failures into account. Individuals who relapse can revisit the contemplation stage and make plans for action in the future (Kritsonis, 2004–2005).

Social Cognitive Theory (Social Learning Theory)

- In social cognitive theory, self-efficacy is the most important characteristic and must be present for successful change. "Self-efficacy is defined as having the confidence in the ability to take action and persist in the action" (Kritsonis, 2004–2005, p. 6).
- Social cognitive theory proposes that behavioral change is affected by environmental influences and personal factors.
- This theory takes into account both external and internal environmental conditions (Grizzell, 2007; Kritsonis, 2004–2005).

Theory of Reasoned Action

- The theory of reasoned action states that a person's actions are determined by his or her intention to perform that action.
- Intention is determined by two major factors:
  1. The person's attitude toward the behavior or change (i.e., beliefs about the outcomes of the behavior and the value of these outcomes).
  2. The influence of the person's social environment or subjective norms (i.e., beliefs about what other people think the person should do, as well as the person's motivation to comply with the opinions of others (Grizzell, 2007; Kritsonis, 2004–2005).

Theory of Planned Behavior

- The theory of planned behavior expands upon the theory of reasoned action by including the concept of the individual's perceived control over the opportunities, resources, and skills necessary to perform a behavior or change. This perception of control is believed to be a critical facet of behavior change processes (Grizzell, 2007).
- As with the social cognitive theory, self-efficacy is an important characteristic and must be present for successful change.

Diffusion of Innovation Theory

Rogers's diffusion of innovation theory provides insight into the process by which new ideas are disseminated and integrated. It can be both spontaneous and planned. "The main elements in the diffusion are

1. An innovation
2. That is communicated through certain channels
3. Over time
4. Among the members of a social system" (Rogers, 2003, p. 35)

In order for diffusion to be successful, it is absolutely essential to have key people and policy makers interested in the innovation and committed to its implementation. This theory further identifies the five steps in the process of innovation diffusion as:

1. Knowledge—the decision-making unit is introduced to the innovation and begins to understand it.
2. Persuasion—an attitude, favorable or unfavorable, forms toward the innovation.
3. Decision—activities lead to a decision to adopt or reject the innovation.
4. Implementation—the innovation is put to use, and reinvention or alterations may occur.
5. Confirmation— "The individual or decision-making unit seeks reinforcement that the decision was correct. If there are conflicting messages or experiences, the original decision may be reversed" (White, 2004, pp. 50–51).

Rogers (2003) describes diffusion as a "kind of social change, defined as the process by which alteration occurs in the structure and function of a social system. When new ideas are invented, diffused, and adopted or rejected, leading to certain consequences, social change occurs" (p. 6). Berwick (2003) uses Rogers's theory to explain the rate of change and states that the rate correlates to the following:

1. Perceptions of the innovation/change
   - Perceived benefit of the change.
   - Compatibility with the values, beliefs, history, and current needs of individuals.
   - Level of complexity of the proposed innovation or change. The rate of change for simpler changes is generally faster than those that are more complex.
   - "Re-invention" of the innovation or change (the adaptability of the change). The capability of making local (or point of use) modifications, which often involve simplification, is a common characteristic of successful dissemination.
   - Changes spread faster when they have these five perceived attributes: benefit, compatibility, simplicity, trialability (ability to "test the waters"), and observability.

2. Characteristics of the people who either adopt the innovation or do not:
   - The curve of adoption of the innovation or change over time generally takes an S-shape, characterized with an early slow phase affecting a very few individuals (early adopters), a rapid middle phase with widespread adoption, followed by a slow third phase, typically ending with incomplete adoption. It has been described as being similar to the epidemic curve of a contagious disease.

- Rogers's (2003) diffusion of innovation theory includes five levels of adoption (for more information, see Figure 13.1):
  1. Innovators
  2. Early adopters
  3. Early majority
  4. Late majority
  5. Laggards

Figure 13.1 Rogers's (2003) adopter areas.

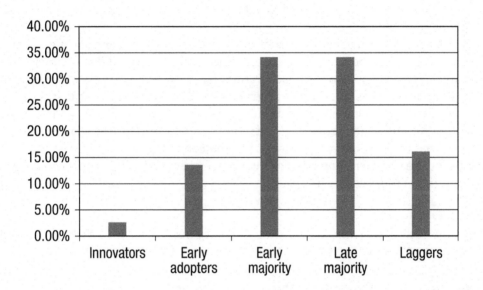

Contextual factors include situational/environmental factors associated with a particular organization or social system, such as management, leadership, communication, or incentives that can either "encourage and support, or discourage and impede, the actual processes" of diffusion (Berwick, 2003, p. 1972).

Davis's Technology Acceptance Model

Davis's technology acceptance model (TAM) is an extension of the theory of reasoned action (described earlier in the chapter). The TAM model provides a mechanism to view how external factors influence the intention to use technology. Specifically, the model considers the external factors that influence (a) perceived usefulness and (b) perceived ease of use as key factors influencing an individual's attitude toward use and in turn, how that influences the actual use (Figure 13.2).

Figure 13.2 Davis's technology acceptance model.

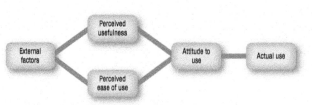

Chaos theory of change or diffusion is a theory that deals with dynamic instability of complex systems such as nursing educational units. The basic premise is that one small change can affect, over time, many larger changes in a system because they are sensitive or dependent on the initial condition. An often-used illustration of chaos theory is that the flap of butterfly wings in one part of the world can cause a random effect that may eventually turn out to be a tornado in another part of the world (Gleick, 1987).

Complexity theory is also discussed in nursing as a change process that has its roots in the physical sciences. Similar to chaos theory, the organization structure must be viewed as a whole that is composed of multiple systems. Decisions are made in relation to human-to-human interactions and may appear random and unrelated, but in the larger scheme of things, make sense within the context in which they were made. It expands the theoretical notions that changes have causes and effects that can always be predetermined (Yoder-Wise, 2011).

◎ **Critical Thinking Question**

Using chaos theory, what may happen to the learners by their senior year if a change was made in the fundamentals class to include a simulation scenario on communication?

 ## CULTURAL SENSITIVITY WHEN ADVOCATING FOR CHANGE

The American Association of Colleges of Nursing (AACN) (2017) states that to "improve the quality of nursing education, . . . the values and principles of diversity, inclusion, and equity must remain mission central" for nurse educators (p. 3). Inclusion, according to the AACN, "represents . . . cultures in which faculty, students, staff, and administrators with diverse characteristics thrive" (2017, p. 1). An important consideration is that an inclusive environment requires "intentionality to embrace differences, not merely tolerate them" with a focused effort to "ensure the perspectives and the experiences of others are invited, welcomed, acknowledged and included" (Breslin, Nuri-Robins, Ash & Kirschling, 2018, p. 104).

Individuals' ethnic identities and cultural backgrounds strongly influence their attitudes, values, and practices. When advocating for change, it is essential that the nurse educator consider these factors and act in a culturally sensitive manner and create an environment that is inclusive and accepting of diversity. Schmidt, MacWilliams and Boylan (2016) state exclusionary behaviors such as "incivility, bullying, and workplace violence, discriminate and isolate individuals and groups who are different whereas inclusive behaviors encourage diversity" (p. 102). The AACN (March 20, 2017) states that "inclusive environments require intentionality and embrace differences, not merely tolerate them. Everyone works to ensure the perspectives and experiences of others are invited, welcomed, acknowledged, and respected in inclusive environments" (p. 1).

Cultural considerations must be incorporated in any efforts to influence change. Rationales for including higher-level cultural competence skills/strategies in health organization policies include:

1. Response to current and projected demographic changes
2. Elimination of long-standing health disparities among people from diverse racial, ethnic, and cultural backgrounds
3. Improvement of the quality of and access to health services (National Center for Cultural Competence, n.d.)

Saha, Beach, and Cooper (2008) observed that cultural competence has become an "all-encompassing approach to address interpersonal and institutional sources of racial and ethnic disparities in healthcare. Though the concept of cultural competence has changed over time and continues to evolve, it has always contained at its core the principles of patient-centered health care delivery" (pp. 6–7). When applying these concepts broadly to efforts to influence change, key considerations would include:

- Sensitivity to others' beliefs and values
- Sensitivity to individual/group needs, preferences, and experiences
- Tailoring communication/materials to the appropriate level, language, and literacy
- Openness and flexibility

Breslin, Nuri-Robins, Ash, & Kirschling (2018) discuss a shift away from the term "cultural competency" to the term "cultural proficiency" a mechanism to communicate a more expansive approach to diversity and inclusion. The authors maintain that shifting the language to "cultural proficiency signals to those familiar with the term cultural competence that we are focusing on something more than diversity. A focus on becoming culturally proficient denotes a commitment to examine policies and practices of the organization as well as the values and behaviors of the individual" (p. 104). The authors present a cultural proficiency continuum framework in which includes the following stages:

- Cultural Destruction: Destroy differences
- Cultural Intolerance: Demean differences
- Cultural Reduction: Discount differences
- Cultural Precompetence: Accommodate differences
- Cultural Competence: Collaborate with differences
- Cultural Proficiency: Co-create a healthy environment (Breslin, Nuri-Robins, Ash & Kirschling, 2018).

TEACHING GEM A transformative teacher is one who models caring to his or her students at all times in order for the students to reflect on themselves as caring people (Diekelmann, 1995).

Nelson, Anis-Abdellatif, Larson, Mulder, and Wolff (2016) acknowledge that a diverse classroom has significant benefits in education—providing multiple perspectives to the learning experience—but point out that there are often gaps in new faculty orientation as well as ongoing faculty development that leave them unprepared to function effectively in the diverse classroom. The authors advocate for ongoing diversity and inclusiveness training within higher education to ensure cultural competency.

The essential cultural competencies relevant to the process of advocating for change include:

- Awareness and sensitivity to the differences that individuals, groups, and organizations may have in their experiences and responses to the change
- Ability to recognize differences and to identify similar patterns of responses to change among individuals, groups, and organizations
- Avoidance of stereotyping by acknowledging variations among individuals, groups, and organizations
- Awareness that communication is inextricably interwoven with culture
- Awareness of how language (preference, level of comfort, and proficiency) influences an individual's perception and ability to understand, develop meanings, and make sense out of the world
- "Knowledge of diversity in communication patterns, styles, and protocols, and of how language and communication may influence the development of trust in relationships" (Meleis, 1999, p. 12)

▶ STRATEGIES FOR PLANNED CHANGE

Successful change involves making a compelling case for the change and then putting into place measures to manage change risk to protect the organization and its stakeholders (Kee & Newcomer, 2008). Strategies for leading change include:

1. Diagnosing change risk and organizational capacity
2. Strategizing and making a case for change
3. Implementing and sustaining change
4. Reinforcing change by creating a change-centric learning organization (p. 5)

Strom (2001) identifies the top eight effective change implementation strategies:

1. Multiple interventions—comprehensive interventions that take into account the many characteristics of the organization as well as the external environment
2. Outreach visits—intensive support by a change agent who provides education, feedback, practical support, reminders, and praise for progress
3. Opinion leaders—recruit individuals who are recognized by peers as influential educators to promote the change
4. Reminders—prompt healthcare professionals to perform a patient-specific clinical action (behavioral approach), which is generally effective across a range of clinical behaviors; this is less effective if used for routine items of care or if too many prompts are presented at the same time
5. Feedback—auditing and providing feedback of summarized clinical performance
6. Interactive (computer-based)—Using computer information systems to support practice, such as teleconferencing, chat-room techniques, and information sharing through listservs

7. Interactive (educational)—customized, phased, educational interventions designed specifically to mitigate potential barriers, including user resistance and teaching new skills

8. Administrative intervention—clinical effectiveness and successful change can be achieved by using a continuous quality improvement (CQI) or quality-management approach, focusing on the core processes as the centerpiece of the initiative

● POLITICAL ACTION

◎ **Critical Thinking Question**

The American Nurses Association believes that advocacy is a pillar of nursing. Nurses instinctively advocate for their patients, in their workplaces, and in their communities, but legislative and political advocacy is no less important to advancing the profession and patient care (ANA, n.d.). What are some a nurse educator can engage in legislative or political advocacy?

Effective leadership skills are essential in efforts to leverage nursing's potential to make a difference in healthcare and reform. To build the capacity of nurse leaders to effectively influence policy, it is important to understand the attributes that support them to function effectively at senior policy levels (Jivraj Shariff, 2015; Rafferty, 2018). The nurse educator has an obligation to function as a role model to others in active engagement in the political processes on a local, regional, national, and global level. By virtue of the role of educator, the nurse educator is uniquely positioned to influence other nurses (and aspiring nurses) to become politically active. Opollo, Bond, Gray, and Lail-Davis (2012) stress the importance of this involvement by pointing out that "both the ANA and the ICN [International Council of Nurses] call on nurses to collaborate with other health professionals and the public to promote community, national, and international efforts to meet health needs" (pp. 77–78). The authors identify four key rationales for nursing involvement:

1. The successful attainment of the United Nations Millennium Development Goals will require strong global partnerships and collaborations.
2. Equipping nurses with culturally relevant competencies is important for promoting the delivery of effective, culturally appropriate healthcare globally.
3. Key tools for engaging in global health efforts include partnerships, education, media outreach, and grassroots, and grasstops approaches.
4. Nurses are strategically positioned to influence global health research, education, policy, and practice by participating in continuing education programs, interprofessional exchanges, and volunteerism with a global health focus (Opollo et al., 2012, p. 79).

Wilson, Anafi, Kusi-Appiah, Darko, Deck, and Errasti-Ibarrondo (2020) point out that nurses are not fully leveraging their potential to influence policy, stating that "nurses have important insights, values, and knowledge of great relevance to public policy. In the future, many more nurses with the aptitudes and skills should be politically active and effective at public policy agenda setting and policy-making" (p. 7). The authors stress that the importance of nurse educators in preparing, mentoring, and encouraging future generations to be politically active.

▶ POLITICAL ACTION RESOURCES

- Professional organizations (e.g., AACN and NLN)
- Political organizations (e.g., American Civil Liberties Union [ACLU])
- Federal, state, and local government agencies (e.g., Occupational Safety and Health Administration [OSHA])
- Electronic political information organizations (e.g., Electronic News Media, Political Information Search Engine: www.politicalinformation.com)
- Government representatives (e.g., contact federal, state, and local representatives via U.S. government websites such as www.usa.gov/Contact/Elected.shtml)

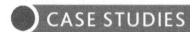 CASE STUDIES

CASE STUDY 13.1

St. Mary's Hospital, a midsized community hospital, initiated a hospital-wide clinical improvement project. An interdisciplinary team of healthcare professionals was recruited to serve on the clinical improvement project panel. One area identified for improvement was to reduce the number of patient falls. A comprehensive, 40-page clinical guideline published by the U.S. Agency for Health Care Research and Quality (AHRQ) was selected for implementation. However, the project team determined that full implementation of these guidelines was too complex and time-consuming for the staff, and therefore would not likely be successful. The panel identified two changes that could be easily implemented and would likely have a significant impact on fall incident rates. A nurse representative from each inpatient unit was recruited to serve as unit leader for the implementation of these changes. A targeted information campaign was designed, and staff in-services were conducted on all units for all shifts. Those two simple innovations, not the larger, more detailed and complex guidelines, reduced the rate of falls in vulnerable patients by 75%.

What strategies for change were utilized by the panel to implement this clinical improvement project? How was Rogers's theory of diffusion applied? How would the principles of leadership support the process? How can evaluation criteria for organizational effectiveness be applied in this scenario? Which criteria would be relevant?

CASE STUDY 13.2

The nursing programs of Drexel University, the Community College of Philadelphia, Bloomsburg University of Pennsylvania, and Howard University entered into a collaborative agreement to incorporate the use of technology in their respective undergraduate and graduate nursing programs. Drexel University, College of Nursing and Health Professions (DUCNHP), with Dr. Linda Wilson as the project director, will be the lead school and will share its technology expertise and resources by working jointly with the faculty of the collaborating schools to ensure faculty competence in selected technologies used by DUCNHP to enhance nursing education curricula and teaching processes. Topics that fall under this initiative include the following: "incorporation of the personal digital assistant into didactic courses and in clinical, development, and implementation of cases and evaluation methods for human simulation including the use of standardized patients and patient simulators, the use of web-based courseware, and the development of a server repository/portal for various interactive learning modules for use by the collaborating nursing programs" (Wilson, 2007, p. 1).

How can the principles of good community–campus partnerships be applied to this initiative to increase the likelihood of success? What strategies for change must be considered? Discuss this initiative from the perspective of organizational culture. What factors must be considered?

1. The novice nurse educator requires additional mentorship when they state that Davis's technology acceptance model involves:

   A. External factors
   B. Ease of use
   C. Perceived usefulness
   D. Thought leaders

2. A leader who establishes an employee development system in which employees focus on developing different skills and competencies is demonstrating which leadership style?

   A. Autocratic
   B. Coaching
   C. Transformational
   D. Bureaucratic

3. The nurse educator understands that Donabedian conceptualizes evaluation into three dimensions that include:

   A. People
   B. Processes
   C. Places
   D. Constructs

4. The dean is a transactional leader, so faculty expect the dean to:

   A. Enlist others in a common vision by appealing to shared aspirations
   B. Share power and decision-making
   C. Experiment and take risks
   D. Use a rewards/punishment system

5. The nurse educator understands that a priority source of motivational influence includes:

   A. Creating social support
   B. Linking to mission and values
   C. Overinvesting in skill building
   D. Changing the environment

6. There are things that a manager can do to "manage" organizational culture. These include which of the following?

   A. Purposeful recruitment, selection, and replacement
   B. Conduct a performance needs assessment
   C. Establish partnerships outside one's usual circles
   D. Plan and implement policies and procedures

1. D) Thought leaders

The Davis's technology acceptance model includes external factors, ease of use, and perceived usefulness, not thought leaders.

2. B) Coaching

A leader who uses the coaching style focuses on building a team where each employee has an expertise or skillset in something different. The goal of this leader is to create strong teams that can communicate well and embrace each other's unique skillsets in order to get work done. Autocratic leaders make decisions without input from or consideration for the impact on team members. Transformational leaders create intellectually stimulating environments to support development and maximize performance outcomes. Bureaucratic leaders make decisions based on company policies and established practices.

3. B) Processes

Donabedian's model conceptualizes evaluation into three dimensions that include structure, processes, and outcomes.

4. D) Use a rewards/punishment system

A transactional leader would use a patriarchal award and punishment system that is dehumanizing. Transformational leaders develop a common vision, take risks, and share power.

5. B) Linking to mission and values

A significant source of influence is being able to link to mission and values. Overinvesting, changing, and creating social supports are not top motivators.

6. A) Purposeful recruitment, selection, and replacement

Purposeful recruitment, selection, and replacement is an effective strategy to manage organizational culture because each individual contributes to the organizational culture. Conducting a performance needs assessment is not interventional. Establishing partnerships outside one's usual circles is not focused on internal culture. Planning and implementing policies and procedures are managerial tasks and do not usually affect culture.

7. The theory that describes change as a dynamic balance of forces working in opposing directions is:

   A. Lippitt's Phases of Change Theory
   B. Prochaska and DiClemente's Change Theory
   C. Theory of planned behavior
   D. Lewin's Three-Step Change Theory

8. The theory that describes change from the perspective of the person moving through stages of change is:

   A. Social cognitive theory
   B. Prochaska and DiClemente's Change Theory
   C. Theory of reasoned action
   D. Theory of planned behavior

9. The novice nurse educator needs additional understanding of contextual factors of the change process when they include:

   A. Situational/environmental factor
   B. Leadership
   C. Communication or incentives
   D. Personal traits

10. For academic institutions to remain viable, competitive, and adaptive to change, which of the following competencies are essential for nurse leaders?

    A. Fiscal acumen
    B. Maintaining operations
    C. Communication through chain of command
    D. Innovative planning

(See answers next page.)

7. D) Lewin's Three-Step Change Theory

Lewin's Three-Step Change Theory includes consideration of opposing forces. Lippitt's Phases of Change Theory discusses specific stages. Prochaska and DiClemente's Change Theory discusses innovation. The theory of planned behavior is a systematic theory.

8. B) Prochaska and DiClemente's Change Theory

Prochaska and DiClemente's Change Theory considers change from the perspective that a person moves through stages of change. The stages are: (1) precontemplation, (2) contemplation, (3) preparation, (4) action, and (5) maintenance. Social cognitive theory discusses influences of change. Theory of reasoned action discusses intentions to change. Theory of planned behavior links beliefs to behavior.

9. D) Innovative planning

Innovative planning is essential for academic institutions to remain viable, competitive, and adaptive to change, because, in order to "achieve a more innovative culture, nurse leaders will need to role model, teach, and foster competencies necessary for a creative workforce" (Snow, p. 311).

10. D) Personal traits

Situational/environmental factor, leadership, and communication or incentives are factors that vary and affect the change process. Situational/environmental factors change; leadership also changes as it is not individualized; and communication/ incentives can also vary. Personal traits should not be considered; change should consider the mission of the organization.

● REFERENCES

American Nurses Association (2018). ANA leadership competency model, Author, https://www.nursingworld.org/~4a0a2e/globalassets/docs/ce/177626-ana-leadership-booklet-new-final.pdf

American Association of Colleges of Nursing (2017). *Position statement: Diversity, inclusion, & equity in academic nursing.* Author. http://www.aacn.nche.edu/media-relations/AACN-Position-Statement-Diversity-Inclusion.pdf.

Anderson, M. H. & Sun, P. Y. T. (2017). Reviewing leadership styles: *Overlaps and the need for a new "Full-Range" theory. International Journal of Management Reviews, 19,* 76–96. 10.1111/ijmr.12082

Arruda, W. (November 15, 2016). 9 differences between being a leader and a manager, Forbes https://www.forbes.com/sites/williamarruda/2016/11/15/9-differences-between-being-a-leader-and-a-manager/?sh=309bda674609

Becker, B. (2020). The 8 most common leadership styles & how to find your own. Hubspot Blog. https://blog.hubspot.com/marketing/leadership-styles

Berwick, D. M. (2003). Disseminating innovations in health care. *Journal of the American Medical Association, 289*(15), 1969–1975.

Breslin, E. T., Nuri-Robins, K., Ash, J. & Kirschling, J. M. (2018). The changing face of academic nursing: Nurturing diversity, inclusivity, and equity. *Journal of Professional Nursing, 34,* 103–109.

Carroll, T. L. (2005). Leadership skills and attributes of women and nurse executives. *Nurse Administrator, 29*(2), 146–153.

Casida, J. (2008). Linking nursing unit's culture to organizational effectiveness: A measurement tool. *Nursing Economics, 26*(2), 106–110.

Cheng, Y. C. (1996). *School effectiveness and school-based management: A mechanism for development.* Routledge.

Clark, D. R. (2008). Concepts of leadership. http://www.nwlink.com/~donclark/leader/leadcon.html

Cooper, R. B., & Jayatilaka, B. (2006). Group creativity: The effects of extrinsic, intrinsic, and obligation motivations. *Creativity Research Journal, 18*(2), 153–172. 10.1207/s15326934crj1802_3

Craig, D. J. (2019). "If not us, then who? if not now, then when?" – nurses as change agents. *The Future of Nursing in Michigan, 5*(2),4-4,9. http://ezproxy2.library.drexel.edu/login?url=https://www-proquest-com.ezproxy2.library.drexel.edu/trade-journals/if-not-us-then-who-now-when-nurses-as-change/docview/2243618107/se-2?accountid=10559

Clyatt, C. (2017). Life as a cat herder: Leadership vs. management. *Leadership Excellence Essentials, 34*(4), 8.

Delgado, C., & Mitchell, M. M. (2016). A survey of current valued academic leadership qualities in nursing. *Nursing Education Perspectives, 37*(1), 10–15. 10.5480/14-1496

Denti, L. (2016). Top six components of a creative climate, innovation psychology. http://www.innovationmanagement.se/2013/05/22/top-six-components-of-a-creative-climate/

Dickenson-Hazard, N. (2004). Notes from the chief executive officer. *"I have experienced this before." Reflections on Nursing Leadership*, 30(2), 4, 38.

Diekelmann, N. L. (1995). Reawakening thinking: Is traditional pedagogy nearing completion? *Journal of Nursing Education*, 34(5), 195–196.

Donabedian, A. (2005). Evaluating the quality of medical care. *Millbank Quarterly*, 83(4), 691–729.

Dye, C. F., & Garman, A. N. (2006). *Exceptional leadership: 16 critical competencies for health care executives*. Health Administration Press.

Eads, M. (2016). The clinical nurse as an agent of change. *Medsurg Nursing*, 25(3), 173–175.

Eva, N., Robin, M., Sendjaya, S., van Dierendonck, D. & Liden, R. C. (2019). Servant Leadership: A systematic review and call for future research. *The Leadership Quarterly*, 30(1), 111–132, 10.1016/j.leaqua.2018.07.004. (http://www.sciencedirect.com/science/article/pii/S1048984317307774)

Faber, H. (2016). Three box solution for sustainable innovation, innovation psychology. http://www.innovationmanagement.se/2016/04/21/three-box-solution-for-sustainable-innovation

Frankel, A. (2011). What leadership styles should senior nurses develop? *Nursing Times*, 104(35), 23–24.

Getha-Taylor, H., Fowles, J., Silvia, C., & Merritt, C. C. (2015). Considering the effects of time on leadership development. *Public Personnel Management*, 44(3), 295–316. 10.1177/0091026015586265

Giddens, J. (2015) The innovation paradox. *Journal of Professional Nursing*, 31(4), 271–272.

Giddens, J. & Thompson, S. A. (2018). Preparing academic nursing leaders for today… and the future. *Journal of Professional Nursing*, 34, 73–74.

Glasgow, M. E. S., & Cornelius, F. H. (2005). Benefits and costs of integration of technology into an undergraduate nursing program. *Nursing Leadership Forum*, 9(4), 175.

Gleick, J. (1987). *Chaos: Making a new science*. New York, NY: Penguin Books.

Grant, A. B., & Massey, V. H. (1999). *Nursing leadership, management & research*. Springhouse Corporation.

Green, C. A. (2019). Workplace incivility: Nurse leaders as change agents. *Nursing Management*, 50, 51–53. https://doi.org/10.1097/01.NUMA.0000550455.99449.6b

Green, D. A. (2006). A synergy model of nursing education. *Journal for Nurses in Staff Development*, 22(6), 277–283.

Grenny, J., Maxfield, D., & Shimberg, A. (2008). How to have influence. *MIT Sloan Management Review*, 50(1), 47–52. http://sloanreview.mit.edu/article/how-to-have-influence

Grizzell, J. (2007). Behavior change theories and models. http://www.csupomona. edu/%7Ejvgrizzell/best_practices/bctheory.html#Reasoned%20Action

Hechanova, C. (2018). Implicit change leadership, change management, and affective commitment to change: Comparing academic institutions vs business enterprises. *Leadership & Organization Development Journal, 39*(7), 914–925. https:// doi.org/10.1108/LODJ-01-2018-0013

Hossain, K. A. (2015). Leadership qualities for 21st century leaders. *Pearl Journal of Management, Social Science and Humanities, 1*(1), 18–29.

Isaksen, S. G. (2009). Exploring the relationship between problem-solving style and creative psychological climate. In J. Funke, P. Meusburger, & E. Wunder (Eds.), *Knowledge and space: Milieus of creativity* (pp. 169–188). Springer Science+Business Media.

Isaksen, S. G., Aerts, W. S., & Isaksen, E. J. (2009). *Creating more innovative workplaces: Linking problem-solving style and organizational climate.* The Creative Problem Solving Group. http://www.cpsb.com/research/articles/featuredarticles/ Creating-Innovative-Workplaces.pdf

Isaksen, S. G., & Akkermans, H. J. (2007). *An introduction to climate.* Creative Problem Solving Group.

Jivraj Shariff, N. (2015). A Delphi survey of leadership attributes necessary for national nurse leaders' participation in health policy development: an East African perspective. *BMC Nursing, 14*(1), 13–13. https://doi.org/10.1186/ s12912-015-0063-0

Kee, J. E., & Newcomer, K. E. (2008). Why do change efforts fail? *Public Manager, 37*(3), 5–12.

King, W. (2011). What qualities must a leader have? *National Driller, 32*(2), 56.

Kritsonis, A. (2004–2005). Comparison of change theories. *International Journal of Scholarly Academic Intellectual Diversity, 8*(1), 1–7. http://www.nationalforum. com/Electronic%20Journal%20Volumes/Kritsonis,%20Alicia%20Comparison%20 of%20Change%20Theories.pdf

Ma Regina, M. H., Caringal-Go, J., & Magsaysay, J. F. (2018). Implicit change leadership, change management, and affective commitment to change. *Leadership & Organization Development Journal, 39*(7), 914–925. http://dx.doi.org.ezproxy2. library.drexel.edu/10.1108/LODJ-01-2018-0013

Magsaysay, J. F. and Hechanova, M. R. (2017). "Building an implicit change leadership theory", *Leadership and Organization Development Journal*, Vol. 38 No. 6, pp. 834–848.

Mahoney, J. (2001). Leadership skills for the 21st century. *Nursing Management, 9*(5), 269–271.

Martz, W. (2008). Evaluating organizational effectiveness. *Dissertation Abstracts International, 69*(07). Publication No. ATT3323530.

Martz, W. (2010). Validating evaluation checklists using a mixed method design. *Evaluation and Program Planning, 33*, 215–222. 10.1016/ j.evalprogplan.2009.10.005

Mattocks, S. (2019). Influence. *Journal of Trauma Nursing, 26*(6), 271–271. https:// doi.org/10.1097/JTN.0000000000000472

Meleis, A. I. (1999). Culturally competent care. *Journal of Transcultural Nursing*, 10(1), 12.

Meyer, R., & Meijers, R. (2017). Leadership agility: Developing your repertoire of leadership styles. ProQuest Ebook Central https://ebookcentral-proquest-com. ezproxy2.library.drexel.edu

Mumford, M. D., Scott, G. M., Gaddis, B., & Strange, J. M. (2002). Leading creative people: Orchestrating expertise and relationships. *Leadership Quarterly*, 13, 705–750.

Muteswa, R. P. T. (2015) Qualities of a good leader and the benefits of good leadership to an organization: A conceptual study, European Journal of Business and Management www.iiste.org ISSN 2222-1905 (Paper) ISSN 2222-2839 (Online) Vol.8, No.24, 2016. https://core.ac.uk/download/pdf/234627475.pdf

National Center for Cultural Competence. (n.d.). The compelling need for cultural and linguistic competence. http://nccc.georgetown.edu/foundations/need.html

Nauheimer, H. (2005). *Taking stock: A survey on the practice and future of change management*. Change Source.

Nelson, A., Anis-Abdellatif, M., Larson, J., Mulder, C., & Wolff, B. (2016). New faculty orientation: Discussion of cultural competency, sexual victimization, and student behaviors. *Journal of Continuing Education in Nursing*, 47(5), 228–233.

Nelson, D., Godfrey, L., & Purdy, J. (2004). Using a mentorship program to recruit and retain student nurses. *Journal of Nursing Administration*, 34(12), 551–553.

Ogbonna, E., & Harris, L. C. (2000). Leadership style, organizational culture and performance: Empirical evidence from UK companies. *International Journal of Human Resource Management*, 11(4), 766–788.

Olanrewaju, O. I., & Okorie, V. N. (2019). *Exploring the Qualities of a Good Leader Using Principal Component Analysis, Journal of Engineering, Project, and Production Management*, 9(2), 142–150. https://doi.org/10.2478/jeppm-2019-0016

Opollo, J. G., Bond, M. L., Gray, J., & Lail-Davis, V. J. (2012). Meeting tomorrow's health care needs through local and global involvement. *Journal of Continuing Education in Nursing*, 43(2), 75–80.

Pesut, D. J. & Thompson, S. A. (2018) Nursing leadership in academic nursing: The wisdom of development and the development of wisdom. *Journal of Professional Nursing*, 34.

Pillay, R., & Morris, M. H. (2016). Changing healthcare by changing the education of its leaders: An innovation competence model. *The Journal of Health Administration Education*, 33(3), 393–410.

Pullen, R. L. (2016). Leadership in nursing practice. *Nursing Made Incredibly Easy*, 14(3), 26–31.

Rafferty, A. M. (2018). Nurses as change agents for a better future in health care: The politics of drift and dilution. *Health Economics, Policy and Law*, 13(3-4), 475–491. http://dx.doi.org.ezproxy2.library.drexel.edu/10.1017/ S1744133117000482

Rogers, E. M. (2003). *Diffusion of innovations* (5th ed.). Free Press.

Rohrich, Rod & Durand, Paul. (2020). Mentors, Leaders, and Role Models: *Same or Different? Plastic & Reconstructive Surgery*, 145, 1099–1101. https:// doi.org/10.1097/PRS.0000000000006702

Ross, E. J., Fitzpatrick, J. J., Click, E. R., Krouse, H. J., & Clavelle, J. T. (2014). Transformational leadership practices of nurse leaders in professional nursing associations. *Journal of Nursing Administration, 44*(4), 201–206.

Rowlings, M. (2016). Innovative workplace benefits: Perks employees look for, innovation psychology. http://www.innovationmanagement.se/2016/03/15/innovative-workplace-benefits-perks-employees-look-for

Rubino, L. (2011). Leadership. In S. B. Buchbinder & N. H. Shanks (Eds.), *Leadership, in introduction to health care management* (2nd ed.). Jones & Bartlett Learning.

Saha, S., Beach, M., & Cooper, L. (2008). Patient centeredness, cultural competence and health care quality. *Journal of the National Medical Association, 100*(11), 1275–1285.

Sandeen, C. A. (2010). Fostering creativity and innovation in the workforce: An annotated bibliography. *Continuing Higher Education Review, 74*, 93–100.

Schmidt, M. (2017). Becoming Inclusive: A Code of Conduct for Inclusion and Diversity. *Journal of Professional Nursing, 33*(2), 102–107. https://doi.org/10.1016/j.profnurs.2016.08.014

Shahzad, F., Luqman, R. A., Khan, A. R., & Shabbir, L. (2012). Impact of organizational culture on organizational performance: An overview. *Interdisciplinary Journal of Contemporary Research in Business, 3*(9), 975–985.

Sims, J. M. (2009). Styles and qualities of effective leaders. *Dimensions of Critical Care Nursing, 28*(6), 272–274.

Snow, F. (2019). Creativity and innovation: An essential competency for the nurse leader. *Nursing Administration Quarterly, 43*, 306–312. https://doi.org/10.1097/NAQ.0000000000000367

Strom, K. (2001). Quality improvement interventions: What works? *Journal for Health Care Quality, 23*(5), 4–14.

Thibodeaux, M. S., & Favilla, E. (1996). Organizational effectiveness and commitment through strategic management. *Industrial Management & Data Systems, 96*(5), 21–25.

Thompson, S. A. & Miller, K. L. (2018). Disruptive trends in higher education: Leadership skills for successful leaders. *Journal of Professional Nursing, 34*, 92–96.

Udod, S. & Wagner, J. (2018). *Common change theories and application to different nursing situations in Leadership and influencing change in nursing*, University of Regina Press, ISBN 9780889775480 https://leadershipandinfluencingchangeinnursing.pressbooks.com/front-matter/about-the-book/

Vaidyanathan, S. (2012). Fostering creativity and innovation through technology. *Learning & Leading With Technology, 39*(6), 24–27.

Veenema, T. G., Griffin, A., Gable, A. R., MacIntyre, L., Simons, N., Couig, M. P., . . . Larson, E. (2015). Nurses as leaders in disaster preparedness and response: A call to action. *Journal of Nursing Scholarship, 48*(2), 187–200. 10.1111/jnu.12198

Weber, E., Ward, J. & Walsh, T. (2015). Nurse leader competencies: A toolkit for success. *Nursing Management, 46*, 47–50. https://doi.org/10.1097/01.NUMA.0000473505.23431.85

White, A. (2004). Change strategies make for smooth transitions. *Nursing Management, 35*(2), 49–52.

White, K. (2021). *Change theory and models: Framework for translation. In Translation of evidence into nursing and healthcare* (3rd ed.). Springer Publishing Company.

Willcoxson, L., & Millett, B. (2000). The management of organisational culture. *Australian Journal of Management & Organisational Behaviour*, 3(2), 100–106.

Wilson, L. (2007). 2229-Wilson-PADCNETC_Abstract. Grants.hrsa.gov via https://www.google.com/url?sa=t&rct=j&q=&esrc=s&source=web&cd=3&ved=0ahUKEwi_9OfTrL3QAhUn44MKHZ8uDd4QFggiMAI&url=https%3A%2F%2Fgrants.hrsa.gov%2F2010%2Fweb2Internal%2FInterface%2FCommon%2FPublicWebLink-Controller.aspx%3FGrantNumber%3DU1KHP09542%26WL_WEBLINK_ID%3D1&usg=AFQjCNH93vnTW60vyypAzoWqwh49JyepTg

Wilson, D. M., Anafi, F., Kusi-Appiah, E., Darko, E. M., Deck, K., & Errasti-Ibarrondo, B. (2020). Determining if nurses are involved in political action or politics: A scoping literature review, *Applied Nursing Research*, 54, ISSN 0897-1897, https://doi.org/10.1016/j.apnr.2020.151279.

Yoder-Wise, P. S. (2011). *Leading and managing in nursing* (5th ed.). Elsevier.

Engaging in the Scholarship of Teaching

14

Diane M. Billings and Susan H. Kelly

Education is the most powerful weapon which you can use to change the world.
—Nelson Mandela

▶ LEARNING OUTCOMES

This chapter addresses the Certified Nurse Educator Exam Content Area 6B: Engage in the Scholarship of Teaching (Content Area 6, which includes 6A, 6B, and 6C, makes up 15% of the examination, approximately 22 questions). For the Certified Nurse Educator Novice Exam it is Content area 7 and makes up 4% of the exam approximately 6 questions

- Discuss the meaning of scholarship in the nurse educator role
- Identify the four types of scholarship outlined by Boyer
- Differentiate between the scholarship of teaching and the scholarship of teaching–learning and being a scholar
- Exhibit a spirit of inquiry about teaching, learning, and evaluation
- Identify the attributes of the science of nursing education
- Learn how to participate in research activities related to nursing education
- Appreciate the knowledge developed from evidence in education
- Demonstrate integrity as a scholar

INTRODUCTION

Being a scholar and engaging in scholarship is an important aspect of the role of nurse educator. This chapter defines Boyer's model of scholarship and the Carnegie Foundation's work in promoting the scholarship of teaching and learning (SoTL). This chapter also discusses the ways nurse educators can engage in scholarship and develop the science of nursing education by participating in research activities and demonstrating integrity as a scholar.

SCHOLARSHIP IN NURSING AND NURSING EDUCATION

A scholar is a person who has particular knowledge in an area of specialization. A scholar has a spirit of inquiry and is able to think logically and communicate effectively. Scholarship is a hallmark of nursing and is an expectation of all nurse educators. The American Association of Colleges of Nursing (AACN; 1999) defined scholarship in nursing as those activities that systematically advance the teaching, research, and practice of nursing through rigorous inquiry that (a) is significant to the profession, (b) is creative, (c) can be documented, (d) can be replicated or elaborated, and (e) can be peer-reviewed through various methods. Scholarship in nursing education is an inquiry process that results in outcomes; for example, innovations such as simulation-based education; strategies used in developing competency; developing and redeveloping courses, teaching–learning strategies; the development of courses, new technologies to administer course materials and/or curricula; and the development of measures to assess and evaluate student learning. Scholarship in nursing education is recognized by peer reviews of the outcomes of teaching–learning practices, awards for teaching excellence, receipt of grants, and invitations to consult or share the scholarly work with others. While scholarship is recognized by presentations, it is the dissemination and peer-reviewed publications that garner the critical need to be shared for the public to review and critique (Oermann, 2017).

 ## THE SCHOLAR'S ROLE

The role of the nursing scholar is to develop and disseminate evidence for best practices in nursing education. The scholarly role is expected of nurse educators who work in schools of nursing. The scholar's role is demonstrated by:

- Critiquing evidence for practice in nursing education
- Using evidence for teaching and learning in one's own practice
- Identifying current and relevant issues for research in teaching and learning outcomes and curriculum impact
- Conducting research in areas to strengthen teaching and learning outcomes curriculum impact
- Disseminating research findings for publication in peer-reviewed journals
- Appointments to committees of professional organizations
- Appointments on editorial boards of journals related to teaching and learning

 ## BOYER'S MODEL OF SCHOLARSHIP

Boyer's model of scholarship is a model that is used in many schools of nursing and institutions of higher learning to guide the work of faculty. This model, proposed by Ernest Boyer (1990), describes four types of scholarship that form the basis of scholarly work and contribute to effective teaching and learning. Although distinct, in practice, the four types of scholarship are often integrated. Boyer's four types of scholarship are:

- Scholarship of discovery (knowing)—research or discovery of new knowledge, systematic inquiry, validation of existing knowledge, and the use of methods to develop a strong basis for practice-related knowledge. Discovery may be disseminated through various methods; however, for teaching to be considered scholarship, it must be clearly documented, peer-reviewed, and disseminated (Acorn & Osborn, 2013)

Example: A nurse educator is using podcasting as a teaching-learning strategy with senior baccalaureate students. The nurse educator conducts a study to determine whether the use of podcasting is appropriate for students with specific types of learning styles.

■ Scholarship of integration—interpretation and synthesis of knowledge; may cross the disciplinary boundaries allowing for new connections. This allows information from different perspectives and requires critical analysis of the research findings.

Example: A nurse educator reviews the health sciences literature about using simulation-based education (SBE) for teaching students to manage a patient in a diabetic crisis. The nurse educator develops a multidisciplinary SBE for students in nursing, pharmacy, and allied health sciences. The collaboration would allow for an evidence-based study to be disseminated for publication in other peer-reviewed journals.

■ Scholarship of application—engagement of the scholar in service-related activities resulting in tangible outcomes. Connects theory and practice; seeks to apply knowledge to significant problems; is a translational work, which assists end users to integrate the findings into their practices; application is also evident in service to the profession.

Example: A nurse educator who has an area of expertise in team-based learning presents the outcomes of the work at a national meeting and then consults with schools to help them integrate the method into their own academic programs and classrooms.

■ Scholarship of teaching—the use of evidence to facilitate learning; the scholarship of teaching also involves identifying a problem, testing strategies, and making teaching and learning public through self-reflection, peer review, and the dissemination of work in appropriate disciplinary journals

Example: A nurse educator collaborates with other nurse educators to develop a method to assess student learning and outcomes on medication administration. The educators use various pedagogical methods in the classroom and lab, which results in an improvement in student learning, higher test scores, and positive feedback from students. The nurse educators develop a manuscript to share the findings of this pedagogical approach for better student outcomes. The manuscript is accepted for publication for wider dissemination and the potential to further the evaluation methods.

▶ THE USE OF BOYER'S MODEL

Boyer's model is used in nursing education as a framework for:

■ Appointment
■ Performance evaluation
■ Demonstration of merit for awards and pay increases
■ Promotion and tenure guidelines
■ Organizing the professional portfolio

EVIDENCE-BASED TEACHING PRACTICE

Fang and Mainous (2019) studied the percentage of deans (2001–2011) who left their positions before 5 years and found that it was 41%. The results of this quantitative study demonstrated that deans in the smaller program have a more likely chance of leaving before five years. Other variables that increased turnover were; age 60 or older, deans with a title as Chair, Director, or Department Head, deans schools without a tenure system, and deans in baccalaureate or associate degree-granting programs.

SCHOLARLY TEACHING, SCHOLARSHIP OF TEACHING, SoTL, AND BEING A SCHOLAR

Educators make a distinction among good teaching, scholarly teaching, scholarship of teaching, SoTL, and being a scholar.

- Good teaching—good teaching is typically defined by student satisfaction and positive student ratings of teaching (Allen & Field, 2005). It involves understanding the students and using effective teaching–learning practices.
- Scholarly teaching—scholarly teaching refers to nurse educator's use of practice wisdom, reflections on the effectiveness of one's own approach to teaching and evaluation, and the use of evidence to guide teaching practice (Allen & Field, 2005). Scholarly teaching involves a systematic study of teaching and learning practices and may result in the dissemination of knowledge through presentations and publications.
- Scholarship of teaching—scholarship of teaching refers to teaching that extends beyond the classroom (Allen & Field, 2005). Scholarship of teaching may include the development of products (simulations, books, games, and podcasts) that can be used by learners and others, development of teaching models that can be shared and replicated, or development of innovative curricula that are implemented state-wide or serve as examples of curriculum development for others. Scholarship of teaching also involves using evidence-based teaching practices (EBTPs) and conducting research about teaching and learning. Nurse educators demonstrate scholarship of teaching when they publish their work in peer-reviewed journals; disseminate their work in poster or podium presentations at local, national, and international meetings; obtain peer review from colleagues; and are recipients of grants.
- The SoTL—the SoTL is an initiative of the Carnegie Foundation (2013) that builds on Boyer's model of scholarship to enhance the value of teaching, advocate for student learning, and bring recognition to teaching as scholarly work. Many campuses have communities of faculty who collaborate to explore, share, and recognize each other's work to develop the SoTL.
- Being a scholar—This involves developing habits of inquiry and intellectual persistence. Scholars seek truth, challenge assumptions, demonstrate integrity, continually learn, and seek review of their work. Being a scholar is a prerequisite for scholarly teaching, using evidence-based teaching, and developing the science of nursing education.

DEVELOPING A SPIRIT OF INQUIRY ABOUT TEACHING, LEARNING, AND EVALUATION

Nurse educators develop a spirit of inquiry by reflecting on their own practice; being open to new ideas; reviewing the literature for evidence of best practices in teaching, learning, and evaluation; and determining whether the use of evidence warrants changes in their own teaching practices. Nurse educators also demonstrate a spirit of inquiry when they identify gaps in the literature and conduct or participate in research that will seek answers to problems related to teaching, learning, and evaluation. Nurse educators are lifelong learners who strive to improve their teaching practice by seeking evidence for their practice.

LIFELONG LEARNER

Nurse educators are experts in their clinical field, however, they may need to learn the skill of item-writing. It is a skill that needs to be perfected and can take time to learn. Educators learn and continue to work to perfect their skill to be successful in item writing (Kranz, Love, & Roche, 2019).

THE SCIENCE OF NURSING EDUCATION

The **science of nursing education** refers to the research-based foundation on which the best practices for teaching nursing are developed and tested. Building the science of nursing education involves:

- Defining a significant problem or issue
- Critiquing the literature and identifying gaps
- Developing or using a framework to guide research
- Designing studies using classroom, multisite, and/or multi-methods
- Conducting studies using classroom, multisite, and/or multi-methods
- Disseminating findings by sharing effective teaching or evaluation strategies and summaries of surveys about classroom practices. Dissemination also takes place when nurse educators present findings from research studies. Evidence of dissemination includes publications and presentations. Publications in peer-reviewed and indexed journals are more highly valued than publications in journals with limited circulation or abstracts in conference proceedings and newsletters; the publication of scholarly work is preferred to presentations at scientific meetings. Publication is a learned skill that can be assisted through mentorship of experts (Oermann & Hayes, 2011).
- Using evidence in scholarship and research: The cycle of scholarship and research is complete when nurse educators base their curriculum development, teaching, evaluation, and use of technology on evidence. Evidence can be found in nursing journals that report study findings, at conferences where papers are presented, and at school and university scholarship days where the results of pilot studies and classroom research are presented. Increasingly, nursing education scholarship and research are interdisciplinary, and evidence for nursing education practice is available in a variety of venues. All nurse educators must read the evidence, test it in their classrooms, and then determine the best practices for their own students.

EVIDENCE-BASED TEACHING PRACTICE

Whalen and colleagues (2020) proposed using Inquiry Project Coordinators to assist clinically-based nursing scholars to produce scholarly projects, including evidence-based practice, quality improvement, and research. This project assists with the direct application of scholarship.

DEVELOPING THE SCIENCE OF NURSING EDUCATION

Nurse educators also have responsibilities for developing the science of nursing education by conducting or participating in research and scholarly work. Developing the science of nursing education:

- Can be conducted by educators, regardless of educational preparation, who participate in the research process as leaders or members of a research team
- Requires the researcher and research team to maintain integrity as scholars by ensuring the protection of human subjects, safeguarding data, using ethical approaches to inquiry, and collaborating with others.
- Can involve collaboration with colleagues at the same and other institutions (multisite research) and with colleagues in other disciplines (interdisciplinary research)

TEACHING GEM Seibert and Harper (2020) suggest the scholarship of application can be applied to nursing because they present "an opportunity for academic faculty to showcase knowledge and skills that could promote the health of communities" (p. 152).

DEMONSTRATING INTEGRITY AS A SCHOLAR

Scholarly integrity involves the observance of ethical principles in teaching, service, and the conduct of research while working as an individual faculty member, member of a research team, and while supervising the scholarly work and research conducted by students. Most colleges and universities have policies about maintaining scholarly integrity, procedures for monitoring integrity of faculty and students, and consequences for misconduct. Nurse educators maintain integrity as scholars by:

- Assuming responsibility for the intellectual quality of their work
- Recognizing and citing works of others to avoid misrepresenting them as their own works
- Protecting human subjects when conducting research by seeking approval of an institutional review board (IRB) before conducting and publishing studies
- Safeguarding data when conducting research
- Safeguarding students when implementing or testing new strategies for teaching, learning, or evaluation
- Observing principles of ethics when serving on research teams
- Establishing clear guidelines for ownership of data or products and publication credit prior to initiating a study or project (Oermann & Hayes, 2011)

- Following publication guidelines for authorship credit
- Serving as a role model for students in the use of evidence and conduct of research
- Being a mentor and role model for students and colleagues
- Conducting peer review of teaching, manuscripts, publications
- Observing codes of civility in communications with others

FUNDING THE SCIENCE OF NURSING EDUCATION

Funding for nursing education research comes from a variety of sources. Professional nursing education organizations, such as the NLN (2007), AACN, Sigma Theta Tau International, and a variety of specialty organizations have grant programs to fund nursing education research. Also, most colleges and universities have small funds for classroom research. Funding for projects and research that involves educational reform may be sought from foundations, such as the Robert Wood Johnson Foundation or the Macy Foundation, or federal sources such as the Health Resources and Service Administration (HRSA) or the Department of Education. Nurse educators who are involved in interprofessional research can also seek funding from agencies that are funding collaborative research.

EVIDENCE-BASED TEACHING PRACTICE

EBTP in nursing is the use of evidence to make decisions about developing educational programs, choosing the best teaching–learning strategies to achieve outcomes for a particular group of students in a particular setting, and selecting appropriate methods for evaluation. EBTP:

- draws on research in nursing education, higher education, psychology, and allied health disciplines
- uses wisdom and accepted practices and is guided by theory and empirical testing
- questions existing teaching–learning practices that are unfounded, based in tradition, and have not been tested

---

EVIDENCE-BASED TEACHING PRACTICE

Simmonds et al. (2020) completed a literature review about pedagogical practices that contribute to undergraduate nursing students' professional identity formation. Using a six-stage methodological framework, the researchers analyzed 114 manuscripts and found a wide range of areas that contribute to the multidimensional elements of nursing identity formation. Included in the variables were the pedagogical practices and learning outcomes that guide course design.

TEACHING GEM If a nurse educator is notified by a nurse educator graduate student or established researcher who would like to use his or her learners as subjects, the researcher should be advised to contact the IRB of the university and the departmental chair or dean. IRB approval from the researcher's institution does not automatically translate to IRB approval in the institution of the planned study site.

CASE STUDIES

CASE STUDY 14.1

A team of three nurse educators teaches a nursing skills course in a learning resources center, and each has the responsibility for clinical supervision of 10 students on a medical–surgical nursing unit at the local hospital. One of the educators, an associate professor, has a doctorate in clinical nursing; two of the nurses have MSN degrees in nursing and are clinical instructors. Scholarship is included in the appointment requirements for all faculty at the school of nursing. The teaching team has noticed that students frequently break the sterile field when changing a sterile dressing. The nurse educators would like to conduct a study to determine whether using simulation with a low-fidelity manikin versus using return demonstration would improve the students' ability to change a sterile dressing correctly.

What is the evidence that needs to be obtained to determine the best practices for teaching students to change a sterile dressing? What steps are needed to design the study? What resources will the faculty need to conduct this study? Will conducting the study fulfill requirements for producing "scholarly work" to meet the criteria for their rank? What will be the most appropriate roles on the research team for each of the nurse educators?

CASE STUDY 14.2

A nurse educator with a doctorate is appointed as an assistant professor of nursing. The nurse educator will have to teach nine credits of undergraduate courses each semester and is expected to develop a program of research and provide service to the school. The school uses Boyer's model of scholarship, and within 5 years, the nurse educator will be expected to have published several articles, obtained excellent ratings in the area of teaching, and provided leadership to the school in the nurse educator's area of expertise. The nurse educator's mentor asks the nurse educator to identify an area of expertise for the program of research.

What factors should the nurse educator consider when identifying an area of expertise for developing a program of research? How can the nurse educator best work with a mentor? What strategies should the nurse educator consider when attempting to meet the expectations for excellence in the three primary areas noted in Boyer's model? What goals and priorities should the nurse educator set for the first year?

Is teaching nine credits each semester a reasonable workload, given the other expectations for productivity?

1. A nurse educator has experience with preparing students for standardized exams and the National Council of State Boards Examination (NCLEX). Which of the following would indicate the educator is meeting the expectations for scholarship of discovery?

    A. The educator conducts critical research on student performance on standardized testing

    B. The educator offers a continuing education program to other faculty at the school

    C. The educator serves on a task force for the state board of nursing on developing methods of retention of nurses

    D. The educator presents findings from a survey at a national meeting for nurse educators

2. The promotion and tenure committee at a school of nursing is reviewing a nurse educator's dossier for promotion to associate professor. Which of the following indicates the nurse educator is demonstrating the scholarship of integration? The dossier indicates the nurse educator:

    A. Has received consistently excellent student reviews of teaching over six semesters

    B. Has created and implemented an interprofessional scenario to be used in a simulation

    C. Has improved teaching following a peer review

    D. Has published three articles about innovative teaching in peer-reviewed journals

3. The scholarship of teaching is teaching that extends beyond the classroom. Which response by a new nurse educator would require a better understanding of the scholarship of teaching?

    A. The nurse educator received an award for teaching excellence from a student organization

    B. The nurse educator developed an escape room for senior nursing students

    C. The nurse educator was involved in an innovative curriculum change shared with other institutions

    D. The nurse educator presented her new escape room at a national conference

1. A) The educator conducts critical research on student performance on standardized testing

Conducting research on students' performance in standardized testing is using research or evidence to promote teaching. Continuing education, serving on a task force, and presenting findings are all examples of the scholarship of application.

2. B) Has created and implemented an interprofessional scenario to be used in a simulation

The interprofessional activity demonstrated the scholarship of integration. Student evaluations and process improvement are the scholarship of application, and publishing articles about teaching is the scholarship of teaching.

3. D) The nurse educator presented a new escape room at a national conference

Presenting an innovative teaching technique is the scholarship of teaching. Developing the technique is the scholarship of application, as is sharing a curriculum change. Receiving an award is the scholarship of application.

4. When reviewing an end-of-course evaluation about the faculty's teaching skills, the department chair asks the faculty member to attend a workshop to learn about effective teaching strategies. The faculty member asks the department chair why it is necessary to attend this workshop. What is the best response the department chair can give to the faculty?

   A. Effective teaching means that faculty as scholars are also learners with specialized skills in teaching strategies and evaluation methods

   B. An effective teacher needs to be strong in their specialized clinical area with little regard for scholarship

   C. Effective teaching means that faculty are only scholars focusing on research and scholarship

   D. Faculty must attend continuing education programs, or they will fail to be effective educators

5. A newly employed nurse educator is interested in conducting a study with undergraduate students in a sophomore-level fundamentals course. The educator is not doctorally prepared and informs the mentor that they do not have the qualifications to conduct the study. What response by the mentor is the most appropriate?

   A. It is imperative to be doctorally prepared to conduct any research study

   B. As long as you are pursuing your doctoral degree, you may conduct the research study

   C. Regardless of education preparation, you may conduct a research study

   D. A senior faculty member must conduct the research study with you

6. Boyer's model of scholarship is most appropriately used to guide which of the following decisions?

   A. Determining an area of research to pursue

   B. Awarding promotion and tenure

   C. Selecting a nursing organization to join

   D. Choosing a mentor

7. A nurse educator is seeking funding to conduct a pilot study of the effects of remote testing compared to face-to-face testing in the educator's classroom. The nurse educator should first seek funding from:

   A. The university's research fund for teaching and learning

   B. Health Resources and Services Administration (HRSA)

   C. National Institutes of Health (NIH)

   D. Robert Wood Johnson Foundation

(See answers next page.)

4. A) Effective teaching means that faculty as scholars are also learners with specialized skills in teaching strategies and evaluation methods

Effective teaching requires the ability to engage in research and scholarship. "Faculty must attend continuing education programs, or they will fail to be effective educators" is not an appropriate answer; it is negative and non-supportive. Effective teaching does not always depend on a research focus or clinical competency.

5. C) Regardless of education preparation, you may conduct a research study

All nurses can conduct a research study as long as they understand the IRB process and where to find resources if needed. Research development is not contingent on degree or years of service.

6. B) Awarding promotion and tenure

Boyer's model of scholarship is used to develop promotion and tenure criteria for excellence in teaching that will help the review committee make decisions about appointment, performance review, promotion, and tenure. Boyer's model is not used to determine a research area, selecting a nursing organization, or choosing a mentor.

7. A) The university's research fund for teaching and learning

This pilot study that is confined to one classroom would warrant a small internal grant. Larger foundational and federal grants usually involve much larger projects.

8. A nurse educator administers a standardized learning-style inventory to incoming students and is planning to use the findings to establish a databank for future analysis. The nurse educator should first:

    A. Administer the learning-style inventory and request the GPA for each student from the student services office

    B. Administer the learning-style inventory and ask each student to self-report their GPA

    C. Seek review and approval from the institutional review board (IRB) to conduct this study

    D. Find a colleague with research skills to be a coinvestigator for this project

9. A nurse educator is conducting a study on student's scores on a standardized exam. The nurse educator is using aggregate data from previous students' scores in comparison with current senior nursing students. Which response by the nurse educator about conducting the study would be inappropriate?

    A. All information needs to be kept confidential and not shared with students

    B. IRB approval is not needed to collect the aggregate data from previous students since they have graduated

    C. I will ask a colleague to assist me in conducting this study

    D. I should explain the study and have students sign a letter of consent for the study

10. An educator has developed a simulation-based education (SBE) activity and conducted a study to evaluate student learning and student satisfaction with the simulation. Results indicated improved test scores and high ratings of satisfaction from students. The nurse educator and colleagues develop a manuscript that is published for wide dissemination. Which element of Boyer's Model of Scholarship is this an example of?

    A. Scholarship of Application

    B. Scholarship of Teaching

    C. Scholarship of Integration

    D. Scholarship of Discovery

(*See answers next page.*)

8. C) Seek review and approval from the institutional review board (IRB) to conduct this study

IRB approval is needed to collect data and store the data for future use. It does not say that the data is de-identified. Administering the learning-style inventory and requesting the GPA for each student from the student services office requires IRB approval. Administering the learning-style inventory and asking each student to self-report their GPA is inappropriate if the participants do not consent and are not knowledgeable about why they are divulging the information. The project needs to be approved before finding a colleague with research skills to be a coinvestigator for this project.

9. B) IRB approval is not needed to collect the aggregate data from previous students since they have graduated

IRB approval is needed for all student data. The students should know and consent to data being collected.

10. B) Scholarship of Teaching

The nurse educator uses evidence to facilitate learning and makes it public through dissemination. It is not integration because it does not involve other disciplines, it is not pure discovery because it is applied to teaching specifically, and it is not application because it does not assist the end user outside of teaching.

REFERENCES

Acorn, S., & Osborne, M. (2013). Scholarship in nursing: Current view. *Nursing Leadership (Toronto, Ont.)*, *26*(1), 24–29.

Allen, M. N., & Field, P. A. (2005). Scholarly teaching and scholarship of teaching: Noting the difference. *International Journal of Nursing Education Scholarship*, *2*(1), Article 12. https://www.ncbi.nlm.nih.gov/pubmed/16646906

American Association of Colleges of Nursing. (1999). Defining scholarship for the profession of nursing. http://www.aacn.nche.edu/publications/position/defining-scholarship

Boyer, E. (1990). *Scholarship reconsidered: Priorities of the professoriate*. Jossey-Bass.

Carnegie Foundation. (2013). Carnegie Academy for the Scholarship of Teaching and Learning. http://www.carnegiefoundation.org/scholarship-teaching-learning

Fang, D. & Mainous, R. (2019). Individual and institutional characteristics associated with short tenures of deanships in academic nursing. *Nursing Outlook*, *67*(5), 578–585. 10.1016/j.outlook.2019.03.002

Kranz, C., Love, A., & Roche, C. (2019). How to write a good test question: Nine tips for novice nurse educators. *The Journal of Continuing Education in Nursing*, *50*(1), 12–14.

National League for Nursing. (2021). Certified Nurse Educator (CNE) 2021 candidate handbook. http://www.nln.org/docs/default-source/default-document-library/cne-handbook-2021_revised_07-01-2021.pdf?sfvrsn=2

National League for Nursing. (2021). Certified Nurse Educator Novice (CNEn) 2021 candidate handbook. http://www.nln.org/Certification-for-Nurse-Educators/cne-n/cne-n-handbook

Oermann, M. H. (2017). Building your scholarship from your teaching: Plan now. *Nurse Educator*, *42*(5), 217.

Oermann, M. H., & Hayes, J. C. (2011). *Writing for publication in nursing* (2nd ed.). Springer Publishing.

Seibert, S. A. & Harper, K. J. (2020).The Scholarship of Application: Opportunities within the NOBC. *Teaching & Learning in Nursing*, *15*(2), 152–154. 10.1016/j.teln.2020.01.005

Simmonds, A. Nunn, A., Gray, M., Hardie, C., Mayo, S. Peter, E., & Richards, J. (2020). Pedagogical practices that influence professional identity formation in baccalaureate nursing education: A scoping review. *Nursing Education Today*, *93*. 10.1016/j.nedt.2020.104516

Whalen, M., Baptiste, D., & Maliszewski, B. (2020). Increasing nursing scholarship through dedicated human resources: Creating a culture of nursing inquiry. *Journal of Nursing Administration*, *50*(2), 90–94. 10.1097/NNA.0000000000000847

Functioning Effectively Within the Institutional Environment and Academic Community

Mary Ellen Smith Glasgow

The time is always right to do what is right.
—Martin Luther King Jr.

▶ LEARNING OUTCOMES

This chapter addresses the Certified Nurse Educator Exam Content Area 6C: Function Effectively Within the Institutional Environment and the Academic Community (Content Area 6, which includes 6A, 6B, and 6C, make up 15% of the examination, approximately 22 questions) and the Certified Nurse Educator Novice exam Area 8 which makes up 11% of the exam or approximately 17 questions

- Identify internal and external factors influencing nursing education
- Describe the relationship of the mission of the parent institution with that of the nursing curriculum
- Discuss the impact of the organizational climate on the development of the nurse educator
- Elaborate on the importance of a professional career development trajectory for nurse educators
- Investigate the concepts of mentorship and protégé as they relate to the educator role
- Analyze the nurse educator's leadership role with respect to institutional governance

● INTRODUCTION

This chapter focuses on the nurse educator's roles and responsibilities within the institutional environment and academic community, with particular emphasis on teaching, research/scholarship, and service requirements, as well as internal and external forces affecting nursing education.

INTERNAL AND EXTERNAL FORCES INFLUENCING NURSING AND HIGHER EDUCATION

The faculty role in most institutions of higher education has evolved from that of a single-focused mission of teaching to a triad of teaching, scholarship, and service. Nursing education has evolved over the decades from being housed in the service sector setting to the college and university setting (Finke, 2012). As nursing education entered the university setting, nursing faculty were held to the same research and scholarship standards as their non-nursing academic colleagues. The emphasis on research and scholarship continues to be a benchmark for nursing faculty productivity in most university settings, particularly at research and comprehensive universities. There are many other internal and external forces influencing both nursing education and higher education today. These driving forces include:

- Multiculturalism of society
- Expanding technology, including distance education and simulation
- Interdisciplinary professional education
- Complexity of clinical care (technology, telehealth)
- Limited financial resources
- Nursing faculty shortage
- Regional nursing shortages
- Aging population
- Health disparities
- Knowledge explosion
- Emphasis on the "learner" instead of the "teacher" in relation to pedagogy
- Increased demand for accountability
- Outcomes assessment
- Accreditation requirements
- Federal funding
- Economic climate
- Political landscape
- Healthcare reform
- Global society (information exchange, infectious diseases)

External landmark reports have made strong recommendations to nursing education and the nursing profession in general. Among these, *The Future of Nursing Report: Leading Change, Advancing Health* (Institute of Medicine, 2010) recommended that "nurses should achieve higher levels of education and training through an improved education system that promotes seamless academic progression" (p. 4-1). Such education needs to provide learners with "a better understanding of and experience in care management, quality improvement methods, systems-level change management, and the reconceptualized roles of nurses in a reformed health care system" (p. 4-1). Nurse educators need to create academic programs that are competency-based and interdisciplinary in nature, inspiring lifelong learning, and promoting the diversity of the student population. The report proposes "strategies to shape the future of healthcare by creating models of nursing education focused not only on curriculum changes, but also, on transforming the student population, integrating the science and research in the curriculum and influencing health care policy" (Smith Glasgow, Dunphy, & Mainous, 2010, p. G9). This document also calls for educating nurses to work and lead collaboratively with other healthcare professionals to improve the quality and safety of healthcare delivery, expand access to quality healthcare within our communities, and redesign our healthcare systems to ensure the skills and competencies of nurses are fully utilized to the benefit of patients.

The 2010 Carnegie Foundation study (Benner, Sutphen, Leonard, & Day, 2010) called for educators to transform nursing education. This report noted that "nursing education needs teachers with a deep nursing knowledge who also know how to teach and conduct research on nursing education" (p. 6).

Enrolment, curriculum design, pedagogy, faculty expectations, faculty competencies, and scholarly productivity are all shaped by social, political, and economic forces. For example, societal multiculturalism will continue to shape curricula, and faculty will need to understand and respond to a culturally diverse student body and to teach them how to effectively meet the cultural needs of patients (Diaz, Clarke, & Gatua, 2015; Latham, Singh, & Ringl, 2016; Young & Lu, 2018). Today, changing demographics, culture, and linguistic diversity need to be emphasized in nursing curricula at all levels. Curricula need to be continually re-examined in light of these internal and external forces.

▶ PREPARATION FOR THE FACULTY ROLE

The nurse educator role requires specialized preparation. It is critical that nurse educators are cognizant of teaching, learning, and evaluation and have knowledge and skill in curriculum development, assessment of program outcomes, and being an effective member of an academic community (National League for Nursing, n.d.). Just as one would never be allowed to practice as a nurse practitioner without formal course work and supervised clinical practice, one should not be allowed to practice as an educator without formal course work and supervised teaching practice. Nursing faculty need specialized course work on teaching/learning, learning styles, how the brain works in relation to learning, curriculum development, program evaluation, the multiple demands of the educator role, the dynamics of academe, resolution of student-related issues, course development, effective student advisement, innovative teaching strategies, online pedagogy, and relevant educational research. Nurse educators should be knowledgeable about the nationally endorsed nurse educator competencies (Fitzgerald, McNelis, & Billings, 2020) and certification (NLN's Certified Nurse Educator) available to document one's expertise as an educator (NLN, n.d.; Valiga, 2016; Summer 2017).

EVIDENCE-BASED TEACHING PRACTICE

Fitzgerald, Mc Nelis, and Billings (2020) explored the representation of the NLN Core Competencies for Nurse Educators in Masters of Science in Nursing Education (MSN Ed) and Post-Masters Certificate (PMC) program in course descriptions. A descriptive design using a web scraping technique served to collect study data.

At the time of the study, the AACN listed 484 schools offering master's or postmaster certificate programs in nursing, and the ACEN listed 92 schools. Of the 576 total, the final sample size for the study was 529 schools (92%) and included 317 (60%) programs with MSN Ed programs and 212 (40%) with PMC programs. Schools that offered both the MSN Ed and PMC programs totaled 174, while 143 schools offered MSN Ed only and 38 schools offered PMC only.

Total credit hours in MSN Ed programs ranged from 28 to 65 with a mean of 39 (SD = 5.3); nursing education focus area credit hours ranged from 6 to 47 with a mean of 19 (SD = 7.5). The PMC program credit hours ranged from 3 to 45 with a mean of 15 (SD = 5.2). The majority of both programs (89%) required a practicum course. Almost all practicum hours were reported as credit hours; however, a few practicum courses were reported as clock hours, precluding a consistent method of reporting the actual number of hours of the experience. Nursing education practica credit hours ranged from 1 to 18 for MSN Ed programs and 1 to 14 for PMC programs. Mean practicum credit hours were 4.4 for MSN Ed (SD = 2.2) and 4.6 for PMC programs (SD = 1.9). A total of 23 programs used clock hours when reporting clinical practica requirements for both MSN Ed and PMC programs; clock hours ranged from 60 to 500 with a mean of 186 hours (SD = 101.6). Forty-two (13%) MSN Ed programs used courses from schools outside nursing to fulfill or complement program requirements. Courses in the school of education were used most frequently ($n = 25$); additional courses were from an education subspecialty or other departments, such as statistics, biology, or ethics. Notably, every state in the United States, except Hawaii, offered either an MSN Ed or PMC. Of the 529 MSN Ed and PMC programs, 199 (37%) were completely distance accessible. Only 317 (32%) of the MSN Ed program and 212 (38%) of PMC program websites clearly stated the program prepared graduates to take the CNE exam. In summary, four competencies were well represented (≥85%), and four competencies were poorly represented (<50%) in a sample of 529 schools.

▶ ACCREDITATION

- There are three national professional nursing organizations that currently accredit nursing education programs: the Commission for Nursing Education Accreditation (CNEA), the Accreditation Commission for Education in Nursing (ACEN), and the Commission for Collegiate Nursing Education (CCNE). The NLN's accreditation services, represented by the NLN CNEA, accredits all nursing programs, including licensed practical nursing, nursing diploma, associate degree, baccalaureate degree, master's degree, and doctor of nursing practice (DNP) programs. The ACEN was originally the National League for Nursing Accreditation Commission (NLNAC) but split off from the NLN in 2013 and is now a separate legal entity. ACEN accreditation includes practical, diploma, associate, baccalaureate, master's/post master's certificate, and clinical doctorate programs of nursing education. The American Association of Colleges of Nursing (AACN) represented by the CCNE accredits baccalaureate, masters, and DNP degree programs.
- CCNE accredits DNP programs that focus on advanced practice nursing, nursing leadership/administration, and health policy. In addition, it must be noted that all

BSN to DNP programs that require new licensure (certified nurse midwife, nurse practitioner, and nurse anesthetist) require accreditation as well as specialty accreditation in some instances.

■ Currently, CCNE will not accredit DNP programs that have an educator track as part of their core curriculum. Since 2004, the AACN has been clear that the educator role is not an advanced nursing practice role and requires a research-focused doctorate; they underscored the point with the 2006 publication of *The Essentials of Doctoral Education for Advanced Nursing Practice* (AACN, 2004, 2006). ACEN will accredit DNP program options with a clinical focus; therefore, if the DNP is an educational track, it still needs to have a clinical focus (N. Ard, personal communication, May 2, 2016). It should be noted that AACN Doctoral Essentials are currently under revision.

■ Research-focused doctoral programs (PhD, EdD, DNS, and DNSc) are not subject to accreditation.

■ Baccalaureate nursing education programs or higher can choose to be accredited by CNEA, ACEN, or CCNE; some programs elect to be accredited by more than one organization. Associate degree or diploma programs are accredited by CNEA.

■ The accreditation process provides an evaluative review of all components of the education program with an emphasis on program outcomes. Substantive components considered for accreditation include curriculum, institutional and program governance, fiscal resources, instructional learning resources, student support services, faculty qualifications, student qualifications, faculty and student accomplishments, and a program evaluation plan that guides faculty program reviews and decision-making.

■ The process for CNEA, ACEN, and CCNE accreditation requires an onsite visit from faculty colleagues or peer reviewers from similar institutions.

■ Prior to the onsite visit, faculty members prepare a written self-study report addressing each accreditation standard. It is important for faculty to have a clear understanding of the accreditation standards that guide the nature and execution of their nursing program.

■ The CNEA accreditation standards can be found online at www.nln.org/accreditation-services/overview; the CCNE accreditation standards can be found at www.aacn.nche.edu/Accreditation/index.htm; and the ACEN standards can be located at www.acenursing.org.

THE ACADEMIC SETTING

▶ COLLEGE/UNIVERSITY

The organizational structures of American colleges and universities vary depending on institutional type, culture, and history, yet they also have much in common. Although a private liberal arts and public research university in a state system may differ in terms of mission and focus, the majority of public and private universities are overseen by an institutional or system-wide governing board. Faculty self-governance is common in academia, and faculty members are involved in their campuses' strategic planning, fiscal oversight, curriculum planning, and student affairs.

Historically, the majority of American colleges and universities are nonprofit; however, there is a burgeoning of for-profit universities that deliver predominantly online academic programs. University norms, such as faculty self-governance and full-time faculty composition, are less common in these new for-profit academic organizations as a result of different business and organizational models; however, these institutions need to meet the same accreditation requirements as their nonprofit colleagues if they seek accreditation (Springer & Clinton, 2017).

▶ SCHOOL OF NURSING

- The school of nursing or nursing program's mission, philosophy, program outcomes, and curriculum are based on the college's and university's mission. For example, a faith-based institution's values are expressed in these entities as well as its pedagogy (a mode of teaching and learning).
- The expectations of the internal and external stakeholders need to be considered during program development or evaluation.

▶ MISSION

- According to Thelan (2017), a mission statement is a public statement of what an institution is about and why it exists.
- A mission statement provides direction for the planning of educational activities and provides clarity related to the target constituencies' goals for the institution related to teaching, research, and practice, and the level to which the institution aspires.
- The nursing educational mission is derived from the institution's mission statement, and the two mission statements need to be congruent with one another.
- The nursing educational mission statement describes the unique attributes of the program and provides direction for curriculum development.
- Curricular and structural changes need to consider the missions of both the university and its nursing program.

▶ FACULTY GOVERNANCE

- Finke (2012) describes how faculty have traditionally enjoyed the right of self-governance within the university setting.
- Self-governance includes developing policies related to student affairs, faculty expectations; faculty tenure and promotion guidelines; serving on faculty search committees; and developing, revising, and evaluating the curriculum.
- Faculty in partnership with academic administrators, who also hold a faculty rank in many instances, work collaboratively to address issues facing the university and larger academic community.

▶ ORGANIZATIONAL CLIMATE

- The organizational climate, or culture, is critical to the retention of nursing faculty, enthusiasm for innovation and learning, scholarly productivity, and clinical excellence.
- An organizational culture that encompasses the values and beliefs that the organization wants to promote is integral to any organization's success.
- Successfully balancing multiple expectations related to teaching, scholarship, and service can be challenging for new faculty. Supportive resources for faculty development may assist in easing the role transition and ultimately increasing competency, job satisfaction, and retention of new nurse faculty (Aquino, Lee, Spawn, & Bishop-Royse, 2018). Heavy faculty workloads often preclude having a meaningful life outside of work, leading to emotional exhaustion (Bittner, & Bechtel, 2017; Yedidia, Chou, Brownlee, Flynn, & Tanner, 2014; Candela, Gutierrez, & Keating, 2015). Promoting a healthy workplace in academic nursing settings is vital to recruiting and retaining faculty and enhancing the work life of faculty for optimism and happiness. Renewed attention is needed to focus on the importance of adopting standards to combat incivility, to stay optimistic despite challenges, and to use the tenets of appreciative inquiry (Fontaine, Koh, & Carroll, 2012; Frisbee, Griffin, & Luparell, 2019).
- Leaders need to effect change, promote a positive organizational culture, articulate a vision, implement strategic plans, garner resources, network, and adapt to changing landscapes.
- Leadership wisdom is a function of horizontal (acquisition of information, skills, and competencies) and vertical development (the development of more complex and sophisticated ways of thinking). Principles and practices that promote vertical development in self and others deepen performance expectations of those in the academy and support personal professional development and organizational success (Pesut, & Thompson, 2018).
- The importance of promoting a healthy environment in academic schools of nursing where faculty can flourish cannot be overstated. It is time in nursing's history to focus on a collegial, healthy educational environment, given the increase in retirements of senior faculty. New faculty are seeking a supportive, fulfilling work environment as they learn the nurse educator role (Fontaine et al., 2012).

▶ COMMUNITY OF INQUIRY

As online learning becomes a leading pedagogy resulting from access and convenience factors, Garrison, Anderson, and Archer's Community of Inquiry (CoI) Framework (2000) has been instrumental in understanding online learner engagement and has generated great interest among educational researchers. The CoI framework has been used extensively in the research and practice of online and blended learning, identifying the core elements associated with role adjustment to online learning, namely, cognitive, social, and teaching presence in an online environment. Garrison, Anderson, and Archer (2000) define **cognitive**, **social**, and **teaching presence** as:

■ "Cognitive presence relates to the design and development of instructional materials, enabling students to construct and confirm meaning through related reflection and discourse" (p. 93).

■ "Social presence relates to the establishment of a supportive learning community, providing a venue for communication within a trusted environment where students can express individual identities and establish social relationships. Social presence is defined as the ability of participants in a community of inquiry to project themselves socially and emotionally, as 'real' people (i.e., their full personality), through the medium of 'communication being used'" (p. 94).

■ "Teaching presence relates to the process of design, facilitation, and direction throughout the learning experience in order to realize desired learning outcomes. The three major categories under teaching presence are instructional design and management, building understanding, and direct instruction. Establishing teaching presence means, creating a learning experience for students to progress through with instructor facilitation, support, and guidance" (p. 101).

Five areas of adjustment characterize the move toward competence in online learning: (a) interaction, (b) self-identity, (c) instructor role, (d) course design, and (e) technology (Garrison, Cleveland-Innes, & Fung, 2004). Faculty preparation in online pedagogies is a crucial prerequisite for a successful higher educational experience (Figure 16.1).

Figure 16.1 Elements of an Educational Experience.

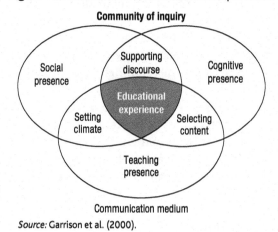

Source: Garrison et al. (2000).

▶ COLLABORATION, PARTNERSHIPS, AND INNOVATION

■ To develop and maintain an innovative curriculum, nurse educators need to lead a cultural paradigm shift in nursing education that welcomes innovation, embraces creativity, and designs novel curricula and pedagogy that will ultimately improve the health and welfare of patients and professional nurses (Smith Glasgow et al., 2010).

- Strategic partnerships are one example of innovation as nurse leaders devise ways to manage the nursing shortage and the nurse faculty shortage and to increase the number of BSN-prepared nurses. Innovative curricular models, such as the Oregon Consortium for Nursing Education, provide a model to facilitate the movement of students through associate degree to baccalaureate degree programs in a seamless fashion, which eliminates duplication and prepares graduates with the competencies needed to meet the needs of the state's aging and ethnically diverse population.
- One example of collaboration is Academic Practice Partnerships. One model is the Professional Nurse-Student Nurse Academic Partnership using a Dedicated Education Unit (DEU). This model for clinical nursing education is a partnership where professional nurses on the staff are trained to mentor and participate closely in the clinical education of nursing students. These strategic models of synergistic collaboration are being used to address issues of both nursing and nursing faculty shortages. Dedicated education units offer a new way to conceptualize the roles of nurse educators, students, and clinical staff during clinical learning experiences (Sebastian et al., 2018). "This new model of education is broader, more inclusive, and seeks to find commonalities in the culture of both service and academe, and may provide the best site for faculty practice as well" (Smith Glasgow et al., 2010, p. G9).
- Collaborative arrangements between academic and healthcare institutions allow partners to combine their respective strengths in achieving their mutual goals of increasing the registered nurse and nursing faculty workforce (Smith Glasgow et al., 2010; Sebastian et al., 2018).
- Typically, the master's-prepared nurse clinician or DNP-prepared advanced practice nurse is selected by the academic and healthcare institution to teach students in the clinical area based on his or her educational preparation, clinical expertise, and desire to teach (Dreher & Smith Glasgow, 2016).
- Leaders need to create a safe, inclusive environment where faculty can feel comfortable regarding the adoption of innovative learning experiences.
- Visionary leaders are successful in developing partnerships in the organization while leading faculty and anticipating the effects of innovation by:
- Staying focused on the educational program's core mission and values while being responsive to trends in the profession
- Identifying innovations of use to the institution

TEACHING GEM Nurse educators should keep an ongoing electronic file and record each activity that adds to the portfolio as soon as the activity is completed. For helpful tips on preparing a portfolio, nurse educators should consider reading *The Academic Portfolio: A Practical Guide to Documenting Teaching, Research, and Service* (Seldin & Miller, 2009).

EVIDENCE-BASED TEACHING PRACTICE

Kalb et al. (2015) conducted a national online study to describe nursing faculty perspectives and practices about evidence-based teaching practice (EBTP). EBTP was defined for this study as the use of evidence by nursing faculty to inform: (a) what to teach, (b) how to facilitate and evaluate student learning, and (c) how to design nursing curricula and programs to promote the education of nurses. Professional standards for nurse educator practice stress the importance of EBTP; however, the use of evidence by faculty in curriculum design, evaluation and educational measurement, and program development has not been reported. Nurse academic administrators of accredited nursing programs in the United States ($N = 1{,}586$) were emailed information about the study, including the research consent form and anonymous survey link, and invited to forward information to nursing faculty. Respondents (551 faculty and nurse academic administrators) described the importance of EBTP in nursing education, used multiple sources of evidence in their faculty responsibilities, and identified factors that influence their ability to use EBTP. Respondents identified ways they have learned about EBTP, most frequently identifying professional journals ($n = 404$, 73%), continuing education programs ($n = 360$, 65%), and faculty development programs ($n = 314$, 57%). EBTP in nursing education requires sustained institutional, administrative, and collegial support to promote faculty effectiveness and student learning.

ACADEMIC RESPONSIBILITIES

▶ TEACHING

Elements of faculty participation in the teaching mission of an institution include:

- Effectiveness in undergraduate and graduate teaching in the classroom and/or clinical area
- Contributions to the curriculum, such as substantial revisions of existing courses, and the development of new courses and techniques for teaching
- Development of student evaluation methods
- Publications related to teaching, such as textbooks, manuals, and articles
- Development of innovative pedagogical methods and materials
- Authorship of a funded external teaching-oriented grant proposal
- Effectiveness as an undergraduate and/or graduate adviser and/or mentor, including dissertation, thesis, or independent study advisement
- Responsiveness to peer review feedback on one's teaching (Mager et al., 2014)
- Teaching is evaluated based on student evaluations of teaching strategies, peer reviews of teaching strategies, evaluation of a teaching dossier, and assessment of student learning and other indicators of teaching excellence (Sauter et al., 2012)

EVIDENCE-BASED TEACHING PRACTICE

McPherson (2019) reviewed the evidence of what is needed for clinical faculty as they assume the faculty role. Using a systematic approach, 19 articles were included in this integrated review. Themes identified included Mandatory/Structured Orientation, Mentoring, Support, and Communication/Connection. Issues of Pay and Compensation and the Transient Nature of Year-to-Year Contract Work were also themes found in this review. Clinical education is imperative to developing safe, competent new nurses. Identifying the needs of clinical faculty hired to reduce the impact of the faculty shortage is needed for continued program stability and ensuring continuity of the nursing faculty workforce. The need to adequately clinical nursing faculty for their role continues to be a persistent problem for nursing programs. Identifying the learning and developmental needs of clinical faculty is essential to ensuring that nursing programs are fully staffed and may lead to graduating safe, competent new nurses.

▶ RESEARCH/SCHOLARSHIP

Elements of faculty participation, particularly for tenure-track and tenured faculty, in a continuing program of research or other scholarship, include:

- Quantity and quality of research or scholarship, as evidenced by publications, presentations of papers (including invited presentations nationally and internationally), and peer-reviewed scholarship
- Publications related to the advancement of pedagogical theory
- Success in securing intramural (internal or institutional) funding
- Success in securing extramural funding (external federal funding or private funding)
- Effectiveness in directing the research of students
- Originating, participating in, and/or directing research projects (Sauter et al., 2012)

▶ SERVICE

Elements of faculty participation in service to the program, department, school or college, and university, and to the profession at the national and/or international level include:

- Leadership and/or participation in faculty elective bodies and service on committees at the program, department, college or school, and university levels
- Faculty mentoring
- Service to individual students and/or student organizations
- Promotion of the university through extramural activities, such as recruitment events, alumni affairs, and so on
- Other forms of service to the profession and society, such as serving on editorial boards, national organizations, and grant-review panels (Finke, 2012)

APPOINTMENT, PROMOTION, AND TENURE

▶ FACULTY APPOINTMENT

- Potential faculty candidates are invited to interview by a faculty search committee appointed by a dean or other university administrator. Faculty candidates may be asked to conduct a presentation about their research agenda or to demonstrate teaching competency during the interview process. Potential faculty candidates may also be interviewed by the department chair, associate dean for research, and dean, depending on the academic rank.
- Once considered for appointment, the faculty candidate's vita is reviewed by the appointment, promotion, and tenure committee or another appropriate committee for the recommendation of faculty rank to the dean. The academic ranks of instructor, assistant professor, associate professor, and professor are typically appointed based on the faculty candidate's teaching, research, and service experience and expertise (O'Connor & Yanni, 2013).
- More recently, there has been an increase in the number of faculty appointed to clinical-track positions. These faculty members may enjoy the same promotion in rank as their tenure-track and tenured colleagues but are usually not eligible for tenure. Faculty who are hired into a clinical-track position typically have the designation **clinical** before their academic rank and are hired for their clinical knowledge and expertise. Many of these clinical faculty members may have joint appointments with a healthcare institution, which involves an adjustment and negotiation in workload.

▶ ACADEMIC RANKS

- Finke (2012) noted that appointment ranks, or tracks, have been developed to specify the responsibilities of faculty members in relation to teaching, scholarship, and service.
- Ranks include **tenure, clinical,** or **research scientist**. Clinical and research faculty have a designation before their academic rank (e.g., clinical assistant professor or research associate professor). Tenure-track and tenured faculty titles have no prefix.
- Tenure-track faculty are considered tenure probationary until they achieve tenure. The tenure track is established for faculty whose primary responsibilities are teaching and research.
- The clinical faculty track was developed for those faculty members whose primary responsibilities are clinical practice or clinical supervision of students and is generally a contingent faculty role with a defined annual or multiyear contract.
- The research scientist track is for faculty whose primary responsibilities are generating new knowledge and disseminating research findings and is generally a contingent faculty role based on extramural funding.
- Adjunct faculty role was developed for part-time faculty. Adjunct faculty typically teach in the clinical environment but can also teach in the classroom, lab, or online. They generally do not hold a professorial rank.

▶ NONTENURE APPOINTMENTS

Clinical and research faculty are generally nontenured positions and are considered contracted faculty. Faculty members receive contracts on an annual or multiyear basis.

▶ THE APPOINTMENT, PROMOTION, AND TENURE PROCESS

- The contemporary concept of tenure in U.S. colleges and universities can be traced to the "Statement of Principles of Academic Freedom and Tenure," which was adopted in 1940 by the American Association of University Professors (AAUPs) and the Association of American Colleges, where the basic principles of tenure as a system to protect the academic freedom of faculty members were first articulated.
- Criteria for promotion and tenure are based on a university's overall mission and the Carnegie Foundation's university classification system; therefore, requirements vary among institutions from tribal colleges to doctoral universities. Doctoral universities are assigned to one of three categories based on a measure of research activity. Nurse educators should evaluate their research productivity/skills in lieu of these categories when seeking tenure and promotion.
- **Promotion** refers to advancement in rank. To be considered for promotion, a faculty member must submit a dossier as evidence of excellence in teaching, scholarship, and service.
- The criteria for tenure and/or promotion are established by the school/college and are evaluated by a committee of peers, school and university administrators, and the university board of trustees or other governing body.
- In most schools of nursing, a tenure-track faculty member is appointed as an assistant professor and can expect to be promoted to the rank of associate professor at the time when tenure is granted.
- The AAUP can serve as a resource related to faculty rights pertaining to tenure and promotion. Their website is www.aaup.org/aaup.

● CAREER DEVELOPMENT FOR NURSE EDUCATORS

Both new and experienced faculty need clear guidelines on career development and advancement in their respective academic institutions (Seldin & Associates, 2006; Seldin & Miller, 2009; Seldin, Miller, Seldin, & McKeachie, 2010).

▶ PORTFOLIO/DOSSIER DEVELOPMENT

- The professional portfolio/dossier is typically used to display one's work when applying for appointments, promotions, and tenure. A portfolio or dossier should include sample publications, grant submissions, awards, syllabi, teaching evaluations, and recommendation letters. A portfolio or dossier is a practical way to reflect on and document one's teaching, research, and service (Seldin & Associates, 2006; Seldin & Miller, 2009; Seldin et al., 2010; Wittmann-Price, 2012).

■ In recent years, electronic portfolios have come into use in academic institutions as a means for students to display their work and demonstrate competency related to writing, clinical objectives, and so on.

■ Some academic institutions are also using electronic portfolios for faculty to construct and display their promotion and tenure dossiers.

▶ DEVELOPING A CAREER TRAJECTORY

Successful faculty members have often developed a career development plan for themselves. Such a plan may include the following elements:

■ Developing career goals
■ Short-term career goals
■ Long-term career goals
■ Using effective time management
■ Identify the most productive intellectual time and protect it
■ Maximize the value of scholarship and research time
■ Understanding of the trajectory and stages of an academic career and the goals at each stage
■ Mastery of negotiation and conflict-resolution skills
■ Developing a teaching portfolio
■ Developing collaboration skills and the ability to maximize the benefits of collaboration while maintaining autonomy and boundaries
■ Valuing the benefits of being mentored
■ Developing a primary mentor–protégé relationship
■ Appreciation for the need for lifelong learning
■ Consulting a coach to deal with any issues and barriers effectively (Feldman et al., 2015; Weinstock & Smith Glasgow, 2016)

▶ CAREER STAGES

Distinct academic accomplishments are associated with various levels of faculty appointments during progressive career stages. These can generally be described for each faculty level as follows:

1. Instructor
   ● Develop skills in the scholarship of discovery (research or discovery of new knowledge)
   ● Develop skills in the scholarship of teaching
   ● Develop skills in scholarship of integration (interpretation and synthesis of knowledge across discipline boundaries in a manner that provides new insights)
   ● Develop skills in the scholarship of application of knowledge (connects theory and practice; Boyer, 1997)
   ● Understand the responsibilities of protégé and mentor

2. Assistant Professor
   - Develop an area of expertise
   - Pose and address an important question or focus in that area that has the potential for significant findings or impact (scholarship or research)
   - Develop oneself autonomously within this area or develop an interdisciplinary research team and bring your area of expertise to the team
   - Develop one's own laboratory for evaluating these questions, whether the laboratory is a wet-bench laboratory; the skills, staff, and resources for clinical, population-based, or teaching investigation; or another setting (i.e., demonstrating the ability to function scientifically as an "independent" investigator or "collaborative" investigator)
   - Lead or collaborate in the development and evaluation of an innovative educational program
   - Present findings from this work at appropriate national meetings and/or publish the results of this work in peer-reviewed journals
   - Obtain external, peer-reviewed funding to support this work
   - Become nationally recognized for this body of work, whether it be clinical research or education
   - Initiate or continue to compile the teaching portfolio (Seldin & Miller, 2009)
   - Provide faculty teaching and service to the nursing department (Wittmann-Price, 2012)

3. Associate Professor
   - Continue research/scholarship in one's area of expertise as an autonomous investigator and in publication productivity
   - Become an interdependent investigator and/or leader
   - Continue with the activity of developing and evaluating innovative educational programs
   - Establish a body of contributions that one can make in one's defined area; become nationally and internationally recognized for this work
   - Take on responsibility for an area important to one's own institution, becoming a resource and leader recognized beyond one's department
   - Mentor junior faculty in a productive manner
   - Demonstrate peer-reviewed awards, honors, or other indications of excellence
   - Demonstrate peer-reviewed support for research or program development
   - Become involved at the national level through involvement in societies reflective of one's expertise
   - Serve on national committees such as study sections
   - Serve on departmental and university functions, particularly some time-consuming committees

4. Professor
   - Continue to demonstrate leadership in research, teaching, and service at a national and international level
   - Become internationally recognized for this body of work, whether it be clinical research or educational research
   - Function as a role model and enhance the mentoring role and, in particular, assist junior faculty in their career development

▶ CHOOSING A MENTOR

- A faculty mentor either can be assigned to the protégé, or the mentor and protégé can mutually agree upon the relationship. The mentoring relationship is generally consultative and constructive in most institutions; however, some schools have a more prescriptive approach (Sauter et al., 2012).
- Jeffers & Mariani (2017) discuss the positive effect of a formal mentoring program on career satisfaction and intent to stay in the faculty role for novice nurse faculty. The mentor provides support and guidance during times of stress while assisting in the development and enhancement of the novice nurse faculty's knowledge and skills.

Some organizations have more formalized mentoring programs for junior faculty, such as Sigma Theta Tau International/Elsevier Nurse Faculty Leadership Academy (NFLA). The Sigma Theta Tau/Elsevier NFLA is an intense international leadership development experience designed to (a) facilitate personal leadership development; (b) foster academic career success; (c) promote nurse faculty retention and satisfaction; and (d) cultivate high-performing, supportive work environments in academe (Sigma Theta Tau International Inc., 2016).

- The mentor helps the protégé learn the political landscape, expand his or her network, gain professional insight, and foster personal and professional growth.
- An authentic mentor invests a great deal of time and effort into the advancement of his or her protégé. The mentor–protégé relationship is conscious, purposeful, and typically lasts for a number of years.
- It is important for the protégé to set goals, track progress, and obtain feedback from the mentor on his or her development plan.
- A mentor looks for the following attributes in the protégé:
  - Intelligence
  - Strong work ethic
  - Initiative
  - Integrity
  - Professional demeanor
  - Commitment
  - Ability to accept feedback
  - Intellectual curiosity
- A protégé looks for the following attributes in the mentor:
  - Intelligence
  - Someone who is willing to invest in him or her
  - Willingness to give feedback
  - Strong networking capabilities
  - Professional contacts
  - Ability to motivate
  - Integrity

▶ FACULTY ORIENTATION AND DEVELOPMENT

New nursing faculty members struggle to meet the individual needs of an increasingly diverse and growing population of nursing students while simultaneously attempting to balance the research, scholarship, and stewardship requirements of their institutions. To meet these demands, a formal, robust faculty orientation is essential. During a faculty orientation, new nursing faculty members begin the process of socialization into the academy. Novice faculty need to understand the expectations for tenure and promotion and the socio-political issues of the institution upon assuming their new role as educators (Sauter et al., 2012; Suplee & Gardner, 2009).

- Nurse educators need to understand the mission and goals of the institution, the nature of the curriculum, academic policies and procedures, the organization of the program, the school and how it fits into the university, and the structure and charges of the various nursing and university committees.
- Seasoned nurse educators should be involved in these orientation and development sessions to facilitate collegial relationships, impart knowledge and expertise, and encourage mentor–protégé relationships.
- The use of travel monies to attend conferences, seminars, and research colloquia is critical to faculty development.
- Nurse educators who need to maintain clinical certification as an advanced practice nurse should negotiate practice time as part of their faculty role.
- Tenure-track or tenured faculty who need to secure external funding should negotiate start-up funds to assist in research productivity (e.g., graduate assistant, statistical support, research software, peer review, editorial support, and research space and equipment).
- New faculty should also discuss teaching load – the equivalent of 12 credits per semester is customary for nontenure track faculty, while the equivalent of 6–9 credits per semester is customary for tenure track or tenured faculty. Faculty should negotiate a reduced teaching load their first year.
- It is essential that the novice faculty member have an "action plan" to develop his or her career that is realistic and is congruent with the promotion and tenure guidelines of the institution.

TEACHING GEM It is important for the novice nurse faculty member to keep continuous track of accomplishments and maintain a current, comprehensive curriculum vitae (CV) in addition to uploading teaching evaluations, publications, continuing education certificates, and so forth in an electronic portfolio for tenure and/or promotion.

Finke (2012) stated that ongoing support and professional development are needed for nurse educators throughout their careers in the following areas:

- Curriculum development and teaching, using teaching, learning, information resources, and evaluating student outcomes
- Professional practice
- Relationships with learners and colleagues

- Service and faculty governance
- Scholarship
- Mentoring

▶ THE CURRICULUM VITAE

- A curriculum vitae—often called a CV or vita—is used for academic positions. Thus, vitae tend to provide great detail about academic and research experiences. Although résumés tend toward brevity, vitae lean toward detail (Seldin et al., 2010). A sample CV format can be found in Exhibit 16.1.

EXHIBIT 15.1 Sample Curriculum Vitae

A curriculum vitae should include the following items:
1. Name in full
2. Current home and mailing address, telephone number, fax number, and email address
3. Education
    A. List of degrees, with the last degree listed first
    B. For each degree, include the name of the college/university, year degree was granted, major(s)/concentration(s), minor(s), title of dissertation/thesis, if applicable
    C. Postgraduate training
        i. List chronologically, starting with most recent position
        ii. Give years, institutions, and type of training
4. Employment history
    A. List chronologically, starting with the most recent position held and including consulting positions, if applicable
    B. Indicate each place of employment and years employed
5. Certification and licensure (including recertification)
6. Military service
7. Honors and awards
    A. Starting with the most recent, list chronologically by name of the award
    B. Include each awarding institution and/or organization
    C. Indicate the nature of each award if not apparent
8. Memberships and offices in professional societies
9. Professional committees and administrative service
    A. Institutional: Committees on which you have served or chaired, including years of membership
    B. Extramural (local, regional, national, and international). Include:
        i. Membership on editorial boards
        ii. Editorship of symposia volumes, texts, or journals
        iii. Service as an examiner for a professional organization
        iv. Reviewer of grants for extramural funding sources
        v. Reviewer of manuscripts for journal publications
        vi. Convener of symposia, conferences, or workshop in one's field and/or profession
    C. Name of each organization or publication, your role, and years of service
10. Community service (service not related to the institution but provided by you, either in your profession or in some other capacity)
    A. List chronologically, earliest first
    B. Give your role and the organization

11. Educational activities
    A. Courses/clerkships/programs taught, coordinated, or developed
    B. Advising/mentoring/tutoring: For each of the aforementioned areas, include course title, audience, and years of involvement
    C. Educational materials: List texts, atlases, manuals, evaluation tools, and so on, developed that were used only within the institution
12. Clinical activities
    A. Outline of major clinical activities, including rounds, clinics, development and/or implementation of clinical programs and quality assessment of programs
    B. Healthcare education in the lay community
13. Support
    A. List past and present extramural support received
    B. List past and present intramural support received. Include role in the project, title of study, funding agencies, including appropriate ID number, effective dates, and total amount of award
    C. List grant applications already submitted and still pending, with the same information as aforementioned
14. Graduate students, postdoctoral fellows, and postgraduate trainees
    A. List the graduate students who have received advanced degrees (master's, PhD) with you as their supervisor; give the name of each student and years of study, thesis title, date when degree was awarded, program/department in which study was done, and institution awarding degree
    B. List postdoctoral fellows and postgraduate trainees and visiting scientists who have been under your direct supervision for their training; give names, years, research or clinical study, and means of support (if training grant or NRSA)
15. Publications in the lay press
    A. Published full-length papers
        1. Provide a chronological list with complete citations, including:
            i. Names and initials of all authors
            ii. Titles of the articles
            iii. Name of journal, volume, page numbers, year
        2. Indicate whether peer-reviewed by using an asterisk before the citation
    B. Books and chapters in books, including page numbers; provide complete citations, including press and city of printing
    C. Communications, such as videotapes, disks, slide atlases, and computer programs, and so on, used by others outside the institution
    D. Book reviews, letters to editors (if these are not articles, which they can be, as in *Nature* [London] or *Journal of Molecular Biology*); provide complete citations
    E. Abstracts (optional, but if included, provide complete citations). Indicate by asterisk whether peer-reviewed
16. Presentations
    A. By invitation: May include invited seminar presentations (except those for job interviews) and presentations at conferences, society meetings, and professional boards
    B. By competition or peer review
    For each presentation, provide type, full title, date and place presented, and the auspices presented under (program, department, college, university, society, etc.); wherever possible, use American Psychological Association (APA) style
17. Bibliography
    To be listed under the following separate headings and according to APA style

    N.B.: Items "accepted for publication" and/or "submitted for publication" should be so indicated and should include, together with the following information, the expected date of publication and/or date of submission
    (Christenbery, 2014).

CASE STUDY

CASE STUDY 15.1

A new PhD graduate, who completed a postdoctoral fellowship but has limited teaching experience, is interviewing at a very high-activity research university.

What questions would you want to ask this faculty candidate regarding her career trajectory plan? What is important to convey to this faculty member given her early developmental stage as a nurse educator? Should you advise this faculty member to apply for a tenure track or nontenure track position? What are important items for this new faculty member to negotiate?

1. A new PhD graduate, who completed a postdoctoral fellowship, is interviewing at a very high-activity research university for a tenure track position. What are important items for this new faculty to negotiate?

   A. A research start-up package
   B. Faculty office
   C. Tenure year
   D. Vacation time

2. Which of the following would developing a curriculum based on external forces best include?

   A. Emphasis on the teacher
   B. Political affiliation
   C. Universal healthcare
   D. Health disparities

3. The Future of Nursing Report: Leading Change, Advancing Health, (Institute of Medicine, 2010) recommended all of the following except:

   A. Nurses should achieve higher levels of education and training through an improved education system that promotes seamless academic progression
   B. Educate nurses to work and lead collaboratively with other healthcare professionals
   C. Nurse educators should create curriculum models that transform the student population
   D. All nurse educators should obtain a doctorate

4. The following professional organizations accredit nursing education programs except:

   A. CCNE (Commission of Collegiate Nursing Education)
   B. ACEN (The Accreditation Commission for Education in Nursing)
   C. NLN (The National League for Nursing)
   D. CNEA (The Commission for Nursing Education and Accreditation)

5. The 2010 Carnegie Foundation study called for nurse educators to transform nursing education by:

   A. Increasing the number of nurse practitioners
   B. Increasing nurse educators scholarly productivity
   C. Conducting research on nursing education
   D. Distinguishing outcomes of the DNP and PhD

1. A) A Research Start-up Package

A Research Start-up Package will help facilitate the faculty member's success and is something the PhD graduate can control. Faculty offices are typically assigned, and tenure year and vacation time are usually standard in a university.

2. D) Health disparities

Health disparities is an important contemporary topic that is external and needs consideration to be included in the curriculum. Emphasis should not be on the teacher but on the learner, and political affiliations are not important. Universal healthcare is an important topic but not a current external force.

3. D) All nurse educators should obtain a doctorate

The recommendation was to double the number of doctorates, not 100% of the educator workforce obtain a doctorate. The Institute of Medicine's (2010) recommendations did include higher levels of education, promote interprofessional collaboration, and redesign nursing curricula to promote quality practice.

4. C) NLN (The National League for Nursing)

The NLN is professional nursing organization for nursing faculty and not an accrediting body. CCNE, ACEN, and CNEA are the three specialty accreditation organizations for nursing education.

5. C) Conducting research on nursing education

More research is needed about nursing education to promote evidence-based teaching practices. Increasing the number of nurse practitioners does not necessarily affect nursing education. Increasing nurse educator's scholarly activity is an asset in academia, but it is not always scholarship about nursing education. Distinguishing between the DNP and PhD is not the focus because both doctorates teach in academia.

6. The novice nurse educator needs additional mentorship when they place a section in the promotion package labeled:

   A. Teaching
   B. Collegiality
   C. Scholarship
   D. Service

7. Which academic nursing programs are not normally subjected to a specialty accreditation process?

   A. Doctor of Philosophy in Nursing
   B. Associate of Science in Nursing
   C. Bachelor of Science in Nursing
   D. Doctor of Nursing Practice

8. Which aspects of organizational climate are detrimental to the retention of nursing faculty?

   A. Autonomy
   B. Productive
   C. Leadership
   D. Incivility

9. The novice nurse educator needs a better understanding of Community of Inquiry Framework concepts when they identify the following element is associated with role adjustment to online learning:

   A. Online presence
   B. Teaching presence
   C. Social presence
   D. Cognitive presence

10. Teaching portfolios usually include all the following items except:

    A. Curriculum vitae (CV)
    B. Student work
    C. Examples of syllabi
    D. Teaching philosophy

6. B) Collegiality
Collegiality is not a separate category if evaluated teaching, scholarship, and service are commonly evaluated as criteria for promotion and tenure in an academic organization.

7. A) Doctor of Philosophy in Nursing
Research-focused doctorates are not subject to accreditation. Associate of Science in Nursing, Bachelor of Science in Nursing, and Doctorate of Nursing Practice programs are most likely accredited.

8. D) Incivility
Faculty, administrative, or student incivility is one of the main reasons nurse educators leave academia. Nurse educator autonomy is a positive organizational climate element. Productivity is a nurse educator's expectation, and leadership in an organization is usually not the reason for attrition.

9. A) Online presence
There is no core element that calls for online presence. Core elements include teaching presence or being engaged and available to students, social presence or being responsive to students' situations, and cognitive presence or understanding the best method to present information.

10. B) Student work
Teaching portfolios usually do not include exemplars of student work unless they are above and beyond what is normally completed as classroom assignments. A CV, examples of syllabi, and a written teaching philosophy are normally included.

REFERENCES

American Association of Colleges of Nursing. (2004). AACN position statement on the practice doctorate in nursing. http://www.aacn.nche.edu/DNP/pdf/DNP.pdf

American Association of Colleges of Nursing. (2006). Essentials of doctoral education for advanced nursing practice. http://www.aacn.nche.edu/DNP/pdf/Essentials.pdf

Aquino, E., Lee, Y.-M., Spawn, N., & Bishop-Royse, J. (2018). The impact of burnout on doctorate nursing faculty's intent to leave their academic position: A descriptive survey research design. *Nurse Education Today, 69,* 35–40.

Benner, P., Sutphen, M., Leonard, V., & Day, L. (2010). *Educating nurses: A call for radical transformation.* Jossey-Bass/Carnegie Foundation for the Advancement of Teaching.

Bittner, N. P., & Bechtel, C. F. (2017). Identifying and describing nurse faculty workload issues: A looming faculty Shortage. *Nursing Education Perspectives, 38*(4), 171–176.

Boyer, E. L. (1997). *Scholarship reconsidered: Priorities of the professoriate.* Jossey-Bass.

Candela, L., Gutierrez, A. P., & Keating, S. (2015). What predicts nurse faculty members' intent to stay in the academic organization? A structural equation model of a national survey of nursing faculty. *Nurse Education Today, 35*(4), 580–589.

Christenbery, T. L. (2014). The Curriculum Vitae. *Nurse Educator, 39*(6), 267–268. 10.1097/NNE.0000000000000083.

Diaz, C., Clarke, P. N., & Gatua, M. W. (2015). *Cultural competence in rural nursing education: are we there yet? Nursing Education Perspectives (National League for Nursing), 36*(1), 22–26.

Dreher, H. M., & Smith Glasgow, M. E. (2017). *DNP role development for doctoral advanced nursing practice.* Springer Publishing Company.

Feldman, H. R., Greenberg, M. J., Jaffe-Ruiz, M., Kaufman, S. R., & Cignarale, S. (2015). *Hitting the nursing faculty shortage head on: Strategies to recruit, retain, and develop nursing faculty. Journal of Professional Nursing, 31*(3), 170–178.

Finke, L. M. (2012). Teaching in nursing: The faculty role. In D. Billings & J. Halstead (Eds.), *Teaching in nursing: A guide for faculty* (4th ed., pp. 1–14). Elsevier Saunders.

Fitzgerald, A., McNelis, A. M., & Billings, D. M. (2020). NLN Core competencies for nurse educators: *Are they present in the course descriptions of academic nurse educator programs? Nursing Education Perspectives, 1,* 4–9.

Fontaine, D., Koh, E., & Carroll, T. (2012). Promoting a healthy workplace for nursing faculty and staff. *Nursing Clinics of North America, 47*(4), 557–566. http://www.aana.com/resources2/professionalpractice/Pages/Promoting-a-Culture-of-Safety-and-Healthy-Work-Environment.aspx

Frisbee, K., Griffin, M. Q., & Luparell, S. (2019). Nurse educators: incivility, job satisfaction, and intent to leave. *Midwest Quarterly, 60*(3), 270–289

Garrison, D. R., Anderson, T., & Archer, W. (2000). Critical inquiry in a text-based environment: Computer conferencing in higher education. *Internet and Higher Education, 2*(2–3), 87–105.

Garrison, D. R., Cleveland-Innes, M., & Fung, T. (2004). *Student role adjustment in online communities of inquiry: Model and instrument validation.* Journal of Institute of Medicine. (2010). *The future of nursing: Leading change, advancing health.* National Academies Press.

Jeffers, S., & Mariani, B. (2017). The effect of a formal mentoring program on career satisfaction and intent to stay in the faculty role for novice nurse faculty. *Nursing Education Perspectives, 38*(1), 18–22.

Kalb, K. A., O'Conner-Von, S. K., Brockway, C., Rierson, C. L., & Sendelbach, S. (2015). Evidence-based teaching practice in nursing education: Faculty perspectives and practices. *Nursing Education Perspectives, 36*(4), 212–219.

Latham, C. L., Singh, H., & Ringl, K. K. (2016). Enhancing the educational environment for diverse nursing students through mentoring and shared governance. *The Journal of Nursing Education, 55*(11), 605–614.

Laurencelle, F. L., Scanlan, J. M., & Brett, A. L. (2016). The meaning of being a nurse educator and nurse educators' attraction to academia: A phenomenological study. *Nurse Education Today, 39,* 135–140. 10.1016/j.nedt.2016.01.029

Mager, D. R., Kazer, M. W., Conelius, J., Shea, J., Lippman, D. T., Torosyan, R., & Nantz, K. (2014). Development, implementation and evaluation of a peer review of teaching (PRoT) Initiative in Nursing Education. *International Journal of Nursing Education Scholarship, 11*(1), 113–120.

McPherson, S. (2019). Part-time clinical nursing faculty needs: An integrated review. *Journal of Nursing Education, 58*(4), 201–206.

National League for Nursing. (2021). Certified Nurse Educator (CNE) 2021 candidate handbook. http://www.nln.org/docs/default-source/default-document-library/cne-handbook-2021_revised_07-01-2021.pdf?sfvrsn=2

National League for Nursing. (2021). Certified Nurse Educator Novice (CNEn) 2021 candidate handbook. http://www.nln.org/Certification-for-Nurse-Educators/cne-n/cne-n-handbook

O'Connor, L. G., & Yanni, C. K. (2013). Promotion and tenure in nursing education: Lessons learned. *Journal of Nursing Education and Practice, 3*(5), 78.

Pesut, D. J., & Thompson, S. A. (2018). Nursing leadership in academic nursing: The wisdom of development and the development of wisdom. *Journal of Professional Nursing, 34*(2), 122–127.

Sauter, M. K., Gillespie, N. N., & Knepp, A. (2012). Educational program evaluation. In D. Billings & J. Halstead (Eds.), *Teaching in nursing: A guide for faculty* (4th ed., pp. 503–549). Elsevier Saunders.

Sebastian, J. G., Breslin, E. T., Trautman, D. E., Cary, A. H., Rosseter, R. J., & Vlahov, D. (2018). Leadership by collaboration: Nursing's bold new vision for academic-practice partnerships. *Journal of Professional Nursing, 34*(2), 110–116.

Seldin, P., & Associates. (2006). *Evaluating faculty performance: A practical guide to assessing teaching, research, and service.* Anker Publishing.

Seldin, P., & Miller, E. J. (2009). *The academic portfolio: A practical guide to documenting teaching, research, and service*. Jossey-Bass.

Seldin, P., Miller, J. E., Seldin, C. A., & McKeachie, W. (2010). *The teaching portfolio: A practical guide to improved performance and promotion/tenure decisions*. San Francisco, CA: Jossey-Bass.

Sigma Theta Tau International. Honor Society of Nursing. (2016). Sigma Theta Tau International Nurse Faculty Leadership Academy (NFLA). http://www.nursingsociety.org/learn-grow/leadership-institute/nurse-faculty-leadership-academy-%28nfla%29

Smith Glasgow, M. E., Dunphy, L. M., & Mainous, R. O. (2010). Innovative nursing educational curriculum for the 21st century. Transformational models of nursing across different settings. In Institute of medicine report on the future of nursing: Leading change, advancing health (G8–G12). National Academies Press.

Smith Glasgow, M. E., Niederhauser, V., Dunphy, L. M., & Mainous, R. O. (2010). Supporting innovation in nursing education: Regulatory issues. *Journal of Nursing Regulation*, 1(3), 23–27.

Springer, R. A., & Clinton, M. E. (2017). 'Philosophy Lost': Inquiring into the effects of the corporatized university and its implications for graduate nursing education. *Nursing Inquiry*, 24(4), 1–8.

Summers, J. A. (2017). Developing competencies in the novice nurse educator: An integrative review. *Teaching and Learning in Nursing*, 12(4), 263–276.

Suplee, P. D., & Gardner, M. (2009). Fostering a smooth transition to the faculty role. *Journal of Continuing Education in Nursing*, 40(11), 514–520.

Thelan, J. R. (2017). *American Higher Education: Issues and Institutions*. Routledge Publishing.

Valiga, T. (2016). The role of the educator: Reflective response. In H. M. Dreher & M. E. Smith. Glasgow (Eds.), *DNP role development for doctoral advanced nursing practice*. Springer Publishing.

Weinstock, B., & Smith Glasgow, M. E. (2016). Executive coaching to support doctoral roletransitions and promote leadership consciousness. In H. M. Dreher & M. E. Smith Glasgow (Eds.), *DNP role development for doctoral advanced nursing practice*. Springer Publishing.

Wittmann-Price, R. A. (2012). *Fast facts for developing a nursing academic portfolio*. Springer Publishing.

Yedidia, M. J., Chou, J., Brownlee, S., Flynn, L., & Tanner, C. A. (2014). Association of faculty perceptions of work-life with emotional exhaustion and intent to leave academic nursing: Report on a national survey of nurse faculty. *Journal of Nursing Education*, 53(10), 569–79.

Young, S. & Lu, K. (2018). Educational interventions to increase cultural competence for nursing students. *International Journal of Organization Theory & Behavior*, 21(2), 85–97.

Practice Test

1. A former student requests that a nurse educator write a letter of recommendation for an application to a doctoral program. The nurse educator remembers this student very well and is happy to write a strong letter of support, which includes:

   A. A copy of a graded paper the student submitted in class
   B. A description of personality traits that contributed to the student's success
   C. A student's overall grade point average
   D. A list of courses that students took with the professor to depict the rigorous content

2. Contrasting the appropriate Standards of Practice and Code of Ethics to various practice situations is an example of a Level _____ Program Objective.

   A. One
   B. Two
   C. Three
   D. Four

3. A student repeatedly does not identify the patient during medication administration. What is the clinical instructor's best action?

   A. Accompany the student to each medication administration event
   B. Correct the student at the patients' bedside
   C. Inform the course chair of the student's behavior
   D. Refer the student to the Student Remediation Laboratory

4. To make a course accessible, faculty should provide:

   A. Instructions articulate or link to the institution's accessibility policies and services
   B. An overview of technologies utilized in the course
   C. Information on how learners can protect their data and privacy
   D. Alternative means of access to multimedia content

5. Rationales for including higher-level cultural competence skills/strategies in health organization policies include:

   A. Consideration of individual/group needs and preferences
   B. Elimination of long-standing health disparities
   C. Monitoring the quality of and access to health services
   D. Needing to be sensitive to others' beliefs and values

6. Which of the following would be considered an internal force that influences both nursing education and higher education?

   A. Global and domestic terrorism
   B. Economic recession
   C. Emerging infectious diseases
   D. The curriculum

7. A nurse educator uses a vodcast to remotely introduce themselves to the class because it provides:

   A. An audio recording that can be uploaded into a Learning Management System (LMS)
   B. A social media website that can be incorporated into a course
   C. A video recording that can be uploaded into an LMS
   D. An App that can be incorporated into a course

8. According to the VARK (Visual, Auditory, Reading/Writing Preference, and Kinesthetic) basic categories of learning styles, which type of learner would prefer lectures and small group discussions?

   A. Aural learners
   B. Kinesthetic learners
   C. Visual learners
   D. Read/write learners

9. Which of the following would be considered an external force that influences both nursing and higher education?

   A. Mission and purpose
   B. Philosophy and goals
   C. Regulations and accreditation
   D. Library and academic resources

10. A student states, "I never understand what exactly my assignment is for the day." The best response by the clinical nurse faculty member is:

    A. "That is because you did not read your assignment"
    B. "Did you complete your assigned readings?"
    C. "You need to discuss this with your classroom instructor"
    D. "I will help you make an appointment with the counseling center"

11. Which of the following statements by students provide evidence that a service-learning trip was beneficial?

    A. "I really gained a personal understanding of how underprivileged some cultures are"
    B. "It was a great way to see the world and other cultures"
    C. "It made me realize how good I have it here at home"
    D. "It was a great way to fulfill my graduation requirement"

12. The best classroom management procedure to address two students in the back of the room who exchange comments via texting while seated six feet apart is to:

    A. Request that they move their seats further apart
    B. Tell all students in the low residency classroom to place their phones visibly on their desks
    C. Request the two students remain after class and speak to them about their behavior
    D. Provide the entire class with a survey about what is the most engaging learning activity

13. Which of the following actions by a nurse educator is an example of fair use?

    A. Showing a copyrighted motion picture to class for instructional purposes
    B. Making three copies of a textbook and place them on reserve in the library for the class
    C. Copying excerpts of textbooks and journals from various sources to place in a coursepack
    D. Delivering a presentation to a community audience that displays photographs for which permission was not obtained

14. Regarding educational technology, the faculty is expected to:

    A. Be a super user of at least one technology
    B. Know technology resources
    C. Expect that students find their own technology support
    D. Be an expert on most types of technology

15. Which of the following leadership styles is most effective in facilitating the change process?

    A. Transformative
    B. Servant
    C. Autocratic
    D. Democratic

16. Which of the following is a national professional nursing organization that currently accredits nursing education programs?

    A. Sigma Theta Tau International (STTI)
    B. Commission for Collegiate Nursing Education (CCNE)
    C. American Association of Critical Care Nurses (AACN)
    D. National Institute for Nursing Program Certification (NINPC)

17. Which of the following activities would be an effective teaching method in the psychomotor domain?

    A. Skills demonstration
    B. Concept mapping
    C. Computer-assisted instruction
    D. Case studies

18. While developing online instruction, a nurse educator wants to promote critical thinking. The best method to do so would be to:

    A. Provide questions intermittently during the voice-over PowerPoint presentation
    B. Ask students to join a discussion board and answer questions and respond to peers
    C. Assign students a case study using a rubric to highlight the pathophysiology
    D. Develop a concept map of a patient's condition and ask a group to explain links

19. Which is the best example of nursing faculty striving toward a better system of self-governance?

    A. Choosing to have courses assigned
    B. Serving on a faculty search committee
    C. Taking part in a community outreach program
    D. Attending a university faculty meeting

20. Which of the following is crucial for a nurse educator to become successful?

    A. Understanding of learning styles and evaluation methods
    B. Budgetary knowledge
    C. Knowledge of student's social communication skills
    D. Background history of good faculty peer evaluations

21. When preparing an exam for students who have English as their additional or second language (EAL/ESL) the educator should:

    A. Use complex sentences
    B. Highlight key words
    C. Use proper medical terminology
    D. Use statements that need completion

22. Considering the analysis of the items below, which statement is accurate?

Exam Item	Difficulty Factor (*p*-value	Item discrimination (point biserial index)
1	.02	0.89
2	.96	0.25
3	1.00	0.00

A) Item 3 was too easy and needs revision
B) Item 1 was too easy and needs revision
C) Item 2's discrimination was better than item 1
D) The difficulty of all items is in an acceptable range

23. Which of the following programs would enable a student to spend a semester in a university in another country?

A. Global classroom
B. Service learning
C. Study abroad
D. Independent practicum

24. Which of the following would be an example of a formative evaluation?

A. A concept map of their patients' overall assessment
B. An essay on the process of acute renal failure
C. Socratic questioning about content just covered
D. A comprehensive final exam

25. A student nurse took a picture of a new mother and her baby and posted it on a social media site. This is a violation of the:

A. American Nursing Association Code of Ethics
B. Health Insurance Portability and Accountability Act (HIPAA)
C. Code of Federal Regulations (45 CFR)
D. Family Educational Rights and Privacy Act (FERPA)

26. The novice nurse educator needs a better understanding of leading change when they state that effective change leaders possess:

A. Strategic competence
B. Technical competence
C. Perseverance competence
D. Execution competence

27. Which of the following is the best example of providing a positive organizational climate for promotion and tenure?

    A. Nursing faculty come to campus to teach and have online office hours
    B. A mentorship program includes a mentor from another discipline only
    C. Having monthly social events and all nursing faculty are invited
    D. Providing a three-credit download in work effort for scholarship

28. When planning to incorporate technology for course teaching and effectiveness, the faculty should incorporate

    A. Technology that is available in the course
    B. At least one new technology each week of the course
    C. Only technology that the learners are familiar with
    D. The technology that best supports the learning outcomes

29. The nurse educator understands that creating this teaching element is not permissible by a student under *Fair Use*:

    A. Creating a presentation that incorporates copyrighted music into the background for a face-to-face class
    B. Creating a presentation that incorporates copyrighted music into the background for a virtual class meeting
    C. Creating and recording a presentation that incorporates copyrighted music into the background, which will be posted in the learning management system for students to view and comment on
    D. Creating a presentation that incorporates copyrighted music into the background, which will be shown at a school fund-raising event

30. Which of the following distractors needs revision in the item below, for which Response C is the correct answer?

Question #5	Response A	Response B	Response C	Response D
# Students answering it correctly	8	0	52	12

    A) A
    B) B
    C) C
    D) D

31. A nurse educator is applying for a full-time faculty position and is revising their curriculum vitae (CV). After listing the identifying data, the nurse educator should include:

    A. Current position and years of service in the position
    B. Certifications and active dates of the certifications
    C. Year of original RN licensure and state
    D. Year and degree of all education

32. Which of the following methods would be best to develop cultural competence in the classroom?

    A. Record all lectures
    B. Discuss cultural norms
    C. Promote independent projects
    D. Speak using local language

33. After a classroom lecture and skills review, "Demonstrate sterile technique with 100% accuracy." is a(n) _____ objective.

    A. Course
    B. Clinical
    C. Leveled
    D. Outcome

34. A student is in the clinical learning environment and refuses to take care of infectious patients even though the student has the proper personal protective equipment (PPE). The clinical nurse faculty member should:

    A. Reassign the student to a non-infectious patient
    B. Refer the student to career counseling
    C. Provide the student with a case study about an infectious patient
    D. Ask the student to leave the clinical learning environment

35. A student nurse states, "I am concerned for the welfare and well-being of my patient and I will strive to advocate for patients in all of my clinical interactions." This is an example of which of the five core values of the American Association Colleges of Nursing's (AACN's) caring, professional nurse?

    A. Altruism
    B. Autonomy
    C. Integrity
    D. Social justice

36. Which of the following can best be used to engage the learners in a course?

    A. A case study of complex patient needs
    B. A problem-based learning exercise
    C. An interactive video discussion board
    D. A topic-based puzzle to complete

37. The novice nurse educator requests information about developing a blog. The mentor explains that a blog is:

    A. A web page with a narrative that is updated by an individual or a group
    B. A social media site for networking with faculty and students
    C. A social media platform for sending out short message about what you are doing now
    D. A web page that can be edited by invited members

38. Analyze the statistic of the item below. Based on this data, which statement is correct?

Item number	Difficulty (p-value)	Overall item Point biserial	Option	Response Proportion	Point biserial of the key correct answer
11	.89	0.31	A	0.27	0.06
			B	0.01	−0.12
			C	0.06	−0.37
			D*	0.86	0.31

    A. More high scoring students selected B than D
    B. Of the students, 89% got the question correct
    C. More low scoring students selected A than C
    D. This is a low overall discriminating question

39. It is essential to provide a healthy and positive nursing education organizational climate because:

    A. It promotes faculty retention
    B. It decreases complaints
    C. It promotes longevity in a rank
    D. It helps reputation

40. Which of the following is an example of a public domain work?

    A. A 2020 publication by the Center for Disease Control (CDC)
    B. Quotes from a webpage that professes social justice
    C. Not-for-profit organization facts about a population
    D. Google Scholar publications

41. A nursing student states, "I realize that I must constantly read what is new so that my practice stays current" is evidence that the student plans to:

    A. Demonstrate culturally relevant practice
    B. Practice within cultural norms
    C. Advocate for access to quality care
    D. Continue to grow as a professional

42. Traditional universities often establish promotion and tenure on the following criteria:

    A. Teaching, scholarship, and service
    B. Teaching, research, and service
    C. Teaching, application, and service
    D. Innovation, teaching, and practice

43. What is the first step in assessing an organization's effectiveness?

    A. Plan and implement the evaluation
    B. Establish the boundaries of the evaluation
    C. Define the criteria of merit
    D. Conduct a performance needs assessment

44. Which of the following characteristics are true about Generation Z'ers?

    A. They prefer to talk on the phone
    B. They are very open about their personal lives
    C. They see education as a means to an end
    D. They value being virtually connected

45. What type of critical scholarship allows an opportunity for the public to review and critique and is highly regarded by the profession?

    A. Dissemination in peer-reviewed publication
    B. Sharing Innovative teaching techniques
    C. Developing measures to write in public journals
    D. Sharing teaching and learning practices

46. The student nurse describes her decision to give her diabetic patient orange juice by saying, "I noticed he was sweating and a bit confused. I know these are signs and symptoms of diabetic shock and that he might have a low blood sugar. I did look at his chart and did check his blood sugar and then got him some orange juice." This is an example of which theory of debriefing?

    A. Critical thinking
    B. Debriefing with good judgement
    C. Debriefing for meaningful learning
    D. Plus/delta

47. A demonstration to life-long learning by a nurse educator is best displayed by:

    A. Joining a professional education organization
    B. Attending continuing education conferences related to academic teaching
    C. Writing exam questions for the certified nurse educator exam
    D. Participating as a journal article reviewer

48. The Simulation Center conducts a simulated health disaster with participants who exhibit both physical and psychological systems. This simulation would be appropriate for which kind of curriculum model?

    A. Conceptual
    B. Integrated
    C. Deconstructed
    D. Interprofessional

49. The novice nurse educator needs additional mentoring when they state, "I understand that in nursing education, issues of enrolment, curriculum design, pedagogy, faculty expectations, faculty competencies, and scholarly productivity are shaped by":

    A. Social forces
    B. Political forces
    C. Economic forces
    D. Administrative forces

50. Which strategy uses technology to support a learning process by embedding repetition and practice to provide students with an opportunity to practice time management and organization?

    A. A problem-based learning exercise
    B. An interactive video discussion board with a challenge question
    C. PowerPoint presentations using the PechaKucha approach
    D. Game-based, self-check learning activity

51. A nurse educator is using Socratic questioning in the classroom setting. When asked by a colleague why they use this strategy, what response best identifies the advantage of this approach?

    A. "This strategy is simple to use and doesn't require additional work"
    B. "Socratic questioning assists with decision-making and can lead to robust discussions"
    C. "Students must be prepared for class in the event they are called on to answer a question"
    D. "This strategy is effective for highlighting the students who know the answers"

52. The American Nurses Association's (ANA's) position is that nurse leaders must possess change management competencies to "facilitate organizational change initiatives and overcome resistance to change" (2018, p. 8). Essential behaviors associated with these competencies include:

    A. Involve key people
    B. Display consistent leadership style
    C. Resist changing external influence
    D. Discount concerns voiced by resisters

53. Content development or revision predicated on external forces may not consider:

    A. Infection control
    B. Childbearing content
    C. Telehealth
    D. Cultural sensitivity

54. A well-managed university student exchange program will:

    A. Mandate that all students must speak the country's primary language
    B. Grant course credits
    C. Divide the tuition and housing costs
    D. Provide specific courses to foreign students

55. When teaching online, module or unit student learning outcomes should be congruent directly with:

    A. Course student learning outcomes
    B. Program outcomes
    C. The syllabus
    D. The mission of the college

56. When interpreting a Kuder-Richardson 20s (KR-20) of four examinations, which of the following statements is accurate about the information provided?

Kuder Richardson (KR-20)
Exam 1 KR=0.19
Exam 2 KR=0.28
Exam 3 KR=0.53
Exam 4 KR-0.70

    A. Exam 3 is the most reliable
    B. Exam 1 is the most internal consistency
    C. Exam 2 is the most discriminating
    D. Exam 4 is the most reliable

57. Which of the following would be an example of implementing a global classroom?

   A. Holding video conferencing with other students for a health policy class
   B. Developing asynchronous lectures for students to watch after work
   C. Having students watch a foreign video and then write a reflective paper
   D. Have students present a research article about nursing in Europe

58. A learning disability would affect which of the areas of learner readiness?

   A. Knowledge
   B. Emotional
   C. Social
   D. Physical

59. An evaluation method based on a summary of accumulated observations of the learner's clinical performance compared to course objectives is a(n):

   A. External review
   B. Anecdotal note
   C. Skills checklist
   D. Rating scale

60. Which of the following would be the best type of activity to help new graduate nurses socialize into the role of nursing?

   A. Role-playing a scenario of an issue that might come up on the hospital unit and discussing following the proper chains of command
   B. Performing a full head to toe assessment in the clinical learning environment
   C. Demonstrate an example of how to properly give report to the next shift
   D. Having the learners write a reflective journal on an incident they witnessed in clinical

61. Nurse educators are encouraged to have specialized courses in all the following areas except:

   A. Teaching and learning principles
   B. Evaluation and assessment methods
   C. Leadership and management
   D. Curriculum development and design

62. Which method would be effective for a teaching method in the affective domain?

   A. Computer-assisted instruction
   B. Lecture with automated response questions
   C. A debrief asking to share feelings after a patient died
   D. Demonstrating how to insert a foley catheter

63. Which course student learning outcome is measurable?

    A. Understand the difference between placenta previa and placenta abruption
    B. Consider the difference between placenta previa and placenta abruption
    C. Contrast the difference between placenta previa and placenta abruption
    D. Remember the difference between placenta previa and placenta abruption

64. Which of the following demonstrates quality improvement in the nurse educator role?

    A. Progressive publications
    B. Multiple student thank-you cards
    C Community service awards
    D. Political activist activities

65. When planning a service-learning project, which of the following should be implemented?

    A. Assigning a course faculty to take the students abroad
    B. Form a planning group for the project
    C. Choose students by faculty recommendation and financial ability
    D. Choose a place that students and faculty want to go

66. Which is the best method for the new faculty to get feedback on one's teaching strategies?

    A. Attend a conference on teaching strategies
    B. Watch teaching videos of faculty with several years of experience
    C. Ask a mentor to sit in on a class and provide feedback
    D. Read a research article on teaching strategies

67. A novice nurse educator wants to join an organization that supports teaching and learning. The best recommendation would be:

    A. Oncology Nursing Society
    B. National League for Nursing (NLN)
    C. National Patient Safety Foundation
    D. Sigma Theta Tau International Honor Society (STTI)

68. A new faculty member has joined the nursing department's Evaluation and Outcomes Committee. In order to prepare for their first meeting, the nurse educator knows that program evaluations are:

    A. Needed only when accreditation is due
    B. Systematic analyses of all aspects of the program
    C. Agreed-upon rules to measure quantity, extent, value, and quality
    D. Standards with which a learner is evaluated for admission into a nursing program

69. Key transformational leadership practices include:

    A. Reinforcing and stabilizing existing processes

    B. Inspiring a shared vision

    C. Establishing a contractual reward system

    D. Display concern for others

70. Specialty accreditation agencies in nursing are predicated on the concept of:

    A. Expert opinion

    B. Curriculum guidance

    C. Regulatory standards

    D. Peer evaluation

71. Which academic rank is appropriate for a nurse educator to hold if they continue to demonstrate leadership in research, teaching, and service at a national and international level as well as become internationally recognized for this body of work, whether it be clinical research or educational research?

    A. Instructor

    B. Assistant Professor

    C. Associate Professor

    D. Professor

72. Point Biserial = .51 = C P value = .78 N = 80 KR20 = .64
Based on this item analysis the faculty should:

Distractor Analysis:#Chosen	A 5	B 2	C* 61	D 11
Point Biserial	−0.30	−0.14	0.51	−0.34
% selected	6.25	2.50	77.50	13.75

    A. Use the question again in future tests

    B. Revise the question stem

    C. Revise the wrong distractors

    D. Remove the question from the test score

73. Analytic technologies can support student learning by:

    A. Generating automatic assignment grading

    B. Providing critical information regarding student learning

    C. Collecting student demographic information

    D. Offers improved access through mobile interfaces

74. A faculty is developing a test blueprint for students in their course. In addition to using the course content that was covered, the faculty should also base questions on the NCLEX blueprint. The highest percent of NCLEX test plan which will cover:

    A. Pharmacological and parenteral therapies
    B. Reduction of risk potential
    C. Psychosocial integrity
    D. Management of care

75. The first assignment in a health assessment course requests the students to map their genealogy. This assignment indicates that the teacher is including which concept in the course?

    A. Anti-racism
    B. Biracial content
    C. Multiculturalism
    D. Genetics

76. A clinical nurse educator is teaching an adult nursing care course at the local hospital. Which of the following assignments is most appropriate assignment for beginning students?

    A. A 56-year-old newly diagnosed diabetic
    B. A 89-year-old with congestive heart failure
    C. A 76-year-old with a broken hip in traction
    D. A 30-year-old recovering from abdominal surgery

77. The most important element of new faculty orientation is discussing:

    A. Expectations of the academic faculty role
    B. Salary of the faculty
    C. Benefits of the faculty
    D. Legal issues in academic education

78. A culture of shared governance can be best described as:

    A. Voices of nurse educators being heard by university administration about issues
    B. Students and nurse educators make decisions and present them to administration
    C. University administration and faculty arrive at decisions by joint consensus
    D. University administration informs faculty of decisions before implementation

79. A nurse educator is role-playing for a leadership class as bureaucratic leader. Which attribute should the nurse educator display in the role?

    A. Make decisions with input from other nurse educators

    B. Make decisions that uphold company policy

    C. Make decision by consensus of committee members

    D. Promotes decisions that are congruent with organizational mission

80. A nurse educator is taking a group of students on a service-learning trip. Which of the following safety items is a priority?

    A. Pack extra clothes in your luggage for rain and cold

    B. Be sure to have cash with you for exchange

    C. Be generous to local children if approached

    D. Have immunizations, passports, and necessary medications

81. Which of the following would the nurse educator recognize as an act of incivility by a learner?

    A. Learners discussing their grades after an examination

    B. A learner using their computer to shop for shoes during class

    C. A learner who is using their cell phone in the hallway between classes and talking loudly

    D. A learner who is questioning an assignment they do not understand seeking clarification as the rubric does not make sense to them

82. The novice nurse educator needs additional mentoring when they state; "I think the best way my students learn is when I …

    A. use PowerPoints that have lots of graphics"

    B. link new material learned to their clinical learning experiences"

    C. take an active role with them in the classroom"

    D. provide assignments that are pertinent"

83. Consideration of the number and the expertise of faculty when redesigning a curriculum and choosing a curriculum model is part of the:

    A. External forces

    B. Budgetary considerations

    C. Internal forces

    D. Workforces pool

84. A novice nurse educator states that using gaming technology can provide students with the following benefits. Which of the following benefits is not attributed to gaming and therefore, the nurse educator needs better understanding of the modality?

    A. Student understanding of content
    B. Student misconceptions
    C. Student technology mastery
    D. Student collaboration preferences

85. Mentorship of new faculty is the responsibility of:

    A. The assigned mentor for the faculty
    B. The informal mentor for the faculty
    C. The chair of the department
    D. All faculty in the department

86. A nurse educator is applying for a full-time position at a University and is told on the interview that it is expected that they obtain a federal grant during their first six years as a faculty member. The nurse educator contributes this criterion to:

    A. The expectations of the nursing discipline
    B. The Carnegie Classification of the institution
    C. The Dean of Nursing's initiative
    D. The economic status of the University

87. Which of the following contribute to student motivation and retention?

    A. Extracurricular activities
    B. Clinical learning experiences
    C. Participation in simulation scenarios
    D. Frequent interaction with faculty

88. When the faculty is teaching about appropriate food to include in a diabetic diet for a Latinx patient, they are practicing what kind of education?

    A. Anti-racist
    B. Pro-Latinx
    C. Multicultural
    D. Interdisciplinary

89. An example of participating actively in a professional organization is:

    A. Being a member of the American Association of Colleges of Nursing
    B. Having a subscription to Nursing Education Perspectives Journal
    C. Serving on the governance committee for the local chapter of Sigma Theta Tau International
    D. Critiquing a journal article for a nurse educator colleague

90. A course team is looking at a recent 50-item multiple-choice exam they gave to their students. The KR was 0.37. The faculty's next step is to:

    A. Look at the number of questions on the test
    B. Perform an item analysis of test questions
    C. Review the test key for correctness
    D. Evaluate the testing environment

91. Which of the following is the best mentor for a new academic faculty?

    A. A current faculty member who is a friend of the faculty member
    B. Another new faculty member that can appreciate being new
    C. A faculty member with a similar background and teaching schedule
    D. A faculty member with the same terminal degree

92. To engage students with different learning styles, it is most important for class instructional material to be:

    A. Assessable
    B. Reliable
    C. Varied
    D. Current

93. Garrison, Anderson, and Archer's Community of Inquiry (CoI) Framework discuses "teacher presence." What does "teacher presence" mean?

    A. Being physically in a classroom
    B. Listening to students when they speak
    C. Facilitate the learning experience
    D. Communication in a timely manner

94. The novice nurse educator needs a better understanding of open educational resources (OER) when they state that OER will provide:

    A. Customizable content
    B. A learning management system
    C. Digital textbooks
    D. Research materials

95. Nursing educational programs' mission statements should be derived from the:

    A. American Nurses Association
    B. University or College's mission statement
    C. Philosophy of the faculty and administration
    D. National League of Nursing

96. Organizational culture can be influenced by which of the following management strategies?

    A. Clear chain of command

    B. Specific recruitment

    C. Performance reward system

    D. Flexible policies and procedures

97. The nurse educator assigns the undergraduate students a research article critique. This assignment is most effective in measuring which of the following domains of learning?

    A. Affective

    B. Cognitive

    C. Psychomotor

    D. Formative

98. A nurse researcher is conducting a study that needs IRB approval for her doctoral studies at two different institutions. The mentor explains what important aspect to the graduate student about IRB approval?

    A. IRB approval from the researcher's institution does not automatically translate to the IRB in the institution of study

    B. IRB approval from the researcher institution does automatically translate to the IRB in the institution of study

    C. IRB approval is not necessary unless experiments are being conducted on students under the age of 18

    D. IRB approval is only dependent on the study that is being conducted

99. A nurse educator questions their educational level with whether they may participate in a research study with a team of educators and leaders from the school. What would be an appropriate response to questioning the level of education to participation in the study?

    A. Educational level is required and must be considered when choosing members of the research team

    B. Nurse educators who only have a role in teaching and learning may not be supported in any research studies

    C. Nurses must hold a doctorate to conduct any research for dissemination and publication

    D. Regardless of educational preparation nurse educators and leaders may collaborate in research and scholarly work

100. Point Biserial = 0.05 Correct answer = C p-value = .99 N = 149 KR20 = .37
Based on this item analysis the faculty knows all the following is true except

Distractor Analysis:	A	B	C*	D
Point Biserial	0.00	0.00	0.05	−0.05
% selected	0.00	0.00	98.66	1.34

A. Items that have a point biserial of zero means learners did not select them because the distractor was good

B. Learners probably got the question correct by guessing

C. Negative discriminating power occurs when more learners in the lower group than in the upper group choose the correct answer

D. The item needs to be revised or replaced

101. Which is an appropriate alternate experience for students when the medical-surgical unit census is low?

A. Sending them to the cafeteria to collaboratively study for the next medical-surgical test

B. Sending them to another nursing unit to observe a different cohort of patients

C. Finding observational experiences that are congruent with their clinical objectives

D. Canceling the clinical day and making it up when the census is higher on the nursing unit

102. An item-analysis report for a multiple-choice exam revealed that the KR-20 was 0.78. Based on this statistic, which of the following interpretations can be made regarding this exam?

A. The exam is reliable in measuring learner knowledge of the material

B. There are too few items on the exam

C. The items are poorly written and do not discriminate

D. There is an excess of very easy questions

103. A nurse educator is teaching a lunch and learn on active learning strategies. One of her colleagues remains very resistant to any change from traditional lectures. What statement would have the greatest impact?

A. "Students are passive learners with lecture and little effort is required on their part"

B. "Students are easily bored when they are required to listen for hours on end"

C. "Active learning promotes critical thinking, which is important for NCLEX-RN success"

D. "Lecture is not the best way to teach these millennial students"

104. A nurse educator is planning a skills review in conjunction with the laboratory coordinator. What strategy would be most effective in reviewing skills and evaluating student learning in senior level students?

    A. Demonstration

    B. Vignettes

    C. Imagery

    D. Simulation

105. To be an effective mentor, a nurse educator should have

    A. At least 5 years experience

    B. At least 10 years of experience

    C. A terminal degree

    D. Formal training on how to be a mentor

106. An educator is developing spirit of inquiry about teaching, learning, and evaluation. Which of the following would be an example of spirit of inquiry?

    A. Identifying a gap in the literature and deciding to conduct a research study

    B. Continue to teach using the same methods without inquiry

    C. Decide to use only their student evaluation responses to research problems

    D. Obtain presentation materials from the internet to use as evidence to change practice

107. A novice nurse educator has invited his mentor to observe his pharmacology class because they are concerned with the lack of student participation. After observing his lecture, what useful advice can the mentor provide?

    A. "Giving the students more frequent breaks will keep them awake"

    B. "Breaking up the lecture with activities will keep the students involved"

    C. "With experience, you will learn to make your PowerPoints more exciting"

    D. "Students may prefer to have the lectures recorded so they can view them at a later time"

108. As the lead nurse educator on a service learning, what would be the most important thing to be sure is in place prior to leaving on the trip?

    A. Registration with the U.S. Embassy in the foreign country

    B. A list of student food likes and dislikes of students

    C. Have extra cash in the event it is needed in an emergency

    D. Have layered clothing for weather differences

109. The nurse researcher attends a conference to present her work on outcomes from using standardized testing which are integrated throughout an undergraduate curriculum. The researcher is approached to consult in other schools of nursing as they work to incorporate this approach into their curriculum. Which of the following is the researcher accomplishing?

A. Scholarship of Teaching
B. Scholarship of Application
C. Scholarship of Inquiry
D. Scholarship of Publication

110. A colleague is providing a peer review of a novice nurse educator's adult health course. What statement would be most effective in helping the novice understand the use of humor while teaching?

A. Humor can be effective in providing a sense of belonging for students
B. All students appreciate and understand the use of humor in the classroom
C. Most nurse educators have difficulty in using appropriate humor
D. Humor can be used with any nursing topic

111. Planning learning activities for a class should begin with the following step:

A. Developing the learning outcomes
B. Selecting a teaching strategy
C. Considering implementation strategies
D. Finding a population to meet the objectives

112. A nurse educator is discussing with colleagues how to use games in their classroom. Which statement by a colleague indicates further information is needed?

A. "Using scaffolding, games can incorporate progressively more challenging tasks"
B. "Games are a great way to engage the learners and encourage interaction"
C. "Games are an effective strategy for kinesthetic learners"
D. "Games can also be used as a method of evaluation of individual learning"

113. A novice nurse researcher who has never published decides to disseminate their findings for publication in a peer-reviewed journal. What would be an important aspect of publication for the novice researcher to understand?

A. Publication is based on when the manuscript is submitted
B. Publication in a non-peer reviewed journal will give the same recognition as peer-reviewed
C. Publication is a learned skill that can be assisted through mentorship of experts
D. Publication requires the hiring of an editor to oversee the manuscript

114. What is the best method to secure an online objective exam?

    A. Randomize the order of the answer responses
    B. Set a time limit to complete the online exam
    C. Randomize the order of the questions
    D. Have a remote proctor

115. Which is the best method for the faculty to be available for learners in an online course?

    A. Schedule weekly virtual office hours
    B. Provide an email for learners to contact the faculty
    C. Provide a phone number for learners to contact the faculty
    D. Ask the learners to post any questions on the Q and A Discussion Board

116. A novice clinical educator is talking about her post-clinical conferences. Which statement indicates that the clinical educator needs further mentoring in the role?

    A. "In post-conference today, the students analyzed some ECG strips after learning about them in class this week"
    B. "I try to build up my students in post-conference by highlighting 'well-done' moments from clinical"
    C. "Most weeks, we use post-conference to talk about the skills they completed"
    D. "I plan ahead for post-conferences so we can use our time most effectively"

117. A nurse educator reports to their colleagues that students are expressing significant discontent with the flipped classroom. What statement by the educator could indicate the source of the problem?

    A. "During class time, the students are working in teams to complete case studies"
    B. "I am able to focus on key points for learning in the classroom"
    C. "Instructional technology has been very helpful in working through any issues"
    D. "I posted all of my voice-over PowerPoints for review prior to class"

118. Students place posters advertising a Women's Shelter in the Women's Restrooms at the university. This is an example of which of the following?

    A. An assessment technique to determine if domestic violence exists
    B. The recognition of how cultural factors influence the patterns of domestic violence
    C. Legal and ethical issues in reporting domestic violence
    D. Interventions to reduce vulnerability and increase safety for women

119. Nursing faculty are discussing strategies for assisting students to make the transition from theory to practice. Which learning activity would be most effective?

    A. Collaborative learning
    B. Debate
    C. Case studies
    D. Group discussions

120. A student is trying to become more culturally competent. What would you advise the student to do as a first step to assist in this process?

    A. Listen to the music of that culture
    B. Observe the way of dress of the culture
    C. Learn the slang language and how they talk in that culture
    D. Soul search for your own biases and stereotypical ideas

121. A novice nurse educator is engaged in process improvement and is passionate about taking on the role of scholar. Which of the following would be a method for the educator to begin this role?

    A. Conducting a quick survey of students learning preferences
    B. Creating a poster on immunizations to be displayed in the school
    C. Conducting an IRB research project in areas of strength of teaching
    D. Joining a journal club critiquing articles on standardized testing

122. A student needs further understanding of the assigned preceptor experience when the student verbalizes:

    A. "I follow their preceptor's schedule"
    B. "They will assist me to learn procedures"
    C. "The preceptor will not have much time to teach me"
    D. "My preceptor will assign me to appropriate patients"

123. Nurse educators learn about Boyer's Model as a framework of scholarship and research. Which of the following responses regarding the four dimensions of the model made by a nurse educator would be most appropriate?

    A. Educational sabbatical leave is assessed and decided using this model
    B. Workload decisions for nurse educators are based on the model
    C. Appointment and performance evaluation are integral frameworks to the model
    D. Student performance and evaluations are integral frameworks to the model

124. A nurse educator wants to help a struggling student in his Med-Surg II course and has scheduled an appointment to meet with the student. To prepare for these meetings, the most important thing they should do is:

A. Access the student's previous course tests from Med-Surg I
B. Consult with the faculty who taught the student in Med-Surg I
C. Review student's assignments/tests submitted in the course
D. Send the student to the college's tutoring center

125. Which factor creates a barrier to creativity and innovation?

A. Trust
B. Conflict
C. Challenge
D. Established norms

126. After administering an exam, the nurse educator is reviewing the item analysis for each of the multiple-choice questions. One question yielded the following statistics for the items:

Point Biserial = 0. 43		= A		Total Group = 57%	
Distractor Analysis	A	B	C	D
Point Biserial	0.43	−0.15	0.00	−0.48
Frequency	57%	23%	0%	20%

Based on this analysis, what action should be taken by the nurse educator?

A. Revise right answer A
B. Revise distractor B
C. Revise distractor C
D. Revise distractor D

127. According to Boyer's Model of Scholarship, which of the following is the best description of scholarship of integration?

A. Interpretation and synthesis of knowledge
B. Validation of existing knowledge
C. Connection of theory to practice
D. Use of evidence to facilitate learning

128. The student nurse states, "Now I understand how all this ties together; how one body system effects another." The teaching technique that helped her realize this is a(n):

    A. Concept map
    B. Discrepant event
    C. Appropriate analogy
    D. Short quiz

129. A nurse educator who has a spirit of inquiry and knowledge in a particular area of specialization and pursues the research would be considered a(n):

    A. Clinician
    B. Teacher
    C. Academic
    D. Scholar

130. The nurse educator is preparing to teach a group of learners with previous education experiences or degrees. What is important when teaching this group of students?

    A. Be prepared and know the content well
    B. Avoid having them share previous experiences
    C. Realize these students lack motivation
    D. Engage them in clinical experiences

131. The student states, "I can't believe that I learned so much today. All of this just fits together and makes sense." This is an example of:

    A. Reflective learning
    B. Evidence-based learning
    C. Critical thinking
    D. Integrating theory and practice

132. A nurse educator has assigned readings from several journals available in the library which is on the other side of campus. The nurse educator wants to make it easy for students to get the article. Which of the following is in compliance of Fair Use for educational purposes?

    A. Make copies of the articles to distribute in class
    B. Post a pdf of the article in the LMS for students to access and print
    C. Post instructions and a direct link to the library e-journal in the course
    D. Make arrangements with the library to duplicate and provide the article

133. The nursing program's Progression Committee members were reviewing their goals and policies to ensure they were congruent with institutional standards and found which policy should be updated:

   A. All students need a minimum GPA 3.0 to progress, or otherwise be placed on academic probation

   B. If a students received a C or lower in any nursing course they must repeat that course and obtain a grade of C+ or better. If a student fails the course for a second time, or fails any additional course, they will be dismissed from the program

   C. A student may take a leave of absence for up to 2 years. If a student's fails to contact the nursing department, or goes beyond 2 years, they will need to reapply to the program

   D. Achievement of a minimum grade of 850 on standardized achievement tests is needed to progress

134. In online and hybrid learning it is important for learning tools to be:

   A. Innovative

   B. Accessible

   C. Individualized

   D. Free

135. In setting up a course's evaluation method that matches the objectives, a faculty member wants students to demonstrate a higher level of cognitive thinking that evaluates the affective domain and connection of concepts. The faculty evaluates all the following assignments, except:

   A. Reflective journal response to a discussion board post

   B. One Minute Paper at the end of class

   C. Concept map to address the interrelated concepts of primary concepts

   D. Oral presentation of the impact a course concept and the profession of nursing

136. A clinical adjunct faculty member is planning their orientation to the unit with the students and knows that students should not be confused or anxious at the end of the semester if they will pass or not. They plan on having weekly informal meetings recapping their performance. This type of evaluation process is known as:

   A. Summative

   B. Normed

   C. Achievement assessment

   D. Formative

137. Sigma Theta Tau International/Elsevier Nurse Faculty Leadership Academy (NFLA) was developed and designed directly to assist:

    A. The advancement of nursing research
    B. Junior faculty assimilation into academia
    C. Seasoned faculty promotion and tenure
    D. Development of deans as leaders

138. Alignment of student learning outcomes facilitates:

    A. Connecting course materials with assessment
    B. Making a course easier to navigate
    C. Organizing content for learner support
    D. Creating authentic learning opportunities

139. Why are progression policies important to have in an undergraduate nursing program?

    A. They set a "norm" and minimum level for where students should be performing
    B. They compare students against each other to identify the better learners
    C They predict which students will definitely pass the NCLEX exam
    D. They help identify students who may need additional resources

140. The student says, "I always read the most current journal articles about my patients before I go to my clinical day so that I can use the most current techniques to care for them." This demonstrates which of the following NLN Competencies for Graduates of Baccalaureate Programs?

    A. Human flourishing
    B. Nursing judgment
    C. Professional identity
    D. Spirit of inquiry

141. Cultural proficiency is a new term selected to convey a more expansive approach to diversity and inclusion. According to the model, a cultural proficient individual will:

    A. Accommodate differences
    B. Collaborate with differences
    C. Incorporate cultural artefacts into the environment
    D. Examine policies and practices of an organization

142. Item analysis of an exam question revealed the following statistics:

Point Biserial = 0. 40	= A		Total Group = 72%	
Distractor Analysis	A	B	C	D
Point Biserial	0.40	0.03	0.04	0.12
Frequency	72%	6%	15%	7%

How should the nurse educator interpret these results?

A. This question needs to be revised as too many learners answered it correctly
B. High-scoring learners answered the question correctly
C. Lower scoring learners answered the question correctly
D. There is inadequate discrimination of the distractors

143. Which of the following actions by faculty would be a proactive course management strategy?

A. Reaching out to students who have missed submission deadlines
B. Offer opportunities for student to schedule appointments
C. Monitor assignment submissions and remind students of due dates
D. Provide a comprehensive syllabus and due dates at the start of the course

144. The new Next Generation NCLEX (NGN) items that faculty devise uses unfolding case studies that assist clinical decision-making. The first question pertaining to the unfolding case study is developed to assist students to:

A. Recognize cures
B. Analyze cues
C. Develop a hypothesis
D. Take action

145. Upon returning from an international service-learning trip, what is the most important thing for the students to do to gain the maximal learning from this experience?

A. Tell all their family and friends about the experience
B. Do a role-play activity to demonstrate to peers a situation that occurred on the trip
C. Participate in a debriefing session to explore feelings and perceptions of the experience
D. Have the students write a paper about the experience

146. The new Next Generation NCLEX (NGN) items that faculty devise use unfolding case studies that assist clinical decision-making. The last question pertaining to the unfolding case study is developed to assist students to:

A. Recognize clues
B. Develop a hypothesis
C. Evaluate outcomes
D. Take action

147. Review of an item on a test reveals the following statistics:

Point Biserial = 0.13		= D		Total Group = 82%	
Distractor Analysis	A	B	C	D	
Point Biserial	0.02	0.19	0.01	−0.13	
Frequency	12%	5%	1%	82%	

The likely cause for this frequency distribution is:

A. Higher scoring learners answered the question correctly
B. Higher scoring learners answered the question incorrectly
C. Lower scoring learners answered the question incorrectly
D. The distractors show clear discrimination

148. The new Next Generation NCLEX (NGN) standalone bowtie items that faculty devise assists clinical decision-making. The question is developed to assist students to relate:

A. Manifestations and medications to a disease process
B. Patients' perceptions and psychosocial care to a disease process
C. Nursing actions and monitoring to a disease process
D. Nursing assessment and interventions to a disease process

149. Instructional class materials should be:

    A. Entertaining

    B. Less than five years old

    C. Retrievable

    D. Seminal

150. A nurse educator reports to his mentor that students are complaining about a group project assignment because some students are not participating nor carrying their weight. What suggestion from the mentor would be most helpful?

    A. "Group projects require collaboration among the students"

    B. "Adding a peer evaluation as part of the grade may encourage better participation"

    C. "Students have to learn how to handle conflict"

    D. "I'm sure it is challenging for students to schedule time to work as a group"

Practice Test: Answers

1. B) A description of personality traits that contributed to the student's success
Faculty can include a description of personality traits that contributed to the student's success, but the student's educational record, including grades, GPA, classes, etc., cannot be shared without the student's written permission.

2. D) Four
A Level Four Objective is one of the higher levels of Bloom's Taxonomy and is appropriate behavior for students at the end of their program. Level Four is in the analyzing category and develops connections between ideas. Level Three is applying and uses new information in a different situation. Level Two is understanding and explains ideas or concepts, and Level One is remembering and uses recall.

3. D) Refer the student to the Student Remediation Laboratory
Students who are having problems in the clinical area should be referred to the Remediation Laboratory for help to correct the problem. The first step should be to make an effort to correct any unsatisfactory or unsafe learner behavior in a timely manner.

4. D) Alternative means of access to multimedia content
To make the course accessible to learners, faculty should provide alternative means of access to multimedia content in formats that meet the needs of diverse learners. Providing instructions or links regarding accessibility policies, an overview of the technology, and information on how to protect data does not make the course more accessible.

5. B) Elimination of long-standing health disparities
The underlying rationale for including higher-level cultural competence skills and strategies in health organization policies is to address the overarching goals to improve the quality and eliminate long-standing health disparities. Elimination of long-standing health disparities among people from diverse racial, ethnic, and cultural backgrounds is a national priority. Consideration of individual/group needs, preferences, access to health services, and needing to be sensitive to others' beliefs and values are all parts of eliminating health disparities but do not encompass the overriding policy that is needed.

6. D) The curriculum

The curriculum is an internal force that is made and modified by the faculty within the nursing academic institution. Terrorism, economic recession, and emerging infectious diseases are considered external forces.

7. C) A video recording that can be uploaded into an LMS

A vodcast is a video recording that can be uploaded into a course for learners.

8. A) Aural learners

Aural or auditory learners prefer to listen to sounds, music, and audiotapes to learn. Kinaesthetic learners prefer to learn by doing or hands on. Visual learners prefer pictures, movies, or diagrams to learn. Reading and writing learners prefer print. This print can be in the form of a book or information found on the internet.

9. C) Regulations and accreditation

Regulations and Accreditation is an external force that is external to the nursing academic institution and regulated by a governing body outside of the university. Mission and purpose, philosophy and goal, and library and academic resources are all examples of internal forces that influence nursing and higher education

10. D) "I will help you make an appointment with the counseling center"

The student may need academic or personal counseling to determine why the student is having problems understanding the assignments. The other answers are punitive.

11. A) "I really gained a personal understanding of how underprivileged some cultures are"

A student who now has gained insight on how other cultures live, how underprivileged some people are, and has grown in cultural insight and diversity. The other statements focus on the student, not the experience.

12. C) Request the two students remain after class and speak to them about their behavior

Speak to the two students after class. Since this does not involve everyone in the class, there is no need to tell all students to put their phones on the desks or to take a class-wide survey. Separating the two students will not affect texting.

13. A) Showing a copyrighted motion picture to class for instructional purposes

Using the video for instructional purposes is permissible under Fair Use. Permission is required before reprinting or copying excerpts of textbooks and journals. Images for which permission was not obtained can only be used for instructional purposes, not for the general public.

14. B) Know technology resources
The faculty needs to know what technology resources are available and whom to contact for support. Students are also expected to be able to call for support, and faculty do not have to be experts or super users.

15. A) Transformative
Transformative leadership style is most effective in encouraging change processes that are positive and lead to better outcomes.

16. B) Commission for Collegiate Nursing Education (CCNE)
The Commission for Collegiate Nursing Education (CCNE) is one of three national professional nursing organizations that accredits nursing education programs. The other two are the Commission for Nursing Education Accreditation (CNEA), the Accreditation Commission for Education in Nursing (ACEN).

17. A) Skills demonstration
Skills demonstration would be an example in the psychomotor domain. Concept mapping and computer-assisted instruction would be in the cognitive domain and visual. Case studies would be in the affective domain.

18. D) Develop a concept map of a patient's condition and ask a group to explain links
Explaining how assessment, planning, intervention, and evaluations of nursing care links together promote critical thinking. Concept mapping has demonstrated that it is an effective method to promote critical thinking. Discussion boards, case studies, and answering questions may also promote critical thinking if developed in a method that promotes reflection, but there is less evidence to demonstrate that these methods directly promote critical thinking.

19. B) Serving on a faculty search committee
Serving on a faculty search committee is being part of the interview and decision process to recruit and hire new faculty. This is an example of faculty self-governance.

20. A) Understanding of learning styles and evaluation methods
It is crucial for a nurse educator to be aware of different learning styles and methods for evaluating students to be a successful educator. Understanding the budget, communication modalities, and having peer support is helpful but not required in order to be successful.

21. B) Highlight keywords
Highlighting keywords can assist the student to answer the question correctly and avoid what students describe as "trickery." Questions should also be written in simple terms, using words understood by most people.

22. A) Item 3 was too easy and needs revision

Item 3 was too easy and needs revision; all the students got the question correct. The difficulty factor or p-value was 1.00. So 100 percent of students got the item correct. The point biserial was not discriminating at all, and this question needs revision.

23. C) Study abroad

This would be a study-abroad opportunity. Global classrooms are usually an interactive electronic program, and service learning is usually a shorter experience. An independent practicum is usually a program that houses a student with a foreign family to study abroad.

24. C) Socratic questioning about content just covered

Asking a student a question in class about content just covered enables an instructor to comprehend if the student is comprehending a concept in the process of learning or acquiring a new skill or concept. Simply asking a question and checking if a student is following along is a great way for faculty to be sure they are on track with the teaching method or process.

25. B) Health Insurance Portability and Accountability Act (HIPAA)

HIPAA addresses patient privacy and protection. The other options do not apply to that issue.

26. C) Perseverance competence

Magsaysay and Hechanova (2017) identify the five dimensions of ideal change leaders: (1) strategic/technical competence, (2) execution competence, (3) social competence, (4) character, and (5) resilience. Perseverance is not noted and may not be an attribute if it escalates into bullying.

27. D) Providing a three-credit download in work effort for scholarship

A university that gives faculty a reduced teaching workload and time off so that they can pursue scholarship is an example of a positive organizational climate that is supportive of their faculty. Socials are nice, but they are not the mechanism for satisfaction. Having a mentor in nursing as well as in another discipline may be more effective and having faculty present on campus is not a sure way of promoting career advancement.

28. D) The technology that best supports the learning outcomes

The faculty should only incorporate technology that will support the learning outcomes of the course. There is no need to use technology just because it is available or familiar.

29. D) Creating a presentation that incorporates copyrighted music into the background, which will be shown at a school fund-raising event

This would not be fair use because it is being used for commercial (fund-raising) purposes. Music can be used in classroom (in-person or virtual) for educational instruction.

30. B) B
No students chose this response, so this distractor needs to be revised.

31. D) Year and degree of all education
Education is listed first in reverse chronological order on a CV. Licensure, certifications, and positions are important to list, but educational level is usually the first item that CV reviewers focus on to ensure qualifications.

32. B) Discuss cultural norms
The best way to develop cultural competence in the classroom is to relate content to cultural norms. Discussing how different cultures may respond given specific situations facilitates cultural awareness. Group projects better assist in cultural competence, and recording does not open up discussion. Using local language may be a deficit to students not from the area

33. B) Clinical
The above student learning outcome (SLO) is most appropriate for a clinical skills laboratory experience. The SLO is very specific to the clinical area and would be part of a course that has a much broader content.

34. D) Ask the student to leave the clinical learning environment
The student should be asked to leave the clinical learning environment and report to the college's counseling canter to discuss their rationale. Changing assignment or providing the student with a case study is not necessary if the clinical learning experience is available. Career counseling is inappropriate since the student has decided on nursing, but psychological counseling may be needed to determine underlying fears.

35. A) Altruism
Altruism is what is being professed, the selfless concern for others. While the other options are part of the five core values of the AACN's caring professional nurse, autonomy refers to independence, integrity truth telling and doing the correct thing, and social justice looks at equity for all.

36. C) An interactive video discussion board
An interactive video discussion board will be best to engage the learners with responses. The other methods are static or done solely by the student.

37. A) A web page with a narrative that is updated by an individual or a group
A blog is a web page with a narrative that is updated by an individual or a group. Social media is used for networking, and Instagram is used for tweeting short messages about what is current. A webpage that can be edited is many times attached to a network program.

38. B) Of the students, 89% got the question correct
The correct answer was D*, and 0.86 of the students responded correctly.
The difficulty value (*p*-value) indicates the percentage of students who selected the correct answer. A negative PBS indicates that the low-scoring students elected B more than the high-scoring students; in fact, more high-scoring students selected D instead of B. More high-scoring students selected A than C because it is positive. The overall PBS of 0.32 does discriminate at greater than 0.20 the desired minimum. This question is a highly discriminating question.

39. A) It promotes faculty retention
Having a positive organizational climate is one of the main reasons a university will have less turnover of faculty. This is because faculty will be happier, content, and feel valued. Nursing faculty should be encouraged to be promoted, and complaints are never a positive force. Reputation is also positive but not the most important factor.

40. A) A 2020 publication by the Centers for Disease Control (CDC)
A public domain work is a creative work that is not protected by copyright and which may be freely used by everyone. U.S. government work, ideas, procedures, process and facts are not protected under copyright law. Private companies, published articles, and authored quotes are protected.

41. D) Continue to grow as a professional
NLN (2016) stated that all graduates of any program continually learn and grow as professionals whose practice is supported by evidence

42. A) Teaching, scholarship, and service
Most traditional universities and colleges base promotion and tenure on the traditional criteria of teaching, scholarship, and service in that order.

43. B) Establish the boundaries of the evaluation
The first step in conducting an assessment of an organization's effectiveness is to establish the boundaries of the evaluation. Martz (2010) identifies six steps to use in assessing an organization's effectiveness:
    1. Establish the boundaries of the evaluation
    2. Conduct a performance needs assessment
    3. Define the criteria of merit
    4. Plan and implement the evaluation
    5. Synthesize performance data with values
    6. Communicate and report evaluation findings

44. D) They value being virtually connected
They prefer social media and stay connected by cell phone. They despise talking on the phone. Generally, they are closed about their personal life and are passionate about learning.

45. A) Dissemination in peer-reviewed publications
This garners the most critical method of scholarship, sharing innovative techniques and learning are not as critical as publication.

46. B) Debriefing with Good Judgement
"I saw, I know, I acted" are the hallmarks of Debriefing with Good Judgement. The other options, while theories of debriefing, do not have those characteristics.

47. B) Attending continuing education conferences related to academic teaching
Attending continuing education conferences related to academic teaching. Joining professional organizations, writing examination questions, and reviewing journal articles are all good methods of scholarship and also assist in learning, but conferences are a direct learning format.

48. D) Interprofessional
An Interprofessional Curriculum will prepare all health care professionals together. A health disaster simulation will require many disciplines to work together – medicine, nursing, and psychology.

49. D) Administrative forces
Social, political, and economic forces help share the culture of an organization and that includes enrolment, curriculum design, pedagogy, faculty expectations, faculty competencies, and scholarly productivity. Administration is an internal force and manages the components.

50. C) PowerPoint presentations using the PechaKucha approach
PowerPoint presentations using the PechaKucha approach supports student learning by requiring them to synthesize content into brief presentations consisting of 20 slides and 20 seconds of commentary per slide. This would force students to be brief and to the point, guiding students in a learning process that embeds repetition and practice, provides students with an opportunity to practice time management and organization, and demonstrate their learning creatively.

51. B) "Socratic questioning assists with decision-making and can lead to robust discussions"
Socratic questioning is effective in promoting higher-order thinking and promotes discussion among the group. This type of question is more complex and requires faculty development to learn to ask more than simple yes/no questions. Although students must understand the content to participate, it does not guarantee advanced preparation. Not all students are comfortable speaking in class for fear of being wrong or coming across as a know-it-all.

52. A) Involve key people

ANA identifies the Essential behaviors associated with change management competencies as:
• Leads change by example.
• Adapts plans as necessary.
• Takes into account people's concerns during change.
• Effectively involves key people in the design and implementation of change.
• Adjusts management style to changing situations.
• Effectively manages others' resistance to organizational change.
• Adapts to the changing external pressures facing the organization.
• Is straightforward with individuals about consequences of an expected action or decision.
• Accepts change as positive.

53. B) Childbearing content

Childbirth rates are decreasing in most places. Infection control related to pandemics along with telehealth usage to decrease transmission is important as is cultural sensitivity to increase healthcare assess for all.

54. B) Grant course credits

A well-managed student exchange program will grant both course credits and allow for courses to be transferred. They typically do not mandate that a student must speak only the native language or register for just specific courses.

55. A) Course student learning outcomes

The module or unit student learning outcomes should be congruent with the course students learning outcomes. Indirectly the module or unit student learning outcomes should be congruent with the program outcomes, which are usually benchmarks of graduation, licensure success, and faculty accomplishments. Indirectly the module or unit students learning outcomes should be congruent with the mission of the college also, but they are on a much more specific level. The syllabus is a course overview and many times contains both the course and module or unit student learning outcomes.

Kuder Richardson (KR-20)
Exam 1 KR=0.19
Exam 2 KR=0.28
Exam 3 KR=0.53
Exam 4 KR-0.70

56. D) Exam 4 is the most reliable

A KR measures reliability and internal consistency of an exam. A reliability coefficient of 1.0 indicates perfect reliability, and a reliability coefficient of 0.00 lacks rest reliability. A KR score of 0.60 is acceptable for a teacher-made exam. The higher to 1.0, the more reliable and internally consistent the exam is.

57. A) Holding video conferencing with other students for a health policy class

The best method to implement a global classroom is to have a video conference with other students around the world. This can be done for health policy, research, or other course topics. Having students watch asynchronous lectures, write reflective papers, or present research articles will not allow students to connect and collaborate with others from around the world.

58. A) Knowledge

A learning disability would affect cognitive processing and the knowledge area of learner readiness. An emotional or social disability can affect learning. A physical disability is usually somatically based.

59. D) Rating scale

A rating scale is a summary of accumulated events and observation. An external review is conducted by an observer who has not seen the student previously. Anecdotal note is data collected by observation, and a skills checklist reviews the steps in a process.

60. A) Role playing a scenario of an issue that might come up on the hospital unit and discussing following the proper chains of command

A very good way to assist students socialize into the role of nursing is to help prepare them by role-playing potential scenarios they might experience and show them ways to handle conflict like utilizing the chain of command. Performing an assessment, demonstrating an example, and writing reflective journal pieces will not help with socialization.

61. C) Leadership and management

Although leadership and management are important in nursing education, it is not imperative for novice nurse educators. The necessary courses for nurse educators include understanding teaching-learning principles, learning how to evaluate students and program outcomes, and how curricula are logically developed on sound models.

62. C) A debrief asking to share feelings after a patient died

Asking a reflective question to explore feelings during a debriefing is an excellent way to express the affective domain. Demonstrating how to insert a Foley is in the psychomotor domain, a lecture, and computer-assisted instruction would be examples in the cognitive domain.

63. C) Contrast the difference between placenta previa and placenta abruption

Contrasting can be done using a number of assessment methods to measure while considering, understanding, and remembering are less able to measure learning acquisition.

64. A) Progressive publications

A list of progressive publications is a very important piece to include in a professional portfolio. Other personal activities are not as important but do demonstrate teaching and service.

65. B) Form a planning group for the project

Forming a planning group of volunteers who are interested in the project are ideal. Faculty should never be mandated or forced to go or attend, and the project should be chosen to meet the program goals. Students should be chosen by criteria that considers their passion and interests.

66. C) Ask a mentor to sit in on a class and provide feedback

Ask a mentor to sit in on a class and provide feedback to the faculty member is a great method to receive valuable feedback. Professional development form conferences are always a good way to access new and innovative teaching methodologies, but they need to be enacted. Watching videos of faculty and reading evidence about teaching strategies is also a good learning process, but direct critique assists in individual improvement.

67. B) National League for Nursing (NLN)

NLN is an organization for nurse educators and provides professional development. Oncology nursing is a clinical specialty; the National Safety Foundation is also a clinical resource. STTI is an honor society and also has some professional development activities, but its mission is to recognize leaders in nursing.

68. B) Systematic analyses of all aspects of the program

Program evaluation refers to "systematic assessment and analysis of all components of an academic program" (Billings & Halstead, 2020, p. 513). Evaluations of nursing programs should be continuous and evolving. Standards and guidelines are "Statements of expectations and aspirations providing a foundation for professional nursing. (CCNE [Commission on Collegiate Nursing Education] Accreditation Manual, 2018). Evaluation is a systematic and continuous process in which information is gathered to determine the worth and value of the program, outcomes, and achievement of the learner. (Billings & Halstead, 2020; Fardows, 2011; Keating, 2011).

69. B) Inspiring a shared vision

A transformational leader challenges the established process and inspires a shared vision. A servant leader is characterized by displaying concern for the team members, and a transactional leader will employ a rewards/punishment approach.

70. D) Peer evaluation

Accreditation agencies are organized as a peer-evaluation mechanism to assess if a nursing program meets established standards. Accreditation agencies do not provide expert consult or produce regulatory standards. Such as the boards of nursing. Additionally, accreditation organizations do not dictate curriculum models.

71. D) Professor
A full professor would fulfill all of these qualities.

72. A) Use the question again in future tests
KR20 is between .50 and .80, and the point biserial number is greater than .5 which shows a discrimination index that is maximized. Questions that discriminate well have point-biserial correlations that are highly positive for the and negative for the distractors. This question performed well and should be used again.

73. B) Providing critical information regarding student learning
Analytic technologies can be leveraged by faculty to provide critical information of student learning that is timely and facilitates early faculty intervention to support student success.

74. D) Management of care
NCLEX Test Plan in which patient needs are the basis of the test plan and include four major areas: Safe and effective care environment, Health promotion and maintenance, Psychosocial integrity, and Physiological integrity. These can be further broken down to the following percentages:

> Safe and effective care environment
> - Management of care—20%
> - Safety and infection control—12%
> Health promotion and maintenance—9%
> Psychosocial integrity—9%
> Physiological integrity
> - Basic care/comfort—9%
> - Pharmacological and parenteral
>   therapies—15%
> - Reduction of risk potential—12%
> - Physiological adaptation—14%

75. C) Multiculturalism
A genealogical map is a good way to address cultural differences and promote multiculturalism.

76. D) A 30-year-old recovering from abdominal surgery
The patient recovering from abdominal surgery is the best patient since no complications are noted, and abdominal surgery recovery is routine. A newly diagnosed diabetic needs teaching that is complex, a patient with heart failure needs a nurse who knows signs of complications. A patient in traction would be difficult for a beginning student.

77. A) Expectations of the academic faculty role

The new faculty should receive clear expectations and responsibilities of the academic educator role. Although salary, benefits, and legal issues are all important, understanding the role is a priority.

78. C) University administration and faculty arrive at decisions by joint consensus

In a culture of shared governance, faculty and university administration work together to arrive at answers to issues that affect the organization.

79. B) Make decisions that uphold company policy

Bureaucratic leader makes decisions that 'fit' with company policy or is congruent with established practices. Being congruent with the mission does not mean that the leader has to make the decisions, and they should make decisions based on consensus and nurse educator input.

80. D) Have immunizations, passports, and necessary medications

It is very important to have required immunizations, to always keep your passport with you, and to carry all necessary medications. Do not count on getting medications in other countries, as this might prove problematic. Especially if the medication is a required daily medication. Pack wisely is a good idea, as is having exchange money. Providing money or food to local children is not a good idea, it may promote "begging" which is punishable in some countries.

81. B) A learner using their computer to shop for shoes during class

A learner who is using their computer during class for other activities like shopping would be an example of incivility. Discussing grades and seeking clarification is expected of students to enhance learning. Using a cell phone outside the class is civil.

82. A) use PowerPoints that have lots of graphics"

PowerPoints are passive. Students learn best by linking new material to their experiences. They benefit greatly from case studies. Adult learners are very busy, and they despise busy work or doing assignments they perceive as not being meaningful or having a purpose. Interactions between nurse educators and students facilitate learning.

83. C) Internal forces

Faculty are part of a program's internal forces. Budgetary considerations and workforce pool are important but are part of the external forces of a curriculum development and revision.

84. C) Student technology mastery

Gaming in courses generates data that can reveal insights not only about student success or failure but also about student teamwork and collaboration preferences, learning styles, and a variety of other learning issues. The goal of gaming is not to promote technological knowledge or proficiency.

85. D) All faculty in the department
Mentorship is the responsibility of all the faculty in the department in general. Individual mentors may be assigned, and informal mentors sought, but all faculty create a culture of acceptance, including administration.

86. B) The Carnegie Classification of the institution
The Carnegie Classification of a University usually dictates the expectations of fulltime faculty. Grant writing and attainment is not unusual in research-intensive universities. The nursing discipline expectations are different for each institution, but the standards remain constant, a Dean's initiative is usually in alignment with the mission of the department, and universities should not be counting on grants to maintain their economic base.

87. C) Participation in simulation scenarios
Students who have opportunities to engage in level-appropriate academic challenges, participate actively in collaborative learning, encounter enriching educational experiences, and have frequent interaction with faculty are more likely to be successful and persist. Simulation is the best modality to facilitate academic challenge, collaborative learning, and interaction with peers and faculty.

88. C) Multicultural
Multicultural education aims at the encouragement of diversity and a broader perspective of a world view. Anti-racist education assumes that racism is already present. Interdisciplinary education brings several subjects together around common themes, issues, or problems.

89. C) Serving on the governance committee for the local chapter of Sigma Theta Tau International
Serving on the governance committee for the local chapter of Sigma Theta Tau International is an example of active participation in the organization. The others are examples of passive participation.

90. B) Perform an item analysis of test questions
Factors that lower reliability of test scores can include very easy or very hard questions, so the next step for faculty is to look at the test items for point bi-serial and frequency values. The test environment and subjective scoring are also factors, but more unlikely than too difficult or too easy test items.

91. C) A faculty member with a similar background and teaching schedule
A faculty member with a similar background and teaching schedule is ideal so that the mentor and mentee will have time to meet and work together.

92. C) Varied
Class instructional material should be varied to engage students with different learning styles. It is important that class instructional materials be accessible, reliable, and current, but variety will assist in engaging all types of learners.

93. C) Facilitate the learning experience
Teaching presence relates to the process of design, facilitation, and direction throughout the learning experience in order to realize desired learning outcomes. The three major categories under teaching presence are instructional design and management, building understanding, and direct instruction. Establishing teaching presence means creating a learning experience for students to progress through with instructor facilitation, support, and guidance.

94. B) A learning management system
OER provides teaching, learning, and research materials in any medium – digital or otherwise – that reside in the public domain or have been released under an open license that permits no-cost access, use, adaptation, and redistribution by others with no or limited restrictions. Learning management systems are not included with OER.

95. B) University or College's mission statement
The nursing program's mission statement should be derived from and congruent with the University or College's mission statement. Although it is preferable to also have the nursing program's mission statement congruent with faculty and administration as well as nursing organizations.

96. C) Performance reward system
There are eight key events/interventions that can leverage the opportunity to "manage" organizational culture identified by Willcoxson and Millett (2000). The eight key events/interventions are: strategic recruitment, removal and replacement, socialization, performance management/reward systems, leadership and modeling, participation and development activities, interpersonal communication, and structures, policies, and procedures.

97. B) Cognitive
A critique primarily assesses higher cognitive levels; the cognitive domain addresses intellectual ability. Critiques allow the learner to build critical thinking skills, reinforce expected standards, and promote active learner involvement. They do also assess the affective domain, which focuses on values and attitudes, but this is to a lesser extent. They do not address the psychomotor domain, which addresses motor skills. Formative evaluation is not a domain of learning.

98. A) IRB approval from the researcher's institution does not automatically translate to the IRB in the institution of study

IRB approval from the researcher's institution does not automatically translate to the IRB in the institution of study. An IRB will need to be done for each institution and does not automatically transfer. IRB approval is needed for any research study that is to be conducted.

99. D) Regardless of educational preparation nurse educators and leaders may collaborate in research and scholarly work

A nurse does not need to hold a doctorate to participate in a research study; in fact, educational level is not required. Nurses at many levels may participate in research initiatives.

100. A) Items that have a point biserial of zero means learners did not select them because the distractor was good

Distractors that have a point biserial of zero means learners did not select them and they need to be revised or replaced.

101. C) Finding observational experiences that are congruent with their clinical objectives

Students need to focus on the content they are learning in the classroom and the student learning outcomes (SLOs). Studying, taking care of different types of patients, and canceling do not meet the SLOs.

102. A) The exam is reliable in measuring learner knowledge of the material

This is an appropriate KR-20 for an instructor-made classroom test and reflects the accuracy or power of discrimination of the test.

103. C) "Active learning promotes critical thinking, which is important for NCLEX-RN success"

With the quickly approaching Next Generation NCLEX, students will be increasingly challenged to demonstrate their clinical judgment and decision-making skills. It is important that students are taught to think critically and to practice their decision-making skills. The other statements are accurate, but competency and NCLEX success is a top priority for nurse educators.

104. D) Simulation

Simulation provides an opportunity for students to practice skills in a safe environment. Faculty can also observe whether skills are used safely and competently in a simulated patient situation. Feedback can be provided during debriefing. Demonstration and vignettes provide opportunities for review of procedural steps but lack practice and evaluation time. Imagery allows students to mentally prepare for the skill/procedure, but there is no feedback as part of this strategy.

105. D) Formal training on how to be a mentor

To be an effective mentor, the faculty should have formal training on how to be a mentor. Years of experience may help, but formal education about mentor-mentee expectations is most helpful.

106. A) Identifying a gap in the literature and deciding to conduct a research study

Continuing to teach with the same methods, only using student evaluations or obtaining materials from the internet are not acceptable examples of the spirit of inquiry.

107. B) "Breaking up the lecture with activities will keep the students involved"

Lecture is a passive learning strategy that results in minimal student engagement. Incorporating active learning strategies will keep students involved in their learning. Lecture alone, even with PowerPoints, often results in loss of attention.

108. A) Registration with the U.S. Embassy in the foreign country

The most important thing to do prior to leaving the U. S. when traveling with a group of students to a foreign country is to be sure your group is registered at the U.S. Embassy in that country in the event of a problem or any issues.

109. B) Scholarship of application

Scholarship of application is engagement of scholar in service-related activities resulting in tangible outcomes. Scholarship of teaching is to facilitate learning while inquiry and publication are not defined methods of scholarship for this approach.

110. A) Humor can be effective in providing a sense of belonging for students

Humor is effective in relieving stress and anxiety. It can also make the educator seem more relatable, thus creating an environment that promotes group cohesion. Humor must be used cautiously though because it may be inappropriate with some topics and it could be offensive to some students.

111. A) Developing the learning outcomes
Developing student learning outcomes is the first step to designing a course. While finding a patient population is part of curriculum work, there are many options to assist the learning such as simulation, videos, etc. All of the other activities are vital to implementing the curriculum.

112. D) "Games can also be used as a method of evaluation of individual learning"
It is usually very difficult to evaluate individual student learning when using games. Games are effective for tactile learners and create a fun environment for student learning. Scaffolding increases the challenge associated with the games.

113. C) Publication is a learned skill that can be assisted through mentorship of experts
It is not based upon manuscript submission and does not require hiring an editor. Non-peer reviewed journals do hold the same recognitions as peer-reviewed journals.

114. D) Have a remote proctor
Randomizing the answer responses, randomizing the questions, and setting a time limit for the online exam are all good strategies to secure an online objective exams, but having a remote proctor promotes integrity.

115. A) Schedule weekly virtual office hours
Weekly virtual office hours are very effective for an online course and provide the students with faculty presence. Email, phone calls, and discussion boards are good but not as interactive as virtual office hours.

116. C) "Most weeks, we use post-conference to talk about the skills they completed"
Post-conferences should be a time of continued learning. Listing skills attained is not an effective use of time and sends the message that skills are of primary importance. Post-conferences should be used to connect theory to practice and build confidence. Post-conferences are generally more effective when planned in advance.

117. D) "I posted all of my voice-over PowerPoints for review prior to class"
Students may be discontented when a significant amount of pre-work is required prior to class. It is important for students to be prepared when coming to a flipped classroom, but care must be taken to not overwhelm students with out-of-class work. The flipped classroom also allows the educator to focus the learning on more complex topics while using active learning strategies and team learning.

118. D) Interventions to reduce vulnerability and increase safety for women
AACN recognizes domestic violence as a special form of violence and recommends that faculty ensure that the curricula contain opportunities for all learners to participate in activities that help women, children, and the elderly combat it. Placing posters where women can see them in a safe setting satisfies this goal.

119. C) Case studies
Case studies often provide patient information, e.g., diagnosis, treatment, complications, that promote critical thinking and problem-solving. As students construct their own knowledge, they are able to better translate this knowledge to the practice setting. Collaborative learning, debate, and group discussions all promote teamwork and higher order thinking, but they are not specifically designed to connect didactic learning to practice.

120. D) Soul search for your own biases and stereotypical ideas
The best way to gain cultural competence is to first examine yourself for pre-set biases or stereotypical ideas of any given culture. Although listening to the music, observing the way of dress, and learning the slang language may be helpful in supplementing the student's understanding of the culture, they should not be the first step in building cultural competence.

121. C) Conducting an IRB research project in areas of strength of teaching
Using evidence-based teaching and a research project with IRB approval on strength seeking truth and inquiry. A quick student survey without IRB approval, creating a poster to display at the school or a journal club is not the definition and role of the scholar.

122. C) "The preceptor will not have much time to teach me"
Preceptors have been chosen or volunteered because teaching is a priority. The student will follow the preceptor's schedule and assist them to learn by choosing appropriate patients for the student to care for.

123. C) Appointment and performance evaluation are integral frameworks to the model
Appointment and performance evaluations along with demonstration of merit for awards, pay increase and promotion and tenure guidelines are part of the four dimensions of Boyer's Model. Sabbatical, workload and student performance are not part of the model.

124. C) Review student's assignments/tests submitted in the course
The most important thing to do to prepare for this meeting is to review student performance in the course up to this point to identify areas in which the student can focus for improvement.

125. D) Established norms
Established and entrenched norms and processes can be a significant barrier to creativity and innovation.

126. C) Revise distractor C
No student chose distractor C, so it is not "feasible." The correct answer, A, has a positive point biserial as it should and 57% of the students chose the correct answer. Distractors B and D had negative point biserials and discriminated those students who did not understand the content.

127. A) Interpretation and synthesis of knowledge
Interpretation and synthesis which may cross the disciplinary boundaries. Validation is scholarship of discovery, connection of theory to practice is application, and scholarship of teaching is using evidence to facilitate learning.

128. A) Concept map
A concept map is a diagram that ties concepts together. A discrepant event is a demonstration that produces a surprising or unexpected outcome. An analogy is a comparison of two things. A quiz will test the student's knowledge.

129. D) Scholar
Scholar is a person who has particular knowledge in an area of specialization. The academic is relating to education, the teacher educates and teaches while the clinician is a health care provider.

130. A) Be prepared and know the content well
It is very important to be prepared, know the content well, and be clinical experts in their fields. This group is very motivated and expect a knowledgeable and informed faculty member to teach them. Engaging them in clinical experiences is expected and but for didactic teaching being prepared is paramount.

131. A) Reflective learning
This shows that the student is thinking of what they learned and how this learning has changed their perspective. The remaining options are not examples of reflection.

132. C) Post instructions and a direct link to the library e-journal in the course
Posting instructions meets the requirement of Fair Use and copyright law in that it requires the students to access the articles directly via the library. The other methods violate the law because it is distrusting.

133. D) Achievement of a minimum grade of 850 on standardized achievement tests is needed to progress

Progression policies within the nursing major must be congruent with the program goals and institutional standards and must be clearly identified and published which fall into those goals, creates high stakes testing within a nursing program. The NLN created a task force to develop guidelines for the use of standardized tests as a prerequisite for learner progression in the nursing program (NLN, 2010). Outcomes of this task force included the development of a position statement on fair testing that was approved by the NLN Board of Governors (NLN, 2012b), and the development of Fair Testing Guidelines for Nursing Education (NLN, 2012a). The committee should relook at the policy to see if it is "fail testing" or undue pressure on students.

134. B) Accessible

Tools have to be accessible to the learners in order to increase participation and utilization. Innovation and free of charge tools are great if they are accessible. Usually, class learning tools are not individualized.

135. B) One Minute Paper at the end of class

Evaluation must be selected to assess the effectiveness of learning and the achievement of course and program outcomes in both their theoretical and clinical components. One minute papers evaluate knowledge on a lower level of assessment and is a good indicator for faculty on content that may need to be clarified.

136. D) Formative

Refers to the evaluation of learning while it is occurring, and can identify a learner's readiness to learn and their learning needs and may improve learner's performance before the end of the course or program.

137. B) Junior faculty assimilation into academia

The Sigma Theta Tau International/Elsevier NFLA was developed to mentor junior faculty members into leadership roles in academia. The main purpose was not to promote seasoned faculty or to advance research.

138. A) Connecting course materials with assessment

When these elements are aligned students are able to see how learning activities and materials connect with their assignments and, as a result, have a better learning experience.

139. D) They help identify students who may need additional resources
Progression policies are important so that a minimum competency is maintained to move forward. This enables to identify students who may need additional support services in order that all students are prepared for the demands of the highly complex and technical workforce today and in the future.

140. D) Spirit of inquiry
This assumes the student is acting as a developing scholar who contributes to the development of the science of nursing practice.

141. D) Examine policies and practices of an organization
Cultural proficiency denotes a commitment to examine policies and practices of the organization as well as the values and behaviors of the individual and creating a healthy environment. Although the culturally proficient individual will accommodate and collaborate with differences as well as incorporate cultural artefacts into the environment, they are responsible for examining the cultural needs of an institution.

142. B) Higher-coring learners answered the question correctly
Distractors B, C, and D also need revision because they have a positive point biserial and some of the better scoring students on this test chose them.

143. C) Monitor assignment submissions and remind students of due dates
Proactive Course Management Strategies include monitoring assignment submissions, communicating and reminding students of missed and/or upcoming deadlines, and making course progress adjustments where and when necessary.

144. A) Recognizing cues
Recognizing cues is first step in a six-step unfolding case study process used by NGN. Recognizing cues comes before analyzing the cues and developing a hypothesis. Taking action comes after developing a hypothesis.

145. C) Participate in a debriefing session to explore feelings and perceptions of the experience
It is vital to get the students together once they have returned home to explore feelings and personal experience of the trip. This provides a safe place to discuss, builds cultural awareness, and enables the faculty to tie the experience to learning objectives in the course. Writing a paper is a summary assignment and only a one-way communication tool. A roleplay activity is acting out a given situation and does not allow others to comment. Telling family and friends will not tie the experience back to the course.

146. C) Evaluate outcomes

Evaluating outcomes is the last or sixth question on unfolding case studies and asks the students to evaluate the care they have chosen in the other five questions for effectiveness. Recognizing cures, developing a hypothesis and taking action are all before the evaluation phase.

Point Biserial = 0.13	= D			Total Group = 82%
Distractor Analysis	A	B	C	D
Point Biserial	0.02	0.19	0.01	−0.13
Frequency	12%	5%	1%	82%

The likely cause for this frequency distribution is:

147. B) Higher scoring learners answered the question incorrectly

The right answer had a negative point biserial demonstrating that lower scoring students chose the correct answer as opposed to higher scoring students. Distractors A, B, and C all were incorrect yet had positive point biserials and therefore all answers may need revision.

148. C) Nursing actions and monitoring to a disease process

Standalone bowtie items use disease process as indicators in the middle and use nursing actions on the left and nursing monitoring on the right. The student much drag and drop a nursing action and monitoring to a disease process. This question type facilitates clinical judgement. Standalone bowtie questions do not assess medication, assessment, or psychosocial care.

149. C) Retrievable

It is important that instructional material be current, accurate and retrievable or accessible. It does not necessarily have to be entertaining or seminal. It should be five-years old or less unless it is a classic piece of work.

150. B) "Adding a peer evaluation as part of the grade may encourage better participation"

Peer evaluation may be incentive for students to participate so that their grades are not adversely affected. Group projects require collaboration, conflict resolution, and time management, but simply deflecting this on the students is not helpful.

Index